Teen Health Series

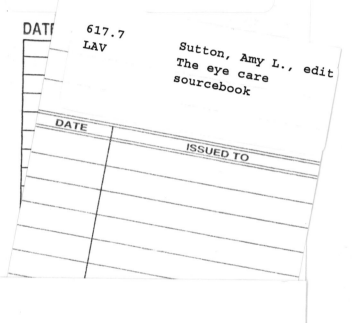

Eye Care
SOURCEBOOK
Second Edition

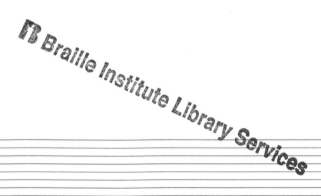

Health Reference Series

Second Edition

Eye Care
SOURCEBOOK

Basic Consumer Health Information about Eye Care and Eye Disorders, Including Facts about the Diagnosis, Prevention, and Treatment of Common Refractive Problems Such as Myopia, Hyperopia, Astigmatism, and Presbyopia, and Eye Diseases, Including Glaucoma, Cataract, Age-Related Macular Degeneration, and Diabetic Retinopathy

Along with a Section on Vision Correction and Refractive Surgeries, Including LASIK and LASEK, a Glossary, and Directories of Resources for Additional Help and Information

Edited by
Amy L. Sutton

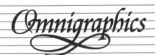

615 Griswold Street • Detroit, MI 48226

Bibliographic Note

Because this page cannot legibly accommodate all the copyright notices, the Bibliographic Note portion of the Preface constitutes an extension of the copyright notice.

Edited by Amy L. Sutton

Health Reference Series

Karen Bellenir, *Managing Editor*
David A. Cooke, MD, *Medical Consultant*
Elizabeth Barbour, *Permissions Associate*
Dawn Matthews, *Verification Assistant*
Laura Pleva Nielsen, *Index Editor*
EdIndex, Services for Publishers, *Indexers*

* * *

Omnigraphics, Inc.

Matthew P. Barbour, *Senior Vice President*
Kay Gill, *Vice President—Directories*
Kevin Hayes, *Operations Manager*
Leif Gruenberg, *Development Manager*
David P. Bianco, *Marketing Consultant*

* * *

Peter E. Ruffner, *Publisher*

Frederick G. Ruffner, Jr., *Chairman*

Copyright © 2003 Omnigraphics, Inc.

ISBN 0-7808-0635-2

Library of Congress Cataloging-in-Publication Data

Eye care sourcebook : basic consumer health information about eye care and eye disorders, including facts about the diagnosis, prevention, and treatment of common refractive problems such as myopia, hyperopia, astigmatism, and presbyopia, and eye diseases, including glaucoma, cataract, age-related macular degeneration, and diabetic retinopathy; along with a section on vision correction and refractive surgeries, including LASIK and LASEK, a glossary, and directories of resources for additional help and information / edited by Amy L. Sutton.-- 2nd ed.
    p. cm. -- (Health reference series)
    Previous ed. published with title: Ophthalmic disorders sourcebook.
    Includes bibliographical references and index.
    ISBN 0-7808-0635-2 (lib. bdg. : alk. paper)
    1. Eye--Diseases--Popular works. 2. Eye--Care and hygiene--Popular works. I. Sutton, Amy L. II. Ophthalmic disorders sourcebook. III. Health reference series (Unnumbered)
RE51 .O64 2003
617.7'1--dc21
                            2002193059

Printed in the United States

Table of Contents

Part II: Vision Correction and Refractive Surgery

Part IV: Pediatric Eye Problems

Part V: Disorders with Eye-Related Complications

Part VI: Other Eye Disorders and Problems

Part VII: Current Research and Clinical Trials

Preface

About This Book

Loss of visual acuity is a widespread health problem throughout the United States. Some difficulties are the result of refractive errors, such as myopia (nearsightedness) and hyperopia (farsightedness). In fact, an estimated 158 million people—more than half the American population—use some type of corrective eyewear to improve their vision, and an increasing number of people are turning to surgical techniques to help them see better. The American Academy of Ophthalmology estimated that 1.8 million refractive surgery procedures would be performed in 2002.

Vision problems can also lead to significant disability. More than one million Americans are blind and 2.4 million are visually impaired—meaning that their corrected vision is worse than 20/40. Statistics suggest that the number of people who suffer from vision loss and blindness will increase—even double—over the next 30 years as the baby boomer generation advances into retirement age.

This book provides important health information about vision problems in adults and children and how to prevent and treat them. Readers will learn essential information about correcting vision with refractive surgery, including new laser surgery techniques such as LASIK and LASEK, as well as how to prevent vision loss from conditions such as glaucoma, cataract, macular degeneration, and other eye disorders. Information about disorders with eye-related complications, such as diabetes and thyroid disease, is included, along with information about current research, a glossary, and a listing of additional resources.

How to Use This Book

This book is divided into parts and chapters. Parts focus on broad areas of interest. Chapters are devoted to single topics within a part.

Part I: General Information about Eye Care provides an overview of the visual system and supplies information about eye care. It explains the differences between various types of eye care professionals and suggests guidelines for when to visit them. Symptoms of common eye problems, refractive errors such as nearsightedness, farsightedness, and astigmatism, and eye protection strategies are also covered.

Part II: Vision Correction and Refractive Surgery reviews vision correction methods, such as eyeglasses and contact lenses, as well as refractive surgery procedures, such as photorefractive keratectomy (PRK), radial keratotomy (RK), orthokeratology (Ortho-K), laser-assisted in situ keratomileusis (LASIK), and laser epithelial keratomileusis (LASEK). A helpful checklist that outlines preoperative, operative, and postoperative expectations of laser eye surgery is also included.

Part III: Age-Related Eye Problems offers information about eye problems that develop with age, such as cataract, ocular hypertension, glaucoma, and macular degeneration. In addition, statistics about vision trends during aging and facts about preventing vision loss are presented.

Part IV: Pediatric Eye Problems describes vision concerns and conditions in childhood, including amblyopia, juvenile macular degeneration, retinitis pigmentosa, retinopathy of prematurity, strabismus, and tear-duct obstruction.

Part V: Disorders with Eye-Related Complications identifies health conditions that may adversely affect vision. Conditions addressed include Behçet's disease of the eye, diabetic retinopathy, histoplasmosis, Sjögren's syndrome, thyroid eye disease, and Usher syndrome. Information about preventing and treating these conditions is offered.

Part VI: Other Eye Disorders and Problems presents information about anophthalmia and microphthalmia, anterior uveitis, blepharitis, color blindness, corneal disease, dry eye, eyelid misalignments, eye allergies and allergic conjunctivitis, macular hole and pucker, retinal detachment, spots and floaters, and other disorders that impact vision.

Part VII: Current Research and Clinical Trials reviews areas of recent and ongoing research in vision preservation, including the effect of vitamins on macular degeneration and cataract; the use of antibiotics to treat chlamydia, a leading cause of blindness at birth; and studies focused on preventing the ocular complications of AIDS.

Part VIII: Additional Help and Information includes a glossary of important terms and a directory of eye care organizations that provide additional information. Resources for people with low vision and blindness are also included.

Bibliographic Note

This volume contains documents and excerpts from publications issued by the following U.S. government agencies: Administration on Aging (AoA)/Department of Health and Human Services (DHHS); Center for Devices and Radiological Health (CDRH); Centers for Disease Control and Prevention (CDC); Federal Trade Commission (FTC); National Cancer Institute (NCI); National Eye Institute (NEI); National Institute of Diabetes and Digestive and Kidney Diseases (NIDDK); National Institutes of Health (NIH); U.S. Department of Labor/Occupational Safety and Health Administration (OSHA); and U.S. Food and Drug Administration (FDA).

In addition, this volume contains copyrighted documents from the following organizations and individuals: American Academy of Ophthalmology (AAO); American College of Allergy, Asthma and Immunology (ACAAI); American Foundation for the Blind; American Macular Degeneration Foundation; American Optometric Association (AOA); American Society of Plastic Surgeons; American Society of Cataract and Refractive Surgery/The Lasik Institute; Cleveland Clinic; Foundation Fighting Blindness; Glaucoma Foundation; Health Communities.com; Lighthouse International; Macular Degeneration Foundation, Inc.; McGraw-Hill Companies; Medem, Inc.; Nemours Foundation; New York Thyroid Center; Prevent Blindness America; Quackwatch; Sjögren's Syndrome Foundation, Inc.; and St. Luke's Cataract and Laser Institute.

Full citation information is provided on the first page of each chapter. Every effort has been made to secure all necessary rights to reprint the copyrighted material. If any omissions have been made, please contact Omnigraphics to make corrections for future editions.

Acknowledgements

Thanks go to the many organizations, agencies, and individuals who have contributed materials for this *Sourcebook* and to medical consultant Dr. David Cooke, verification assistant Dawn Matthews, and document engineer Bruce Bellenir. Special thanks also go to managing editor Karen Bellenir and permissions specialist Liz Barbour for their help and support.

Note from the Editor

This book is part of Omnigraphics' *Health Reference Series*. The series provides basic information about a broad range of medical concerns. It is not intended to serve as a tool for diagnosing illness, in prescribing treatments, or as a substitute for the physician/patient relationship. All persons concerned about medical symptoms or the possibility of disease are encouraged to seek professional care from an appropriate health care provider.

Our Advisory Board

The *Health Reference Series* is reviewed by an Advisory Board comprised of librarians from public, academic, and medical libraries. We would like to thank the following board members for providing guidance to the development of this series:

Dr. Lynda Baker, Associate Professor of Library and Information Science, Wayne State University, Detroit, MI

Nancy Bulgarelli, William Beaumont Hospital Library, Royal Oak, MI

Karen Imarisio, Bloomfield Township Public Library, Bloomfield Township, MI

Karen Morgan, Mardigian Library, University of Michigan-Dearborn, Dearborn, MI

Rosemary Orlando, St. Clair Shores Public Library, St. Clair Shores, MI

Medical Consultant

Medical consultation services are provided to the *Health Reference Series* editors by David A. Cooke, MD. Dr. Cooke is a graduate of

Brandeis University, and he received his M.D. degree from the University of Michigan. He completed residency training at the University of Wisconsin Hospital and Clinics. He is board-certified in Internal Medicine. Dr. Cooke currently works as part of the University of Michigan Health System and practices in Brighton, MI. In his free time, he enjoys writing, science fiction, and spending time with his family.

Health Reference Series *Update Policy*

The inaugural book in the *Health Reference Series* was the first edition of *Cancer Sourcebook* published in 1989. Since then, the *Series* has been enthusiastically received by librarians and in the medical community. In order to maintain the standard of providing high-quality health information for the layperson the editorial staff at Omnigraphics felt it was necessary to implement a policy of updating volumes when warranted.

Medical researchers have been making tremendous strides, and it is the purpose of the *Health Reference Series* to stay current with the most recent advances. Each decision to update a volume will be made on an individual basis. Some of the considerations will include how much new information is available and the feedback we receive from people who use the books. If there is a topic you would like to see added to the update list, or an area of medical concern you feel has not been adequately addressed, please write to:

Editor
Health Reference Series
Omnigraphics, Inc.
615 Griswold Street
Detroit, MI 48226
E-mail: editorial@omnigraphics.com

Part One

General Information about Eye Care

Chapter 1

The Visual System

The human eye is composed of many parts that work together. They receive visual images, focus them properly, and send messages to the brain.

To have vision, you must have three things:

- eyes,
- a brain, and
- light.

Light rays bounce off an object you are looking at. Let's say the object is a dog. The light reflects off the dog's image and comes back to your eye.

Light then enters through the outer part of the eye, called the cornea. The cornea is clear like a window. The cornea helps the eye to focus. 'To focus' means to make things look sharp and clear.

Next, the light rays go through an opening called the pupil. The pupil is the dark round circle in the middle of the colored part of your eye. The colored part is called the iris. The pupil is really a hole in the iris. The iris controls how much light goes into your eye.

When the light is bright, the iris closes the pupil until the right amount of light gets in. When the light is dim, the iris opens the pupil to let in more light. All of this happens automatically. You do not have to tell your eye to do it.

From "Vision—A School Program for Grades 4 to 8," National Eye Institute, available online at http://www.nei.nih.gov, May 2001.

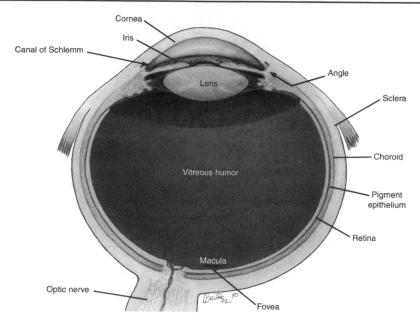

Figure 1.1. *Diagram of the Eye*

Your eye has a lens to focus the rays of light. The lens of the eye is behind the iris. Light passes through the lens on its way to the back of the eye.

The back of the eye is very important. Lining the inside of the eye is the retina. The retina includes 130 million tiny light-sensitive cells that send messages to other cells. These cells come together at the back of the eye to form the optic nerve. The optic nerve is part of the brain.

Fortunately for you, your brain decides how you see. The retina sees the world upside down, but the brain turns it right side up.

When you look at an object, each eye sees a slightly different picture. The brain combines the images, or pictures, that each eye sees and makes them into one picture.

Chapter 2

Eye Examinations

Chapter Contents

Section 2.1

What Is an Ophthalmologist, Optometrist, and Optician?

Medical Information from The Cleveland Clinic

Where do you go when you are having difficulty with your eyesight? Depending on the reason for your doctor visit, your answer may vary. When choosing an eye health professional, you may see an optometrist for simple vision correction. Your optometrist may prescribe eyeglasses or contacts that provide comfort, safety, and reading ease. If you experience more severe vision problems, like eye disease or loss of sight, or if you are looking for permanent vision correction or plastic surgery, you will probably visit an ophthalmologist. Opticians are eye health professionals who work with ophthalmologists and optometrists to provide vision services related to the diagnosis and treatment of vision problems and eye disease. They assist optometrists and ophthalmologists in providing complete patient care, before, during, and after exams, procedures, and surgeries.

What Is an Ophthalmologist?

Ophthalmologists can be either doctors of medicine (MD) or doctors of osteopathy (DO). They specialize in the medical and surgical care of the eyes and visual system, but also in the prevention of eye disease and injury. While medical doctors focus on disease-specific diagnosis and treatment, osteopaths concentrate on the loss of structure in tissue due to disease. Osteopaths give treatment based on the assumption that treating the parts of the visual system with the use

6

of medicines, surgery, diet, and other therapies will therefore treat the eye disorder.

An ophthalmologist has completed four years of premedical undergraduate education, four years of medical school, one year of internship, and three or more years of specialized medical, surgical, and refractive training and eye care experience. As a qualified specialist, an ophthalmologist is licensed by a state regulatory board to practice medicine and surgery, including the diagnosis, treatment, and management of all eye and visual systems. An ophthalmologist is qualified to deliver total eye care, meaning vision services, eye examinations, medical and surgical eye care, diagnosis and treatment of disease, and visual complications that are caused by systemic disease, like diabetes.

What Is a Doctor of Optometry?

Optometrists are doctors of optometry (OD). They examine, diagnose, treat, and manage diseases and disorders of the visual system. The optometrist has completed preprofessional undergraduate education in a college or university as well as four years of professional education at an accredited college of optometry. Some optometrists may have completed a residency, but have not attended medical school.

Like ophthalmologists, optometrists examine the internal and external structure of the eyes to detect diseases like glaucoma, retinal disorder, and cataracts, but do not practice medicine through surgery and are not trained to care for and manage all diseases and disorders of the ocular system. Optometrists diagnose and treat vision conditions like nearsightedness, farsightedness, astigmatism, and presbyopia. They may also test the patient's ability to focus and coordinate the eyes and see depth and colors accurately. Optometrists are state licensed to examine the eyes to determine the presence of vision problems and visual acuity, prescribe eyeglasses, contact lenses, eye exercises, low vision aids, vision therapy, and in some states, medications to treat eye diseases. Optometrists can perform all the services of an optician.

What Is an Optician?

Opticians complete the bridge between optical care and service. They perform dual tasks, providing technical and patient services. With a two-year technical degree, opticians analyze and interpret prescriptions; determine the lenses that best meet the patient's needs;

7

oversee ordering and verification of ophthalmic products from start to finish; dispense, replace, adjust, repair, and reproduce previously ordered contacts, eyeglasses, and frames.

Good eye health is the result of a working partnership between the patient and health care provider. Ophthalmologists, optometrists, and opticians work collectively and with the patient to ensure good ocular health and lifelong vision. You should visit your optometrist or ophthalmologist for an eye exam at least once per year.

Section 2.2

Finding an Eye Care Professional

"Finding an Eye Care Professional," Fact Sheet, National Eye Institute, available online at http://www.nei.nih.gov, December 2001.

The National Eye Institute does not provide referrals or recommend specific eye care professionals. However, you may wish to consider the following ways of finding a professional to provide your eye care.

You can:

- Ask family members and friends about eye care professionals they use.

- Ask your family doctor for the name of a local eye care specialist.

- Call the department of ophthalmology or optometry at a nearby hospital or university medical center.

- Contact a state or county association of ophthalmologists or optometrists. These groups, usually called academies or societies, may have lists of eye care professionals with specific information on specialty and experience.

- Contact your insurance company or health plan to learn whether it has a list of eye care professionals that are covered under your plan.

- At a bookstore or library, check on available journals and books about choosing a physician and medical treatment. Most large libraries have the reference set *The ABMS Compendium of Certified Medical Professionals*, which lists board-certified ophthalmologists, each with a small amount of biographical information. A library reference specialist can also help you identify other books on finding health care professionals or help you seek additional information about local eye physicians using the Internet. In addition, each year, usually in August, the magazine *U.S. News and World Report* features an article that rates hospitals in the United States.

For More Information

- The American Academy of Ophthalmology coordinates Find an Ophthalmologist, an online listing of member ophthalmologists practicing in the United States and abroad. This service is designed to help the general public locate ophthalmologists within a specific region. Website: http://www.eyenet.org.

- The International Society of Refractive Surgery maintains a comprehensive directory of surgeons around the world who are currently performing refractive surgery. Telephone: 407-786-7446. E-mail: isrshq@isrs.org. Website: http://www.isrs.org.

- *The Blue Book of Optometrists* and *The Red Book of Ophthalmologists*, now available online, can be used to find doctors in the United States, Puerto Rico, and Canada. This resource is helpful when you know the doctor's name, but need contact information. Website: http://www.aao.org/news/eyenet.

- Administrators in Medicine and the Association of State Medical Board Executive Directors have launched DocFinder, an online database that helps consumers learn whether any malpractice actions have been taken against a particular doctor. The site provides links to the licensing boards in the participating states. Website: http://www.docboard.org.

- The American Association of Eye and Ear Hospitals (AAEEH) is comprised of the premier centers for specialized eye and ear procedures in the world. Association members are major referral centers that offer some of the most innovative teaching programs and routinely treat the most severely ill eye and ear

9

patients. Telephone: 202-347-1993. A list of member facilities is available online at http://www.aaeeh.org/locations.html.

- The National Eye Institute (NEI), a part of the National Institutes of Health, is the Federal Government's principal agency for conducting and supporting research on the prevention, diagnosis, treatment, and rehabilitation of eye diseases and disorders of the visual system.

Inclusion in this chapter does not imply endorsement by the National Eye Institute or the National Institutes of Health.

Section 2.3

Tips on When to Get an Eye Exam

"How Often to Have an Eye Exam," © 2001 American Academy of Ophthalmology. Used by permission. All rights reserved. For more information, visit www.aao.org.

Many people want to know how often they should have their eyes examined. The answer depends on your age, medical background and risk factors for disease.

In general, Eye M.D.s (ophthalmologists) recommend the following exam schedules:

Children

Screening for eye disease by trained personnel—Eye M.D., pediatrician, or trained screener

- Newborn to 3 months
- 6 months to 1 year
- 3 years (approximately)
- 5 years (approximately)

Adults

Comprehensive medical eye exam by an Eye M.D.

- Once between age 20 and 39
- Age 40 to 64, every two to four years
- Age 65 and older, every one to two years

Some factors may put you at increased risk for eye disease. If any of these factors applies to you, check with your Eye M.D. to see how often you should have a medical eye exam:

- Developmental delay
- Premature birth
- Personal or family history of eye disease
- African-American heritage (African-Americans are at increased risk for glaucoma)
- Previous serious eye injury
- Use of certain medications (check with your Eye M.D.)
- Certain diseases that affect the whole body (such as diabetes or HIV infection)

Protect your family's good vision with thorough exams at appropriate times.

Table 2.1. When to Get an Eye Exam

Age Group	Frequency
Infants and children	By 6 months of age; at 3 years of age, before starting first grade, and every 2 years thereafter
18 years to 40 years	Every 2 to 3 years
41 years to 60 years	Every 2 years
61 years and older	Every year

Source: © 2001 American Optometric Association. Reprinted with permission. For additional information, visit www.aoa.org.

Section 2.4

The Great American Eye Test

Take this simple test to find out if you or someone in your family should have an eye examination. If you answer yes to more than one question, or you have not seen your optometrist in over a year, it's probably time to schedule an appointment. Unique eye and vision conditions exist for seniors, baby boomers, women, and children. This test serves as a quick overview for all populations.

Do you experience:

- difficulty reading small print, sewing, or doing crafts?
- headaches or have tired, burning eyes after reading or working on a computer?
- difficulty seeing at night or seeing street signs while driving?
- irritated, dry, red, or sensitive eyes?
- spots, flashes of light, or floaters in your field of vision?

Do you:

- have diabetes?
- have a family history of glaucoma?
- attend school and have difficulty in reading or learning (or have a child who does)?
- have a family history of lazy eye, weak vision, or eye disease?
- handle chemicals, use power tools, or engage in sports that may be hazardous to your eyes?

Even if you answered no to these questions, keep in mind that symptoms of eye disease and vision problems are not always apparent.

Eye exams by a doctor of optometry can help you be certain that your eyes are healthy and functioning properly.

The American Optometric Association recommends that you visit the optometrist on a schedule depending on your age. You should seek eye care more frequently if new ocular, visual, or systemic health problems develop. Persons with additional risk factors should also be examined more frequently.

Section 2.5

A Checklist for Your Eye Doctor Appointment

Reprinted with permission from Prevent Blindness America. © 2000. For additional information, call the Prevent Blindness America toll-free information line at (800) 331-2020, or visit www.preventblindness.org.

Have you ever left the doctor's office and thought of a dozen questions you meant to ask? We all do that.

This checklist of questions can help you make the most of your next visit to the eye doctor.

When you call to make an appointment:

- Be prepared to describe any vision problems you are having.

- Ask if you will be able to drive yourself home. Will the eye examination affect your vision temporarily?

- Ask how much the exam will cost. Do any of your health insurance plans cover any of the cost? How is payment handled?

Before you go in for your examination, make a list of the following:

- Signs or symptoms of eye problems you have noticed (flashes of light, difficulty seeing at night, temporary double vision, loss of vision, etc.)

- Eye injuries or eye surgery you have had (approximate dates, hospitals where treated, etc.)

- Prescription and over-the-counter drugs you are taking

- Questions you have about your vision
- Your general health condition (allergies, chronic health problems, operations, etc.)
- Family history of eye problems (glaucoma, cataracts, etc.)

Take along the following:

- Your glasses, contact lenses, or both
- Prescription and over-the-counter drugs you are taking
- Medical or health insurance card or your membership certificate

During the examination:

- Ask questions about anything that seems unclear to you, such as the names and purposes of tests you may undergo.
- Ask if there are any changes since your last exam.
- Ask when it is best to call the doctor with questions.
- Find out when you should return for your next exam.

To learn more about preparing for your doctor's visit, please contact Prevent Blindness America or the Prevent Blindness affiliate near you.

Section 2.6

Talking to Your Eye Doctor

"Talking to Your Doctor," Fact Sheet, National Eye Institute, available online at http://www.nei.nih.gov; May 1998.

Today, patients take an active role in their health care. You and your doctor will work in partnership to achieve your best possible level of health. An important part of this relationship is good communication.

Here are some questions you can ask your doctor to get your discussion started:

About My Disease or Disorder

- What is my diagnosis?
- What caused my condition?
- Can my condition be treated?
- How will this condition affect my vision now and in the future?
- Should I watch for any particular symptoms and notify you if they occur?
- Should I make any lifestyle changes?

About My Treatment

- What is the treatment for my condition?
- When will the treatment start, and how long will it last?
- What are the benefits of this treatment, and how successful is it?
- What are the risks and side effects associated with this treatment?
- Are there foods, drugs, or activities I should avoid while I'm on this treatment?

15

- If my treatment includes taking a medication, what should I do if I miss a dose?

- Are other treatments available?

About My Tests

- What kinds of tests will I have?

- What do you expect to find out from these tests?

- When will I know the results?

- Do I have to do anything special to prepare for any of the tests?

- Do these tests have any side effects or risks?

- Will I need more tests later?

Understanding your doctor's responses is essential to good communication. Here are a few more tips:

- If you don't understand your doctor's responses, ask questions until you do understand.

- Take notes, or get a friend or family member to take notes for you. Or, bring a tape-recorder to assist in your recollection of the discussion.

- Ask your doctor to write down his or her instructions to you.

- Ask your doctor for printed material about your condition.

- If you still have trouble understanding your doctor's answers, ask where you can go for more information.

- Other members of your health care team, such as nurses and pharmacists, can be good sources of information. Talk to them, too.

Section 2.7

Financial Aid for Eye Care

"Financial Aid for Eye Care," Fact Sheet, National Eye Institute, http://www.nei.nih.gov; June 2001.

Many state and national resources regularly provide aid to people with vision problems. The National Eye Institute, which supports eye research, does not help individuals pay for eye care. However, if you are in need of financial aid to assess or treat an eye problem, you might contact one or more of the following programs.

You may also contact a social worker at a local hospital or other community agency. Social workers often are knowledgeable about community resources that can help people facing financial and medical problems.

- EyeCare America—National Eye Care Project, coordinated by the American Academy of Ophthalmology (AAO), provides free and low-cost eye exams for U.S. citizens 65 and older who have not had access to an ophthalmologist in the past three years. Telephone: (800) 222-EYES.

- VISION USA, coordinated by the American Optometric Association (AOA), provides free eye care to uninsured, low-income workers and their families. Screening for the program takes place only during January of each year, with exams provided later in the year. Telephone: (800) 766-4466.

- Lions Clubs International provides financial assistance to individuals for eye care through local clubs. There are Lions Clubs in most localities, and services vary from club to club. Check your telephone book for the telephone number and address of your local club. The telephone number for the national office is (630) 571-5466.

- Celebrate Sight: Do You Know Your Glaucoma Risk?, coordinated by the American Academy of Ophthalmology, is a program offering free examinations and treatment for glaucoma to people who do not have medical insurance. Telephone: (800) 391-EYES.

17

- Mission Cataract USA, coordinated by the Volunteer Eye Surgeons' Association, is a program providing free cataract surgery to people of all ages who have no other means to pay. Surgeries are scheduled annually on one day, usually in May. Telephone: (800) 343-7265.

- Knights Templar Eye Foundation provides assistance for eye surgery for people who are unable to pay or receive adequate assistance from current government agencies or similar sources. Mailing address: 5097 North Elston Avenue, Suite 100, Chicago, IL 60630-2460. Telephone: (773) 205-3838. E-mail: ktef@knightstemplar.org. Website: http://www.knightstemplar.org/ktef.

- Sight for Students, a Vision Service Plan (VSP) program, in partnership with national and regional partners, provides eye exams and glasses to children 18 years and younger whose families cannot afford vision care. Telephone: (888) 290-4964. Website: http://www.sightforstudents.org.

- New Eyes for the Needy provides vouchers for the purchase of new prescription eyeglasses. Mailing address: 549 Millburn Avenue, P.O. Box 332, Short Hills, NJ 07078-0332. Telephone: (973) 376-4903.

- The Medicine Program assists people to enroll in one or more of the many patient assistance programs that provide prescription medicine free of charge to those in need. Patients must meet the sponsor's criteria. The program is conducted in cooperation with the patient's doctor. Mailing address: P.O. Box 4182, Poplar Bluff, MO 63902-4182. Telephone: (573) 996-7300. E-mail: help@themedicineprogram.com. Website: http://www.themedicineprogram.com.

- Directory of Prescription Drug Patient Assistance Programs 1999–2000, published by Pharmaceutical Research and Manufacturers of America, identifies company programs that provide prescription medications free of charge to physicians for their needy patients. Telephone: (800) PMA-INFO.

The National Eye Institute (NEI), part of the National Institutes of Health, is the Federal Government's principal agency for conducting and supporting research on the prevention, diagnosis, treatment, and rehabilitation of eye diseases and disorders of the visual system. Inclusion in this chapter does not imply endorsement by the National Eye Institute or by the National Institutes of Health.

Chapter 3

20/20 Vision

20/20 vision is a term used to express normal visual acuity (the clarity or sharpness of vision) measured at a distance of 20 feet. If you have 20/20 vision, you can see clearly at 20 feet what should normally be seen at that distance. If you have 20/100 vision, it means that you must be as close as 20 feet to see what a person with normal vision can see at 100 feet.

20/20 does not necessarily mean perfect vision. 20/20 vision only indicates the sharpness or clarity of vision at a distance. There are other important vision skills, including peripheral awareness or side vision, eye coordination, depth perception, focusing ability, and color vision that contribute to your overall visual ability.

Some people can see well at a distance, but are unable to bring nearer objects into focus. This condition can be caused by hyperopia (farsightedness) or presbyopia (loss of focusing ability). Others can see items that are close, but cannot see those far away. This condition may be caused by myopia (nearsightedness).

A comprehensive eye examination by a doctor of optometry can diagnose those causes, if any, that are affecting your ability to see well. In most cases, your optometrist can prescribe glasses, contact lenses, or a vision therapy program that will help improve your vision. If the reduced vision is due to an eye disease, the use of ocular medication or other treatment may be used.

Chapter 4

Normal Pediatric Vision

Chapter Contents

21

Section 4.1

Your Child's Vision

This information was provided by KidsHealth, one of the largest resources online for medically reviewed health information written for parents, kids, and teens. For more articles like this one, visit www.KidsHealth.org or www.TeensHealth.org. © 2001 The Nemours Center for Children's Health Media, a division of The Nemours Foundation.

There's nothing quite like looking into your child's eyes. But while you're busy gazing at your young one, be sure to pay attention to her eyesight. Early detection and treatment of eye problems are essential to a child's visual health. Here's what to look for.

Check It out

When does your child need her first eye examination? The American Academy of Ophthalmology recommends the following:

- Newborns should be checked for general eye health by a pediatrician or family physician in the hospital nursery.

- High-risk newborns (including premature infants), those with a family history of eye problems, and those with obvious eye irregularities should be examined by an ophthalmologist.

- In the first year of life, all infants should be routinely screened for eye health during well-baby visits with their doctor.

- Around the age of 3 1/2, children should be screened for eye health and tested for visual acuity by their doctor.

- About age 5, children should have their vision and eye alignment evaluated and alignment assessed by their doctor. Children who fail either test should be examined by an ophthalmologist.

- After age 5, further screening exams should be conducted at routine checks at school or at your child's doctor's office, or after the appearance of symptoms such as squinting or frequent headaches. (Many times a teacher will realize the child is not seeing well in class.)

However, children who wear prescription glasses or contacts probably need annual checkups to screen for vision changes, says Byron Demorest, MD, a pediatric ophthalmologist and spokesperson for the American Academy of Ophthalmology.

Signs that a young child may have vision problems include:

- constant eye rubbing
- extreme light sensitivity
- poor focusing
- poor visual tracking (following an object)
- abnormal alignment or movement of the eyes (after 6 months of age)
- chronic redness of the eyes
- chronic tearing of the eyes
- a white pupil instead of black

"A child does not have to be verbal to have an eye examination. We use hand puppets and other devices to evaluate their vision," says Jay Bernstein, MD, a pediatric ophthalmologist and spokesperson for the American Academy of Pediatrics.

In school-age children, watch for other signs such as:

- inability to see objects at a distance
- inability to read the blackboard
- squinting
- difficulty reading
- sitting too close to the TV

Dr. Demorest offers this general piece of advice to parents: "Just watch your child and if there is evidence of poor vision, or if their eyes cross, then they should be examined immediately so that the problem does not become permanent. If caught early, eye conditions can often be reversed."

Newborn Vision

How much can a newborn baby see?

"It's very hard for us to know how well they can see, but it's been estimated that their vision is rather blurry until about 6 months of age, and after that time, it improves rapidly," says Dr. Demorest. "Also, newborns are able to see colors."

When vision begins to improve, infants develop what is called stereo vision, that is, they combine the picture they see with one eye with the picture they see with their other eye.

"[B]abies will begin to look directly at their parent's face and develop depth perception," Dr. Demorest explains.

Common Eye Problems

There are several eye conditions that may affect children. Most of them are detected by a vision screening using an acuity chart during the preschool years.

- **Amblyopia** (lazy eye) is poor vision in an eye that appears to be normal. Two common causes are crossed eyes and a difference in the refractive error between the two eyes. If untreated, amblyopia can cause irreversible visual loss in the affected eye. (By then the brain's programming will ignore signals from that eye.) Amblyopia is best treated during the preschool years.

- **Strabismus** is a misalignment of the eyes; they may turn in, out, up, or down. If the same eye is chronically misaligned, amblyopia may develop in that eye. With early detection, vision can be restored by patching the properly aligned eye, which forces the misaligned one to work. Surgery or specially designed glasses may also help eyes to align.

- **Refractive errors** mean that the shape of the eye doesn't refract, or bend, light properly, so images appear blurred. In addition, refractive errors may also cause eyestrain and/or amblyopia. The most common form of refractive errors is nearsightedness; others include farsightedness and astigmatism.

- **Nearsightedness** is poor distance vision (also called myopia), which is usually treated with glasses.

- **Farsightedness** is poor near vision (also called hyperopia), which is usually treated with glasses.

- **Astigmatism** is imperfect curvature of the front surface of the eye. It is usually treated with glasses if it causes blurred vision or discomfort.

Other eye conditions require immediate attention, such as retinopathy of prematurity (a disease that usually affects premature infants who were on a ventilator for a long period of time after birth) and those associated with a family history, including the following:

- **Retinoblastoma** is a malignant tumor that usually appears in the first 3 years of life. The affected eye may have visual loss and whiteness in the pupil.

- **Infantile cataracts** can occur in newborns. A cataract is a gradual clouding of the eye's lens.

- **Congenital glaucoma** in infants is a rare condition that may be inherited. It is the result of incorrect or incomplete development of the eye drainage canals during the prenatal period. Congenital glaucoma can be treated with medication and surgery.

- **Genetic or metabolic diseases of the eye**, such as inherited disorders that make a child more likely to develop retinoblastoma or cataracts, may make it necessary for a child to have an eye exam at an early age and regular screenings.

Be sure to talk to your child's doctor if your child is at risk for any of these conditions.

Glasses and Contacts

If your child is diagnosed with an eye problem, at what age can she wear glasses or contacts?

"Children of any age, even babies, can wear glasses," says Sharon S. Lehman, MD, a pediatric ophthalmologist.

Keep these tips in mind for a child who wears glasses:

- Allow your child to pick her own frames, since she'll be the one wearing them.

- Plastic frames are best for kids younger than 2.

- If older children wear metal frames, make sure they have spring hinges, which are more durable.

- If your child needs to wear thick lenses, consider plastic frames since these will hold thicker lenses better than metal ones.

- An elastic strap attached to the glasses will help keep them in place for active toddlers.

- Children with severe eye problems may need special lenses called high index lenses that are thinner and lighter than plastic lenses.

- Polycarbonate lenses are recommended for kids who play sports. Polycarbonate is a tough transparent thermoplastic that is used to make thin, light lenses. However, although they are very impact-resistant, these lenses scratch more easily than plastic lenses.

Infants born with congenital cataracts need to have their cataracts surgically removed during the first few weeks of life. "Some children born with that condition wear contact lenses—with their parents inserting them, of course—at 6 months of age," Dr. Demorest says.

Around age 10, children may express a desire for contact lenses for cosmetic purposes or convenience if they play sports. Allowing your child to wear contacts, she says, depends on her ability to insert and remove lenses properly, and faithfully take them out as required and clean them as recommended by her doctor. Soft lenses are easier to adapt to than hard lenses, but not all children are candidates for soft lenses. Talk to your child's ophthalmologist about what type of contact lens is best for your child.

Dispelling Myths

Myth: Sitting too close to a TV is bad for your child's eyes.

Fact: There is no evidence that this damages a child's eyes. Dr. Demorest tells parents with a wink: "TV doesn't damage the eyes of children, it damages their brains!" The American Academy of Ophthalmology says that children can focus up close without eyestrain better than adults, so they often develop the habit of sitting right in front of the television or holding reading material close to their eyes. However, sitting too close to a TV may indicate that a child is nearsighted.

Myth: If you cross your eyes, they'll stay that way.

Fact: No, contrary to the old saying, children's eyes will not stay that way if they cross them.

Myth: If I have poor eyesight, my child will inherit that trait.

Fact: Unfortunately, this one is sometimes true. If you need glasses for good vision or have developed an eye condition (such as cataracts), your child may inherit that same trait. Discuss your family's visual history with your child's doctor.

Myth: Children should eat carrots to improve their vision.

Fact: Although carrots are rich in vitamin A, which is essential for sight, many other foods (asparagus, apricots, nectarines, and milk, for example) also contain vitamin A. So a well-balanced diet, with or without carrots, provides all the vitamin A needed for good vision.

Myth: Using computers damages a child's eyes.

Fact: According to the American Academy of Ophthalmology, working on computers will not harm your eyes. However, when using a computer for long periods of time, the eyes blink less than normal (just as when reading or performing other close work). The reduced rate of blinking makes eyes dry, which may lead to a feeling of eyestrain or fatigue. "The bottom line is that it's probably not the best thing in the world to do for long periods of time, so be sure your child takes breaks from the computer or video games," Dr. Bernstein says.

Myth: Two blue-eyed parents cannot produce a child with brown eyes.

Fact: Two blue-eyed parents can have a child with brown eyes, although it is very rare. Likewise, two brown-eyed parents can have a child with blue eyes, although this, too, is uncommon.

Myth: Only boys can be color-blind.

Fact: About 7% of boys have some degree of color blindness, while only up to 1.5% of girls suffer from the same condition.

Note: All information on KidsHealth is for educational purposes only. For specific medical advice, diagnoses, and treatment, consult your doctor.

Section 4.2

Infant Vision

Your baby has a whole lifetime to see and learn. But, did you know your baby also has to learn to see? As a parent, there are many things that you can do to help your baby's vision develop. First, proper prenatal care and nutrition can help your baby's eyes develop even before birth. At birth, your baby's eyes should be examined for signs of congenital eye problems. These are rare, but early diagnosis and treatment are important to your child's development.

At about age six months, you should take your baby to your doctor of optometry for his or her first thorough eye examination. Things that the optometrist will test for include excessive or unequal amounts of nearsightedness, farsightedness, or astigmatism and eye movement ability as well as eye health problems. These problems are not common, but it is important to identify children who have them at this stage. Vision development and eye health problems can be more easily corrected if treatment is begun early.

Unless you notice a need, or your doctor of optometry advises you otherwise, your child's next examination should be around age three, and then again before he or she enters school.

Between birth and age three, when many of your baby's vision skills will develop, there are ways that you can help.

During the first four months of life, your baby should begin to follow moving objects with the eyes and reach for things, first by chance and later more accurately, as hand-eye coordination and depth perception begin to develop.

To help, use a nightlight or other dim lamp in your baby's room; change the crib's position frequently and your child's position in it; keep reach-and-touch toys within your baby's focus, about eight to twelve inches; talk to your baby as you walk around the room; alternate right and left sides with each feeding; and hang a mobile above and outside the crib.

Between four and eight months, your baby should begin to turn from side to side and use his or her arms and legs. Eye movement and eye/body coordination skills should develop further and both eyes should focus equally.

You should enable your baby to explore different shapes and textures with his or her fingers; give your baby the freedom to crawl and explore; hang objects across the crib; and play patty cake and peek-a-boo with your baby.

From eight to twelve months, your baby should be mobile now, crawling and pulling himself or herself up. He or she will begin to use both eyes together and judge distances and grasp and throw objects with greater precision. To support development don't encourage early walking—crawling is important in developing eye-hand-foot-body coordination; give your baby stacking and take-apart toys; and provide objects your baby can touch, hold, and see at the same time.

From one to two years, your child's eye-hand coordination and depth perception will continue to develop and he or she will begin to understand abstract terms. Things you can do are encourage walking; provide building blocks, simple puzzles and balls; and provide opportunities to climb and explore indoors and out.

There are many other affectionate and loving ways in which you can aid your baby's vision development. Use your creativity and imagination. Ask your doctor of optometry to suggest other specific activities.

Section 4.3

Preschool Vision

During the infant and toddler years, your child has been developing many vision skills and has been learning how to see. In the preschool years, this process continues, as your child develops visually guided eye-hand-body coordination, fine motor skills and the visual motor skills necessary to learn to read.

As a parent, you should watch for signs that may indicate a vision development problem, including a short attention span for the child's age; difficulty with eye-hand-body coordination in ball play and bike riding; and avoidance of coloring and puzzles and other detailed activities.

There are everyday things that you can do at home to help your preschooler's vision develop as it should.

These activities include reading aloud to your child and letting him or her see what you are reading; providing a chalkboard, finger paints, and different shaped blocks and showing your child how to use them in imaginative play; providing safe opportunities to use playground equipment like a jungle gym and balance beam; and allowing time for interacting with other children and for playing independently.

By age three, your child should have a thorough optometric eye examination to make sure your preschooler's vision is developing properly and there is no evidence of eye disease. If needed, your doctor can prescribe treatment including glasses and/or vision therapy to correct a vision development problem.

Here are several tips to make your child's optometric examination a positive experience:

1. Make an appointment early in the day. Allow about one hour.

2. Talk about the examination in advance and encourage your child's questions.

3. Explain the examination in your child's terms, comparing the E chart to a puzzle and the instruments to tiny flashlights and a kaleidoscope.

Unless your doctor of optometry advises otherwise, your child's next eye examination should be at age five. By comparing test results of the two examinations, your optometrist can tell how well your child's vision is developing for the next major step—into the school years.

Section 4.4

School-Age Vision

A good education for your child means good schools, good teachers, and good vision. Your child's eyes are constantly in use in the classroom and at play. So when his or her vision is not functioning properly, learning and participation in recreational activities will suffer.

The basic vision skills needed for school use are:

- Near vision. The ability to see clearly and comfortably at 10 to 13 inches.

- Distance vision. The ability to see clearly and comfortably beyond arm's reach.

- Binocular coordination. The ability to use both eyes together.

- Eye movement skills. The ability to aim the eyes accurately, move them smoothly across a page, and shift them quickly and accurately from one object to another.

- Focusing skills. The ability to keep both eyes accurately focused at the proper distance to see clearly and to change focus quickly.

- Peripheral awareness. The ability to be aware of things located to the side while looking straight ahead.

- Eye/hand coordination. The ability to use the eyes and hands together.

If any of these or other vision skills is lacking or not functioning properly, your child will have to work harder. This can lead to headaches, fatigue, and other eyestrain problems. As a parent, be alert for symptoms that may indicate your child has a vision or visual processing problem. Be sure to tell your optometrist if your child frequently:

- loses his or her place while reading

- avoids close work

- holds reading material closer than normal

- tends to rub his or her eyes

- has headaches

- turns or tilts head to use one eye only

- makes frequent reversals when reading or writing

- uses finger to maintain place when reading

- omits or confuses small words when reading

- consistently performs below potential

Since vision changes can occur without you or your child noticing them, your child should visit the optometrist at least every two years, or more frequently, if specific problems or risk factors exist. If needed, the doctor can prescribe treatment including eyeglasses, contact lenses, or vision therapy.

Remember, a school vision or pediatrician's screening is not a substitute for a thorough eye examination.

Chapter 5

Signs of Possible Eye Trouble

Chapter Contents

Section 5.1

Signs of Possible Eye Trouble in Children

Reprinted with permission from Prevent Blindness America. © 2000. For additional information, call the Prevent Blindness America toll-free information line at (800) 331-2020, or visit www.preventblindness.org.

It is possible for your child to have a serious vision problem without you being aware of it. Any concern about abnormalities in the appearance of the eyes or vision should be investigated. If you have any questions about your child's vision, see an eye doctor. In any case, start early to provide your child with a regular schedule of professional eye exams.

Signs of possible eye trouble in children include:

Behavior

- Rubs eyes excessively
- Shuts or covers one eye
- Tilts or thrusts head forward
- Has difficulty with reading or other close-up work
- Holds objects close to eyes
- Blinks more than usual or is irritable when doing close-up work
- Is unable to see distant things clearly
- Squints eyelids together or frowns

Appearance

- Crossed or misaligned eyes
- Red-rimmed, encrusted, or swollen eyelids
- Inflamed or watery eyes
- Recurring styes (infections) on eyelids
- Color photos of eyes show white reflection instead of typical red or no reflection

Complaints

- Eyes itch, burn, or feel scratchy
- Cannot see well
- Dizziness, headaches, or nausea following close-up work
- Blurred or double vision

If a child exhibits one or more of these signs, please seek professional eye care. A professional eye exam is recommended shortly after birth, by six months of age, before entering school (four or five years old), and periodically throughout school years. Regular eye exams are important since some eye problems have no signs or symptoms.

For more information about children's eye health and safety, contact Prevent Blindness America or the Prevent Blindness affiliate near you.

Section 5.2

Signs of Possible Eye Trouble in Adults

Reprinted with permission from Prevent Blindness America. © 2000. For additional information, call the Prevent Blindness America toll-free information line at (800) 331-2020, or visit www.preventblindness.org.

Any changes in the appearance of your eyes or vision should be investigated further. Some examples include:

- Unusual trouble adjusting to dark rooms
- Difficulty focusing on near or distant objects
- Squinting or blinking due to unusual sensitivity to light or glare
- Change in color of iris
- Red-rimmed, encrusted, or swollen lids
- Recurrent pain in or around eyes

- Double vision
- Dark spot at the center of viewing
- Lines and edges appear distorted or wavy
- Excess tearing or watery eyes
- Dry eyes with itching or burning
- Seeing spots or ghost-like images

The following may be indications of potentially serious problems that might require emergency medical attention:

- Sudden loss of vision in one eye
- Sudden hazy or blurred vision
- Flashes of light or black spots
- Halos or rainbows around light
- Curtain-like blotting out of vision
- Loss of peripheral (side) vision

If you notice any signs of potential eye problems, see an eye doctor for a complete eye exam. Even if you have no signs, regular eye exams are recommended, especially for those with some chronic health conditions such as diabetes and high blood pressure. Early detection and treatment can be the key to preventing sight loss.

To learn more about signs of eye trouble in adults, please contact Prevent Blindness America or the Prevent Blindness affiliate near you.

Chapter 6

What Are Refractive Errors?

For our eyes to be able to see, light rays must be bent or refracted so they can focus on the retina, the nerve layer that lines the back of the eye. The cornea and the lens refract light rays. The retina receives the picture formed by these light rays and sends the image to the brain through the optic nerve. A refractive error means that the shape of your eye doesn't refract the light properly, so the image you see is blurred.

While refractive errors are called eye disorders, they are not diseases. In a normal eye, the cornea and lens focus light rays on the retina.

What Are the Different Types of Refractive Errors?

Myopia (Nearsightedness)

A myopic eye is longer than normal, so that the light rays focus in front of the retina. Close objects look clear but distant objects appear blurred. In myopia, distant objects are blurry because the eye is too long, and images focus in front of the retina instead of on it. Myopia is inherited and is often discovered in children when they are eight to twelve years old. During the teenage years, when the body grows rapidly, myopia gets worse. Between the ages of 20 and 40, there is usually little change.

If the myopia is mild, it is called low myopia. Severe myopia is known as high myopia. If you have high myopia, you have a higher risk of detached retina. It is important to have regular eye examinations by an ophthalmologist (medical eye doctor) to watch for any changes in the retina. If the retina does detach, a surgical operation is the only way to repair it.

Hyperopia (Farsightedness)

A hyperopic eye is shorter than normal. Light from close objects, such as the page of a book, cannot focus clearly on the retina. In hyperopia, the eye is too short for images to focus on the retina, so close objects are blurry.

Like nearsightedness, farsightedness is usually inherited. Babies and young children tend to be slightly hyperopic. As the eye grows and becomes longer, hyperopia lessens.

Astigmatism (Distorted Vision)

The cornea is the clear front window of the eye. A normal cornea is round and smooth, like a basketball. When you have astigmatism, the cornea curves more in one direction than in the other, like a football. Astigmatism distorts or blurs vision for both near and far objects. It's almost like looking into a funhouse mirror in which you appear too tall, too wide, or too thin. You can have astigmatism in combination with myopia or hyperopia.

Presbyopia (Aging Eyes)

When you are young, the lens in your eye is soft and flexible. The lens of the eye changes its shape easily, allowing you to focus on objects both close and far away. After the age of 40, the lens becomes more rigid. Because the lens can't change shape as easily as it once did, it is more difficult to read at close range. This perfectly normal condition is called presbyopia. You can also have presbyopia in combination with myopia, hyperopia, or astigmatism.

How Are Refractive Errors Corrected?

Eyeglasses

Glasses are an easy method to correct refractive errors. They can also help protect your eyes from harmful light rays, such as ultraviolet

(UV) light rays. A special coating that screens out UV light is available when you order your glasses. Bifocals are glasses that are used to correct presbyopia. They have a correction for reading on the bottom half of the lens and another for seeing distance on the top. Trifocals are lenses with three different lens corrections in one set of eyeglasses. If you don't need correction for seeing distance, you can buy over-the-counter reading glasses to correct presbyopia. No exercise or medication can reverse presbyopia. You will probably need to change your prescription from time to time between the ages of 40 and 60, because your lens will continue to lose flexibility.

Contact Lenses

There are now a wide variety of contact lenses available. The type that is best for you depends on your refractive error and your lifestyle. If you want to wear contact lenses, discuss the various options with your ophthalmologist. You may have heard of a process called orthokeratology to treat myopia. It uses a series of hard contact lenses to gradually flatten the cornea and reduce the refractive error. Improvement of sight from orthokeratology is temporary. After the use of the lenses is discontinued, the cornea returns to its original shape and myopia returns.

Refractive Surgery

Radial keratotomy is a surgical operation to improve myopia by changing the curve of the cornea over the pupil. The surgeon makes several deep incisions (keratotomies) in the cornea in a radial, or spoke-like, pattern. The incisions flatten out the cornea and shorten the distance light rays must travel to the retina. In radial keratotomy, incisions are made in the cornea to change its shape and improve myopia. In one large study of RK, 64 percent of people did not wear glasses or contacts five years after their surgery—and 36 percent did, at least for some situations. People with mild myopia have even more satisfactory results. Reading glasses may be necessary for older adults, because RK does not alter the normal aging process of the eye. Complications at the time of surgery are rare but can be serious. After RK, the cornea heals slowly, and concerns remain about the side effects of this delayed corneal healing. There may be:

- Fluctuating vision, especially the first few months after surgery
- A weakened cornea, more vulnerable to rupture if hit directly

39

- Infection

- The need for additional refractive surgery

- Difficulty fitting contact lenses

- Glare or starburst around lights

- Temporary pain

In the past few years a new type of laser surgery has been investigated to correct myopia. In a process called photorefractive keratectomy (PRK), the excimer laser precisely sculpts the surface of the cornea. There are several thousand people in the United States who have had PRK through research studies overseen by the Food and Drug Administration. For mild to moderate myopia, PRK and RK have similar results.

What Is the Best Method of Correcting Refractive Errors?

There is no best method for correcting refractive errors. The most appropriate correction for you depends on your eyes and your lifestyle. You should discuss your refractive errors and your lifestyle with your ophthalmologist to decide on which correction will be most effective for you.

Chapter 7

Low Vision and Blindness

Chapter Contents

Section 7.1

Facts and Figures on Blindness and Low Vision

Every seven minutes, someone in America will become blind or visually impaired. For more facts and figures on the 10 million blind or visually impaired individuals in the United States, see below.

Numbers of Blind and Visually Impaired Americans

Approximately how many blind and visually impaired people are there in the United States?

Although estimates vary, there are approximately 10 million blind and visually impaired people in the United States.

How many legally blind people are there in the United States?

Approximately 1.3 million Americans are legally blind.

How many elderly individuals (aged 65 or older) in the United States are blind or visually impaired?

There are approximately 5.5 million elderly individuals who are blind or visually impaired.

How many visually impaired, blind, and deaf-blind students are served in special education in the United States?

Approximately 93,600 visually impaired or blind students, 10,800 of whom are deaf-blind, are served in the special education program.

How many legally blind children are there in the United States?

There are approximately 55,200 legally blind children.

Getting Around

How many visually impaired and blind people use long canes to get around?

Approximately 109,000 visually impaired people in the United States use long canes to get around.

How many visually impaired and blind people use dog guides to get around?

Just over 7,000 Americans use dog guides. Annually, approximately 1,500 individuals graduate from a dog-guide user program.

Children's Use of Braille

How many legally blind children in the United States use braille most often when reading?

Approximately 5,500 legally blind children use braille as their primary reading medium.

Computer Use

How many blind or visually impaired adults in the United States use computers?

At least 1.5 million blind and visually impaired Americans use computers.

Marital Status

What percentage of blind and visually impaired Americans are married?

Currently, approximately 42 percent of blind and severely visually impaired Americans are married, 33 percent are widowed, 13 percent are separated or divorced, and 13 percent have never married.

Race and Ethnicity

Looking at different racial and ethnic groups, how many blind and visually impaired Americans are there?

Of all blind and visually impaired Americans, approximately 80 percent are white, 18 percent are black, and 2 percent are from other races. Eight percent are of Hispanic origin and could be of any race.

Employment

What percentage of visually impaired working-age Americans (not including those who are blind) are employed?

Approximately 46 percent of visually impaired adult Americans are employed.

What percentage of legally blind working-age Americans are employed?

Approximately 32 percent of legally blind working-age Americans are employed.

Educational Attainment

How much schooling have blind and visually impaired Americans received?

Approximately 45 percent of individuals with severe visual impairment or blindness have a high school diploma, compared to 80 percent among fully sighted individuals. Among high school graduates, those with severe visual impairment or blindness are about as likely to have taken some college courses as those who were sighted, but they are less likely to have graduated.

Does the amount of schooling blind and visually impaired Americans receive vary among different racial and ethnic groups?

Yes. Approximately 62 percent of visually impaired whites complete high school or higher education, compared to 41 percent of visually impaired blacks and 44 percent of visually impaired Hispanics.

Section 7.2

What You Should Know about Low Vision

"What You Should Know about Low Vision," National Eye Institute, available online at http://www.nei.nih.gov, May 2000.

This chapter will help people with vision loss and their families and friends better understand low vision. It describes how to get help and live more safely and independently.

How Do I Know If I Have Low Vision?

There are many signs that can signal vision loss. For example, even with your regular glasses, do you have difficulty:

- Recognizing faces of friends and relatives?
- Doing things that require you to see well up close, like reading, cooking, sewing, or fixing things around the house?
- Picking out and matching the color of your clothes?
- Doing things at work or home because lights seem dimmer than they used to?
- Reading street and bus signs or the names of stores?

Vision changes like these could be early warning signs of eye disease. Usually, the earlier your problem is diagnosed, the better the chance of successful treatment and keeping your remaining vision.

What Is Low Vision?

Low vision means that even with regular glasses, contact lenses, medicine, or surgery, people find everyday tasks difficult to do. Reading the mail, shopping, cooking, seeing the TV, and writing can seem challenging.

Millions of Americans lose some of their vision every year. Irreversible vision loss is most common among people over age 65.

Is Losing Vision Just Part of Getting Older?

No. Some normal changes in our eyes and vision occur as we get older. However, these changes usually don't lead to low vision.

Most people develop low vision because of eye diseases and health conditions like macular degeneration, cataract, glaucoma, and diabetes. A few people develop vision loss after eye injuries or from birth defects. While vision that's lost usually cannot be restored, many people can make the most of the vision they have.

Your eye care professional can tell the difference between normal changes in the aging eye and those caused by eye diseases.

How Do I Know When to Get an Eye Exam?

Regular dilated eye exams should be part of your routine health care. However, if you believe your vision has recently changed, you should see your eye care professional as soon as possible.

Meet Mary, Jim, Crystal, and Mike

By making better use of their remaining vision, people can continue to enjoy doing important daily activities. Here are some examples.

Mary's Story

Mary is slowly losing her straight-ahead vision, which allows her to read and recognize faces. She has age-related macular degeneration, an eye disease that affects central vision.

While Mary's eye care professional has reassured her that she will not lose her vision completely, she is frustrated because she does not see as well as before.

Mary thought that nothing she did would help. Then her eye care professional suggested that she see a specialist in low vision.

A specialist in low vision is an optometrist or ophthalmologist who is trained to evaluate vision. This person can prescribe visual devices and teach people how to use them.

There are a wide variety of devices that help people make the most of their remaining vision. The specialist recommended special magnifying devices for Mary that helped her see things more clearly.

Mary also went to a vision rehabilitation program that taught her new ways of doing tasks. Someone from the program came to Mary's home to see what changes could be made. She also learned about helpful devices, such as talking clocks that tell the time with a press of a button. Large print books and publications made it easier to read and allowed Mary to keep enjoying one of her favorite activities.

Jim's Story

Jim has lost a lot of his side vision because of glaucoma. He found it difficult to do his job.

He made some changes to his office so he could work better. A talking computer keeps him up to date on sales figures. Writing was very difficult until he used better lighting. A vision rehabilitation teacher showed Jim how to use a writing guide to help write clear notes and employee memos.

Learning to get around safely from an orientation and mobility specialist helped him travel independently. He also joined a support group to talk about the challenges, frustrations, fears, and unhappiness that can come from living with low vision. At first, he felt that his vision loss would keep him from doing the things he liked to do. In the end, he found that wasn't true.

Crystal's Story

Crystal lost some vision because of diabetes.

Rather than limit her activities, she chose to look at them as challenges. Crystal met with a vision rehabilitation professional. She received training on how to use certain low vision aids. As a result, Crystal made several changes to her home and simplified her life.

First, raised markings were applied to the most common settings on her microwave dial. This allowed her to more safely adjust the oven.

Better lighting in her stairways, closets, and home workshop made it safer to move about. A magnifier for reading food labels made controlling her diet easy. Special checks with large print and raised markings simplified paying bills. A special needle allowed her to continue sewing, one of her favorite activities.

For Crystal, the result was increased safety, more freedom, and restored confidence.

Mike's Story

Mike also has low vision because of age-related macular degeneration. But he has found ways to adapt to his vision loss.

Mike's doctor referred him to a vision rehabilitation program. As a result of his evaluation, Mike uses a closed circuit television at home. It enlarges the print in letters, bills, newspapers, and magazines. He uses a telescopic lens for getting around his neighborhood. A hand-held magnifier helps him read his mail in his favorite chair and menus at restaurants. Mike learned to adapt, and low vision has not stopped him from enjoying life.

What Can I Do If I Have Low Vision?

Many people with low vision are taking charge. They want more information about devices and services that can help them keep their independence.

Talk with Your Eye Care Professional

It's important to talk with your eye care professional about your vision problems. Even though it may be difficult, ask for help. Find out where you can get more information about services and devices that can help you.

What Jane, Jim, Crystal, and Mike have in common is that they're taking charge of their health. They have different types of vision loss from different eye diseases. Yet each of them asked about available resources that might help them continue to live independently. Each needed specific visual devices and training on how to use them.

Many people require more than one visual device. They may need magnifying lenses for close-up viewing, and telescopic lenses for seeing in the distance. Some people may need to learn how to get around their neighborhoods.

If your eye care professional says, "Nothing more can be done for your vision," ask about vision rehabilitation.

These programs offer a wide range of services, such as low vision evaluations and special training to use visual and adaptive devices. They also offer guidance for modifying your home as well as group support from others with low vision.

Investigate and Learn

Be persistent. Remember that you are your best health advocate. Investigate and learn as much as you can, especially if you have been told that you may lose more vision. It is important that you ask questions about vision rehabilitation and get answers. Many resources are available to help you.

Write down questions to ask your doctor, or take a tape recorder with you.

Rehabilitation programs, devices, and technology can help you adapt to vision loss. They may help you keep doing many of the things you did before.

Know that, like Mary, Jim, Crystal, and Mike, you can make the difference in living with low vision.

Where Can I Get More Information?

For more information about low vision, contact your state or local rehabilitation agency for the blind and visually impaired or the following organizations:.

American Academy of Ophthalmology
P.O. Box 7424
San Francisco, CA 94120-7424
Phone: (415) 561-8500
Website: http://www.aao.org

American Foundation for the Blind
11 Penn Plaza
Suite 300
New York, NY 10001
Toll-Free: (800) 232-5463
Phone: (212) 502-7600
Website: http://www.afb.org

American Optometric Association
243 N. Lindbergh Boulevard
St. Louis, MO 63141
Phone: (314) 991-4100
Website: http://www.aoa.org

Lighthouse International
111 East 59th Street
New York, NY 10022-1202
Toll-Free: (800) 829-0500
TTY: (212) 821-9713
Phone: (212) 821-9200
Website: http://www.lighthouse.org

National Association for Visually Handicapped
22 West 21st Street, 6th Floor
New York, NY 10010
Phone: (212) 889-3141
Website: http://www.navh.org

National Eye Institute
2020 Vision Place
Bethesda, MD 20892-3655
Phone: (301) 496-5248
Website: http://www.nei.nih.gov

What Can I Do about My Low Vision?

Although many people maintain good vision throughout their life-times, people over age 65 are at increased risk of developing low vision. You and your eye care professional or specialist in low vision need to work in partnership to achieve what is best for you. An important part of this relationship is good communication.

Here are some questions to ask your eye care professional or specialist in low vision to get the discussion started:

Questions to Ask Your Eye Care Professional

- What changes can I expect in my vision?

- Will my vision loss get worse? How much of my vision will I lose?

- Will regular eyeglasses improve my vision?

- What medical/surgical treatments are available for my condition?

- What can I do to protect or prolong my vision?

- Will diet, exercise, or other lifestyle changes help?

- If my vision can't be corrected, can you refer me to a specialist in low vision?

- Where can I get a low vision examination and evaluation? Where can I get vision rehabilitation?

Questions to Ask Your Specialist in Low Vision

- How can I continue my normal, routine activities?

- Are there resources to help me in my job?

- Will any special devices help me with daily activities like reading, sewing, cooking, or fixing things around the house?

- What training and services are available to help me live better and more safely with low vision?

- Where can I find individual or group support to cope with my vision loss?

Section 7.3

Living with Low Vision

Reprinted with permission from Prevent Blindness America. © 2000. For additional information, call the Prevent Blindness America toll-free information line at (800) 331-2020, or visit www.preventblindness.org.

Investigate

There are national and local resources available that can help people who have low vision. Information and referrals can be provided by various agencies, organizations, and institutions located throughout the United States. These resources can help educate you on your eye condition, offer support services, and provide rehabilitation services.

Advocate

If you've been told that "nothing more can be done with regular corrective eyeglasses," you may need to have a low vision specialist's evaluation. Vision rehabilitation specialists can prescribe magnifiers, telescopic aids, closed-circuit televisions, and other adaptive equipment that can enhance your existing vision. Ask your ophthalmologist or optometrist for a referral to a vision rehabilitation specialist.

Support

If you are having some difficulty adjusting to your vision loss or want to network with other people who are overcoming vision problems, a support group can be an invaluable resource. Support groups can assist people with vision loss by providing the opportunity to find out how others are coping, learn new ideas on how to do old things new ways, receive information on resources, and receive support in a variety of other ways. If there is no support group available in your community, contact Prevent Blindness America or the Prevent Blindness affiliate near you.

Communicate

Write down questions for your eye doctor before your next visit. Speak frankly with your eye doctor about your questions and concerns. Tell the doctor if you do not understand. Repeat if necessary. Ask a family member or close friend to go with you into the examining room. It helps to be able to confirm information with a family member. Including family members initially helps them get involved and enhances their understanding of your eye condition and future concerns. Family members may surprise you with creative solutions.

Anticipate

If your eye doctor has told you that further vision loss is possible, get prepared. Living with low vision may be viewed either as an obstacle to your independence or more positively, as a challenge. You will need to consider developing new skills in your activities of daily life. Learn as much as you can about resources and rehabilitation services that are available. Learning as much as you can before vision is lost can make your adjustment easier.

Assert Yourself

Don't take no for an answer. Many people who have low vision do not know that help is available. Ask your eye doctor for information and referrals. Remember you are on a mission to maintain your independence.

Educate

Learn everything you can about your eye condition. The more you understand, the less fear you may experience. Educating yourself helps you confront concerns and speak intelligently with your eye doctor and others. Knowledge gives you control.

Determination

Know that many people who have experienced vision loss at first feel anger, grief, and depression. Losing even part of your vision can be devastating. Remain determined and persistent. You can make the most of your remaining vision.

Motivation

Empower yourself with the knowledge that much of what has to be done must be done by you. Take control.

Hope and Research

There are many exciting advances that have been made possible through medical research. This may put an end to many eye conditions and diseases in the future. Support research with your vote. Write to Congressional representatives and stay involved.

To learn more about low vision, contact Prevent Blindness America or the Prevent Blindness affiliate near you.

Section 7.4

Assistive Technology

There is a wide variety of optical devices and adaptive products available to help people with low vision live and/or work more productively and safely. Most people can be helped with one or more of them. Unfortunately, only about 20 to 25 percent of those who could benefit have been seen by a low vision specialist and had treatment options, including low vision devices, prescribed specifically for them. The more commonly prescribed devices are:

- Spectacle-mounted magnifiers—A magnifying lens is mounted in the individual's spectacles or on a special headband. This allows use of both hands to complete the close-up task, such as reading.

- Spectacle-mounted telescopes—These miniature telescopes are useful for seeing longer distances, such as across the room to watch television, and can also be modified for near (reading) tasks.

- Hand-held and stand magnifiers—Serve as supplementary aids. They are convenient for reading such things as price tags, labels, and instrument dials. Both types can be equipped with lights.

- Electro-optical aids—Closed-circuit television (also called CCTVs) enlarge reading material on a video screen. Some are portable, while some can be connected to a computer. The user can adjust the image brightness, size, contrast and background illumination.

In addition, there are numerous other products to assist those with low vision, such as large-type books, magazines, and newspapers, books-on-tape, talking wristwatches, self-threading needles, and more.

Section 7.5

Helping Someone Who Can't See

Excerpted from "What Do You Do When You Meet Someone Who Can't See?" © 1991; updated 2002. Reprinted with permission of Lighthouse International; available online at http://www.lighthouse.org.

On the Street

When someone seems confused or in danger, ask if you can help. Avoid grabbing a person's arm—it's startling, dangerous, and discourteous. Instead, ask if he or she would like to hold your arm at the elbow.

Walk a half step ahead so that your body movements indicate when to change direction, stop or start, and when to step up or down at a curb. Also, provide information verbally about the environment.

Giving Directions

Be specific. For example: "We're on the northeast corner of 59th Street and Park Avenue." Or "We're facing the entrance to the store."

Guide Dogs

Never pet or distract guide dogs. They're working animals. Owners depend on their dog's complete attention for safety.

Safety

Half-open doors are a hazard. Keep doors either closed or wide open.

Handling Money

Coins can be identified by touch, but paper money cannot. Identify each denomination verbally when handing bills to a person who is visually impaired.

Dining out

Ask if you can help guide your dining companion to the table. Once there, place his or her hand on the back of the chair, specifying whether the chair has arms.

If asked, read the menu and describe the locations of food on the plate using an imaginary clock as your reference. For example: "The vegetables are at three o'clock."

In unfamiliar situations, announce your arrival to, and departure from, a room when a person who is blind is present. In a new group setting, address individuals who are blind by name if you wish a reply. Always use a normal tone of voice, and don't feel uncomfortable using such expressions as "See you later."

Chapter 8

Protecting Your Eyes

Chapter Contents

Section 8.1

Ultraviolet Radiation and Your Eyes

"Frequently Asked Questions about UV," reprinted with permission from Prevent Blindness America. © 2000. For additional information, call the Prevent Blindness America toll-free information line at (800) 331-2020, or visit www.preventblindness.org.

What Is UV?

UV is ultraviolet radiation, and is sometimes called the sunburn rays. The sun produces many types of radiation. Some is the light we need for seeing. There is also infrared radiation that is invisible but felt as heat. Ultraviolet radiation is also invisible.

Can UV Radiation Hurt Our Eyes?

More and more scientific evidence shows that long-term exposure to ultraviolet radiation can damage our eyes. With the thinning of the earth's ozone layer and the growing popularity of outdoor activities, there is a strong possibility that UV-related eye disorders will increase within the next decade.

Ultraviolet radiation may contribute to the development of various eye disorders, such as macular degeneration, the leading cause of vision loss among older Americans, and cataracts, a major cause of visual impairment and blindness around the world.

Who Is at Risk?

Everyone—including children—is at risk for eye damage that can lead to vision loss from exposure to UV radiation. Any factor that increases your exposure to sunlight will increase your risk. People whose work or leisure activities involve lengthy exposure to sunlight are at the greatest risk.

How Can We Protect Our Eyes?

Using both a brimmed hat or cap and UV-absorbing eyewear can provide protection from sunlight. A wide-brimmed hat or cap will block roughly 50 percent of the UV radiation and reduce the UV radiation that may enter the eyes from above or around glasses. Ultraviolet-absorbing eyewear provides the greatest measure of UV protection. Examine labels carefully to ensure that the lenses absorb at least 99 to 100 percent of both UV-A and UV-B. Be wary of labels that claim "Provides UV Protection" without specifying exactly what percentage of UV rays the product blocks.

To learn more about protecting your eyes from UV radiation, contact Prevent Blindness America or the Prevent Blindness Affiliate near you.

Section 8.2

Sunglasses

"Frequently Asked Questions about Sunglasses," reprinted with permission from Prevent Blindness America. © 2000. For additional information, call the Prevent Blindness America toll-free information line at (800) 331-2020, or visit www.preventblindness.org.

Why Do We Need Sunglasses?

Sunglasses can help your eyes in two important ways. They enhance the normal light-filtering capabilities of your eyes and they protect against the sun's damaging ultraviolet rays. Good sunglasses will reduce glare, filter out 99 to 100 percent of ultraviolet (UV) rays, provide visual protection, be comfortable, and not distort colors.

Who Is at Risk for Eye Problems Caused by UV Light?

Everyone—even a child—is at risk. No one is immune to sunlight-related eye problems. People who are at higher risk of developing problems from UV rays include those who spend long hours in the sun because of work or recreation, those who have had cataract surgery, and individuals who have certain retinal disorders. Also, some people are more sensitive to UV rays, including those who take certain medications, such as tetracycline, sulfa drugs, birth control pills, diuretics, and tranquilizers that increase the eye's sensitivity to light.

What Types of Sunglasses Are Best?

When your purchase sunglasses, look for a statement on the amount of UV radiation that is blocked from reaching the eye. The rule of thumb is the less UV rays that get through, the better. Experts recommend that to protect your eyes from harmful rays, sunglasses should block 99 to 100 percent of both UV-A and UV-B rays. Since as much as 50 percent of sunlight comes from overhead and gets by many glasses, a brimmed cap or hat should also be worn for maximum protection. Eyewear that wraps around the face also helps minimize the amount of harmful light entering the eyes.

Do Children Need Sunglasses?

Yes. When selecting sunglasses for children, keep these suggestions in mind:

- Check the sunglasses periodically to make sure they fit well and are not damaged.

- Select sunglasses that suit children's active lifestyles. The glasses should be impact resistant (made of polycarbonate), should not pop out of the frames, and the frames should be bendable, unbreakable and/or have snap-on temples.

- The lenses should be large enough to shield the eyes from most angles and to block light that leaks in around the frames.

- Choose a wide-brimmed hat for your child to maximize protection.

To learn more about sunglasses, please contact Prevent Blindness America or the Prevent Blindness affiliate near you.

Section 8.3

What to Look for in a Pair of Sunglasses

"What to Look For in a Pair of Sunglasses," by Michelle Meadows, *FDA Consumer*, U.S. Food and Drug Administration, August 2002.

As you slather on sunscreen to protect your skin this summer, don't forget sunglasses to protect your eyes. The same harmful rays that damage skin can also increase your risk of developing eye problems, such as cataracts—a clouding of the eye's lens that develops over years.

In the short term, people who spend long hours on the beach or in the snow without adequate eye protection can develop photokeratitis, reversible sunburn of the cornea. This painful condition can result in temporary loss of vision. When sunlight reflects off of snow, sand and water, it further increases exposure to ultraviolet (UV) radiation. These invisible high-energy rays lie just beyond the violet end of the visible light spectrum.

Everyone is at risk for eye damage from the sun year-round. The risk is greatest from about 10 a.m. to 4 p.m. Fishermen, farmers, beach-goers, and others who spend time in the sun for extended periods are at highest risk.

UV radiation in sunlight is commonly divided into UVA and UVB, and your sunglasses should block both forms. Don't assume that you get more UV protection with pricier sunglasses or glasses with a darker tint. Look for a label that specifically states that the glasses offer 99 percent to 100 percent UV protection. You could also ask an eye care professional to test your sunglasses if you're not sure of their level of UV protection.

Sunglasses should be dark enough to reduce glare, but not dark enough to distort colors and affect the recognition of traffic signals. Tint is mainly a matter of personal preference. For best color perception, Prevent Blindness America, a volunteer eye health and safety organization dedicated to fighting blindness and saving sight, recommends lenses that are neutral gray, amber, brown, or green. People who wear contact lenses that offer UV protection should still wear sunglasses.

61

Children also should wear sunglasses. They shouldn't be toy sunglasses, but real sunglasses that indicate the UV-protection level just as with adults. Polycarbonate lenses are generally recommended for children because they are the most shatter-resistant.

Sheryl Berman, M.D., a medical officer in the FDA's Division of Ophthalmic and Ear, Nose, and Throat Devices, says that wearing sunglasses reduces the risk of eye damage due to sun exposure, but doesn't completely eliminate it.

"Even when we talk about 100 percent UV protection, light still enters from the sides of sunglasses and can be reflected into the eye," she says. Some people choose sunglasses that wrap all the way around the temples. A hat with a three-inch brim can help block sunlight that comes in from overhead.

The FDA's Center for Devices and Radiological Health regulates nonprescription sunglasses as over-the-counter medical devices. Sunglasses are normally exempt from the FDA's premarket notification procedures. But sunglasses manufacturers who claim their products are of substantial importance in preventing health problems would be required to submit proof to the FDA. The only medical claim manufacturers are allowed to make on sunglasses is that they may reduce eye strain or eye fatigue due to glare.

Even though sunglasses are exempt from premarket notification, they remain subject to several regulations. Sunglasses regulated by the FDA must comply with impact-resistant requirements, for example. This doesn't mean that the glasses are shatterproof, but that they can withstand moderate impact. Sunglasses are not intended to function as protective eyewear in high-impact sports.

Manufacturers of sunglasses also must follow the FDA's labeling regulations. The FDA has issued warning letters to manufacturers about unsubstantiated performance claims, such as those relating to UV-absorbing sunglasses.

Section 8.4

Computers and Their Effects on Your Eyes

"Frequently Asked Questions about Computers and Their Effect on Your Eyes," reprinted with permission from Prevent Blindness America. © 2000. For additional information, call the Prevent Blindness America toll-free information line at (800) 331-2020, or visit www.preventblindness.org.

Are Video Display Terminals (VDTs) Harmful to Your Eyes?

Due to the dramatic increase in computer use—not only in the workplace but also in the home—complaints of eye fatigue and discomfort are common. Many people assume increased computer use is the source of these complaints. But extensive testing in government and private laboratories has not produced scientific evidence that VDTs will harm your eyes. Research has established that VDTs emit little or no hazardous radiation, such as X-ray, or non-ionizing radiation, such as ultraviolet rays.

Can VDTs Cause Eyestrain?

Although people who use VDTs on a daily basis often complain of eye irritation, fatigue, and difficulty focusing, most of these symptoms are caused by conditions surrounding the computer screen, such as poor lighting or improper placement of equipment and supplies. In some instances, a preexisting eye problem may be the cause.

How Can Changes in the Workplace Reduce Eye Discomfort?

Even the most well-planned office layouts can pose circumstances that are not ideal for VDT use. Keep the following checklist in mind when evaluating your workstation:

- Most users prefer a viewing distance of 20 to 26 inches, a little farther away than for reading printed text.

63

- The computer screen should be placed slightly below eye level. Reference material should be placed on a document holder and moved close enough to the screen so that you don't have to swing your head back and forth from the material and the screen. If that happens, your muscles can become stiff and sore, and your eyes have to constantly change focus, which can cause eyestrain or headaches.

- Lighting should be modified to eliminate glare and harsh reflections.

For more information about computers and their effects on your eyes, contact Prevent Blindness America or the Prevent Blindness affiliate near you.

Section 8.5

Eye Protection at Home

"Protect Your Eyes—Ordinary Activities Can Cause Extraordinary Injuries," © 2001 American Academy of Ophthalmology. Used by permission. All rights reserved. For more information, visit www.aao.org.

What do lawnmowers, bungee cords, water balloon slingshots, BB guns, paintball pellets, fireworks, household cleaners, and car batteries have in common?

They're all potentially dangerous to your eyes. Some of the most ordinary activities can cause extraordinary injuries.

According to the U.S. Eye Injury Registry, many eye injuries occur in the home. But a majority of these injuries are preventable if you take safety precautions and use a little common sense.

- Check for rocks and debris before using a lawn mower or trimmer. Stones, twigs, and other small debris can become dangerous projectiles when shot from the blades of a lawnmower. Don't forget to wear your goggles.

- Bungee cords are becoming an increasingly common cause of both severe blunt and penetrating eye injuries, according to a study published in the April 2001 issue of *Ophthalmology*.

- Wear eye protection when using bungee cords.

- Buy safe toys for kids, avoiding those with sharp edges. Water balloon slingshots and BB guns and paintball guns aren't kids' toys.

- Never use fireworks. Even sparklers burn hot enough to melt gold. Attend only professional fireworks displays.

- Keep a pair of safety glasses or goggles with your jumper cables and follow instructions carefully when jump-starting a dead car battery.

- Be safe when handling household chemicals, many are extremely hazardous and can burn your eyes' delicate tissues. Always wear goggles, read instructions carefully, work in well-ventilated areas, and make sure the nozzle is pointed away from you.

- Always wear appropriate, certified eye protection when playing sports, from baseball to paint ball.

- Have fun in the sun, but always wear sunglasses that block 99 percent 100 percent of UV-A and UV-B rays when outdoors for extended periods of time.

   If you sustain an eye injury, here are some tips:

- Sand or small debris: Use eye wash to flush the eye out. Do not rub the eye. If the debris remains, lightly bandage the eye and see an Eye M.D.

- Blows to the eye: Gently apply small, cold compresses to reduce pain and swelling. Don't apply pressure. If you experience reduced vision or discoloration, such as a black eye, see an Eye M.D. If you do sustain significant blunt trauma injury, you may be at increased risk for developing glaucoma. Check with your physician on how frequently you should be examined for glaucoma in the future.

- Cuts or punctures: Don't attempt to wash the eye or remove an object stuck in the eye. A paper cup held over the eye can help protect it until you can get to your Eye M.D. or emergency room.

Section 8.6

Eye Protection in the Workplace

"Eye Protection in the Workplace," U.S. Department of Labor,
Occupational Safety and Health Administration, Fact Sheet No.
OSHA 93-03, January 1993. Reviewed by David A. Cooke, M.D.,
on September 15, 2002.

Every day an estimated 1,000 eye injuries occur in American workplaces. The financial cost of these injuries is enormous—more than $300 million per year in lost production time, medical expenses, and workers compensation. No dollar figure can adequately reflect the personal toll these accidents take on the injured workers.

The Occupational Safety and Health Administration (OSHA) and the 25 states and territories operating their own job safety and health programs are determined to help reduce eye injuries. In concert with efforts by concerned voluntary groups, OSHA has begun a nationwide information campaign to improve workplace eye protection.

Take a moment to think about possible eye hazards at your workplace. A 1980 survey by the Labor Department's Bureau of Labor Statistics (BLS) of about 1,000 minor eye injuries reveals how and why many on-the-job accidents occur.

What Contributes to Eye Injuries at Work?

- Not wearing eye protection. BLS reports that nearly three out of every five workers injured were not wearing eye protection at the time of the accident.

- Wearing the wrong kind of eye protection for the job. About 40 percent of the injured workers were wearing some form of eye protection when the accident occurred. These workers were most likely to be wearing protective eyeglasses with no side shields, though injuries among employees wearing full-cup or flat-fold side shields occurred, as well.

66

What Causes Eye Injuries?

- Flying particles. BLS found that almost 70 percent of the accidents studied resulted from flying or falling objects or sparks striking the eye. Injured workers estimated that nearly three-fifths of the objects were smaller than a pin head. Most of the particles were said to be traveling faster than a hand-thrown object when the accident occurred.

- Contact with chemicals caused one fifth of the injuries. Other accidents were caused by objects swinging from a fixed or attached position, like tree limbs, ropes, chains, or tools, which were pulled into the eye while the worker was using them.

Where Do Accidents Occur Most Often?

Potential eye hazards can be found in nearly every industry, but BLS reported that more than 40 percent of injuries occurred among craft workers, like mechanics, repairers, carpenters, and plumbers. Over a third of the injured workers were operatives, such as assemblers, sanders, and grinding machine operators.

Laborers suffered about one fifth of the eye injuries. Almost half the injured workers were employed in manufacturing; slightly more than 20 percent were in construction.

How Can Eye Injuries Be Prevented?

- Always wear effective eye protection. OSHA standards require that employers provide workers with suitable eye protection. To be effective, the eyewear must be of the appropriate type for the hazard encountered and properly fitted. For example, the BLS survey showed that 94 percent of the injuries to workers wearing eye protection resulted from objects or chemicals going around or under the protector. Eye protective devices should allow for air to circulate between the eye and the lens. Only 13 workers injured while wearing eye protection reported breakage.

- Nearly one fifth of the injured workers with eye protection wore face shields or welding helmets. However, only six percent of the workers injured while wearing eye protection wore goggles, which generally offer better protection for the eyes. Best protection is afforded when goggles are worn with face shields.

- Better training and education. BLS reported that most workers were hurt while doing their regular jobs. Workers injured while not wearing protective eyewear most often said they believed it was not required by the situation. Even though the vast majority of employers furnished eye protection at no cost to employees, about 40 percent of the workers received no information on where and what kind of eyewear should be used.

- Maintenance. Eye protection devices must be properly maintained. Scratched and dirty devices reduce vision, cause glare and may contribute to accidents.

Where Can I Get More Information?

- Your nearest OSHA area office. Safety and health experts are available to explain mandatory requirements for effective eye protection and answer questions. They can also refer you to an on-site consultation service available in nearly every state through which you can get free, penalty-free advice for eliminating possible eye hazards, designing a training program, or other safety and health matters. Don't know where the nearest federal or state office is? Call an OSHA Regional Office at the U.S. Department of Labor in Boston, New York, Philadelphia, Atlanta, Chicago, Dallas, Kansas City, Denver, San Francisco, or Seattle.

- The National Society to Prevent Blindness. This voluntary health organization is dedicated to preserving sight and has developed excellent information and training materials for preventing eye injuries at work. Its 26 affiliates nationwide may also provide consultation in developing effective eye safety programs. For more information and a publications catalog, write Prevent Blindness America, 500 E. Remington Road, Schaumburg, IL 60173, (800) 331-2020; www.preventblindness.org.

Eye Protection Works

BLS reported that more than 50 percent of workers injured while wearing eye protection thought the eyewear had minimized their injuries. But nearly half the workers also felt that another type of protection could have better prevented or reduced the injuries they suffered.

It is estimated that 90 percent of eye injuries can be prevented through the use of proper protective eyewear. That is our goal and, by working together, OSHA, employers, workers, and health organizations can make it happen.

Section 8.7

Eye Protection while Playing Sports

Reprinted with permission from Vinger, PF: A practical guide for sports eye protection. *Phys Sportsmed* 2000, 28 (6): 48-69. © The McGraw-Hill Companies.

Sports eye injuries can be serious but are preventable. Any sport that involves a stick or racket, a ball or other projectile, or body contact presents a risk of serious eye injury. Physicians have an obligation to warn players of potential risk and to recommend appropriate eye protection. Sports eye protection should be designed specifically for the activity or sport. Eye protection that bears the seal of sanctioned organizations should be mandated for high-risk sports.

Eye injuries in sports and recreation are an international problem, widely recognized as preventable with appropriate protective equipment.[1-20] The U.S. Consumer Product Safety Commission (CPSC) estimate of almost 40,000 eye injuries from sports in the United States (Table 8.1)[21] is only a fraction of the total, which also includes eye injuries seen in ophthalmologists' offices and specialty eye hospitals that are not sampled by the CPSC.

Although risk of eye injury exists for many sports, risk can be mitigated with proper eyewear and precautions. Physicians who follow guidelines and prescribe certified eyewear for active patients can help them remain injury-free during participation.

Sports and Risk of Eye Injuries

Sports with the potential of ball (puck, shuttlecock), stick (racket, crosse), or body contact frequently cause eye injuries, but the incidence is difficult to determine because there are few studies in which the actual number of participants at risk is known. Some data are available for selected activities, however.

Statistics

An estimated 5.5 percent of all college varsity athletes sustain some form of eye injury each season.[22] The 25 percent probability that an unprotected squash player will suffer a significant eye injury after 25 years of playing 3 days a week in the Boston area[23] is comparable to an Australian survey of all squash players that showed an incidence of 17.5 eye injuries per 100,000 hours of play.[24] In the latter study, 26 percent of all squash players surveyed reported that they had suffered at least one eye injury. Another racket sport, racquetball, has an incidence of one eye injury for each 1,764 hours of play and hospitalization for eye injury after each 11,760 participation hours.[25,26]

Facial injury (including eye injury) to the unprotected ice hockey player is extremely high—7 percent in the first year of play, increasing to 66 percent after eight seasons, and up to 95 percent for professional players. The average professional hockey player in his career has had 1 facial bone fracture, 2 teeth lost, and 15 facial lacerations that required sutures.[27]

Approximately 1 in 10 college basketball players sustains an eye injury each year.[28] In Massachusetts annually, 1 of every 238 children 5 to 19 years old was treated at a hospital for a baseball-related injury.[29] A 1-year prospective study of eye injuries among 800 major league players from 26 baseball teams showed that 30 percent of the 20 injured players (2.5 percent) missed games because of their eye injury.[30] Women's lacrosse players have a 6.2 percent to 9.9 percent annual incidence of face, eye, and tooth injuries[31]; 22 percent of the players had incurred head or face contact at least once per game.[32] In another study, 6,229 college football players had an eye injury incidence of 0.03 for 1,000 practice or game sessions, and a player on an average college football team had a significant eye injury about once every 62 weeks of participation.[33]

Consequences and Risk Reduction

Eye injuries can be devastating in terms of their total cost: pain, loss of function, and long-term disability. A person who lost one eye at age 16 and faces cataract surgery at age 70 on the remaining eye has far more reason to be anxious than does a person with two good eyes. Eye injuries also affect others besides the injured person. For example, of all the people who visit an eye hospital emergency department for an eye injury, 12.5 percent with severe injury and 5 percent with less severe injury sue someone.[34] Are these litigations justified? Is anyone responsible, or are these injuries the assumed risk that one takes when playing a sport?

The risk of eye injury in a particular sport is proportional to the chance of the eye being hit hard enough to cause injury; however, risk is not correlated with the classification into collision, contact, and noncontact categories. Available eye protectors can reduce the risk of eye injury by at least 90 percent,[35-37] but a principal impediment to the more widespread use of protective eyewear is confusion of all concerned with sports—principals, athletic directors, coaches, umpires, referees, players, and medical personnel—as to which protectors are the most effective.

Table 8.1. Risk Categories for Sports-related Eye Injury for the Unprotected Player

High Risk	*Small, fast projectiles:* Air rifle/BB gun; Paintball
	Hard projectiles, fingers, sticks, close contact: Baseball/softball/cricket; Basketball; Fencing; Field hockey; Ice hockey; Lacrosse, men's and women's; Squash/racquetball; Street hockey
	Intentional injury: Boxing; Full-contact martial arts
Moderate Risk	Fishing; Football; Soccer/volleyball; Tennis/badminton; Water polo
Low Risk	Bicycling; Noncontact martial arts; Skiing; Swimming/diving/water skiing; Wrestling
Eye Safe	Gymnastics; Track and field*

*Note: Javelin and discus have a small but definite potential for injury that is preventable with good field supervision.

Eyewear Safety Certification

Eye safety standards in the United States are primarily the responsibility of two organizations, the American Society for Testing and Materials (ASTM)[38] and the American National Standards Institute (ANSI).[39] The National Operating Committee on Standards for Athletic Equipment (NOCSAE) also writes standards for selected sports. Other countries have their own organizations that set standards and protocols.

Sports Eyewear Safety Standards

The ASTM writes standards for sports eyewear in the United States; the NOCSAE has standards for football face shields and men's lacrosse face shields. Founded in 1898, the ASTM is a not-for-profit organization that provides a forum for users, producers, and those with a general interest (e.g., representatives of government and academia) to meet on common ground and write standards for materials, products, systems, and services in many different fields. ASTM committees are balanced, which means that the number of voting producers (manufacturers) cannot exceed the combined number of voting nonproducers (users and those with general interest). The eye safety subcommittee, a part of committee F-8 on athletics and athletic equipment (one of 134 ASTM standards-writing committees), had its origin in the hockey face shield subcommittee that was formed in 1973.

At present, ASTM has completed the following standards for sports eye protectors:

- ASTM F803: Eye protectors for selected sports (racket sports, women's lacrosse, field hockey, baseball, basketball);

- ASTM F513: Eye and face protective equipment for hockey players;

- ASTM F1776: Eye protectors for use by players of paintball sports;

- ASTM F1587: Head and face protective equipment for ice hockey goaltenders;

- ASTM F910: Face guards for youth baseball; and

- ASTM F659: High-impact resistant eye protective devices for Alpine skiing.

Nonsports Eyewear Standards

ANSI writes standards for protective eyewear in the United States with the exception of sports eyewear. It is the central body responsible for the identification of a single, consistent set of voluntary standards called American National Standards and is the U.S. member of international standards organizations. ANSI follows the principles of openness, due process, and a consensus of those directly and materially affected by the standards.

ANSI standards for eyewear that is *not for sports use* are:

- ANSI Z80.5: Requirements for ophthalmic frames;

- ANSI Z80.1: Prescription ophthalmic lenses—recommendations;

- ANSI Z80.3: Requirements for nonprescription sunglasses and fashion eyewear; and

- ANSI Z87.1: Practice for occupational eye and face protection.

The ANSI Z80 series of standards are for dress eyewear, also called streetwear spectacles. The test requirements are minimal and geared to the desire for a diversity of styles in fashion eyewear. Streetwear spectacles are not appropriate for work or sports with impact potential. Polycarbonate lenses should be used for dress eyewear unless there is a specific reason for another lens material. Streetwear frames are often fragile and have poor lens-retention properties. Significant eye injuries have resulted from frame failure.

The ANSI Z87.1 industrial safety standard is being revised. In its present form, the standard allows for lenses that shatter with relatively little energy. The frame test for spectacles with removable lenses is not strict and allows the substitution of a weaker lens after the frame is tested with a polycarbonate lens. Industrial eye protectors are not satisfactory for sports unless tested to ASTM specifications.

Testing

The NOCSAE has standards for baseball, football, and lacrosse helmets, baseballs and softballs, and face shields for football and men's lacrosse. To determine whether products pass the applicable standards, they are submitted to a testing laboratory. The testing laboratory must comply with the International Organization for Standardization (ISO) and Inter-European Commission (IEC) Guide 25-1990. The American Association for Laboratory Accreditation (A2LA) accredits

Table 8.2. Recommended Eye Protectors for Selected Sports (continued on next page)

Sport	Minimal Eye Protector	Comment
Baseball/softball, youth batter or base runner	ASTM F910	Face guard attached to helmet
Baseball/softball, fielder	ASTM F803 for baseball	ASTM specifies age ranges
Basketball	ASTM F803 for basketball	ASTM specifies age ranges
Bicycling	Helmet plus streetwear ANSI Z80, industrial ANSI Z87.1, or sports ASTM F803 eyewear	Use only polycarbonate lenses; excellent plano industrial spectacles are available that are inexpensive and give good protection from wind and particles
Boxing	None available; not permitted in sport	Sport contraindicated for functionally one-eyed
Fencing	Protector with neck bib	Test requirements of the International Federation of Fencing
Field hockey (both sexes)	Goalie: full face mask; others: ASTM F803 for women's lacrosse	Protectors that pass ASTM F803 for women's lacrosse also pass for field hockey; should have option to wear helmet with attached face mask
Football	Polycarbonate eye shield attached to helmet-mounted wire face mask	
Full-contact martial arts	None available; not permitted in sport	Contraindicated for functionally one-eyed
Ice hockey	ASTM F513 face mask on helmet; goaltenders ASTM F1587	HECC or CSA certified full face shield

Table 8.2. Recommended Eye Protectors for Selected Sports (continued from previous page)

Sport	Minimal Eye Protector	Comment
Lacrosse, men's	NOCSAE face mask attached to lacrosse helmet	
Lacrosse, women's	ASTM F803 for women's lacrosse	Should have option to wear helmet with attached face mask
Paintball	ASTM F1776 for paintball	
Racket sports (badminton, tennis, paddle tennis, handball, squash, and racquetball)	ASTM F803 for specific sport	
Soccer	ASTM F803 for any selected sport	No specific standard for soccer; currently, eye protectors that comply with ASTM F803 for any specified sport are recommended
Street hockey	ASTM F513 face mask on helmet	Must be HECC or CSA certified
Track and field	Streetwear/fashion eyewear	Use only polycarbonate lenses
Water polo/ swimming	Swim goggles with polycarbonate lenses	
Wrestling	No standard is available	Custom protective eyewear can be fabricated

Note: For sports in which a face mask or helmet with eye protector is worn, functionally one-eyed athletes, and those who have had previous eye trauma or surgery, and for whom their ophthalmologists recommend eye protection, must also wear sports protective eyewear that conforms to ASTM F803 requirements all types of laboratories, except medical. A laboratory must be able to provide evidence of the successful completion of the A2LA evaluation process to perform the tests that are relevant to the standard test procedures. A2LA was approved under the Accrediting Body Evaluation Program of the National Institute of Standards and Technology. By the end of 1997, 987 laboratories were accredited and 330 laboratories were in the process of obtaining accreditation.

Eyewear Certification

Eye protectors are often certified, providing the user with the assurance that the protector will afford reasonable protection. The Protective Eyewear Certification Council (PECC; website: http://www.protecteyes.org) certifies protectors complying with ASTM standards (except for ice hockey). The Canadian Standards Association (CSA) certifies products complying with the Canadian racket sport and ice hockey standards, which are similar to the ASTM standards. The Hockey Equipment Certification Council (HECC) certifies ice hockey equipment, including helmets and face shields. NOCSAE does the same for football helmets and face guards, men's lacrosse helmets and face guards, and baseball helmets. The PECC, CSA, HECC, or NOCSAE seals assure users that each protector can be safely used. Categories of eyewear based on their suitability for sports eye protection are listed in Table 8.2.

Choosing Appropriate Eye Protection

The vast majority of sports officials, administrators, and physicians are genuinely concerned about making sports as safe as possible while still maintaining fun and appeal. Most want to protect athletes, but don't know how to proceed or what to buy. They want information on what to use for their athletes, whether they order, specify, or purchase.

The Basic Steps

The basic steps in choosing protective gear for an eye-safety program include (1) knowing the athlete's vision and eye history, (2) using only eye protectors that have been certified to national performance standards, and (3) having professionals assist the athlete in selecting and fitting protective eyewear. The latter point is especially important because various kinds of eye protection and different brands of sports goggles vary significantly in their fit. An experienced ophthalmologist, optometrist, optician, or athletic trainer can help an athlete select appropriate protective gear that fits well. Sports programs should assist indigent athletes in evaluating and obtaining protective eyewear.

Functionally One-Eyed Athletes

It is important to identify athletes who have eye conditions that make them more susceptible to catastrophic injury. One such condition is being functionally one-eyed—having a best-corrected visual acuity of worse than 20/40 in the poorer-seeing eye.[31] A severe injury to the better eye in this person can result in a major handicap, such as the inability to obtain a driver's license in many states.[40] Athletes who are functionally one-eyed must wear appropriate eye protection during all sports and recreational activities, and athletes who have had eye surgery or trauma to the eye may have weakened eye tissue that is more susceptible to injury. Those who have had prior surgery are considered functionally one-eyed if the best corrected vision in either eye is less than 20/40. Athletes who have had surgery may need additional eye protection if the surgery makes them more prone to serious injury from trauma. Some may be restricted from participating in certain sports; however, with proper protection the functionally one-eyed and those with prior eye disease should be able to participate in most sports. The input of the treating ophthalmologist is essential in making the determination.

Additional Recommendations

Several other recommendations also address eyewear choice and should be considered in fitting patients with eye protection:

- Proper fit in children is essential. Because some children have narrow facial features, they may be unable to wear even the smallest sports goggles. A possible solution is to fit these children with impact-resistant 3-mm polycarbonate lenses in ANSI Z87.1 frames designed for children. However, the parents must be informed that this protection is not optimal, and the choice of eye-safe sports should be discussed.

- Protectors with clear lenses (plano [nonprescription] or prescription) should have polycarbonate lenses, which is the strongest lens material available.[41] In the extremely rare instance that a polycarbonate lens cannot be used (e.g., the athlete can tolerate only the optics of a lens with a lower index of refraction than polycarbonate), the athlete who participates in an eye-risk sport should either (1) wear contact lenses plus an appropriate protector, or (2) wear an over-the-glasses eyeguard that conforms to the specifications of ASTM F803 for sports for which an ASTM F803 protector is recommended.

- For sports requiring a face mask or helmet with an eye protector or shield, functionally one-eyed athletes should also wear sports eye protectors that conform to the requirements of ASTM F803 (for any selected sport) to maintain some level of protection if the face guard is elevated or removed (as in ice hockey or football by some players on the bench). The helmet must fit properly and have a properly fastened chin strap for optimal protection.

- Contact lenses offer no protection. Therefore, athletes who wear contact lenses must also wear appropriate eye protection.

- Athletes must replace sports eye protectors that are damaged or yellowed with age, because they may have become weakened.

- Functionally one-eyed athletes and those who have had an eye injury or surgery can participate in almost all sports if they use appropriate eye protection. The exceptions are boxing, for which eye protection is not practical, and full-contact martial arts, for which protection is not allowed. No standards exist for eye protectors in wrestling, but the incidence of eye injuries is low in this sport. Eye protectors that are firmly fixed to the head have been custom made for wrestling, but wrestlers need to know that such protectors may not be sufficient to prevent injury.

Parting Views

There are effective means of protecting the player from injury with products that conform to ASTM, CSA, or NOCSAE specifications. Products that bear a certification seal from PECC, HECC, CSA, or NOCSAE are easily identifiable and are preferred. During several million player-years of use, there have been no eye injuries to any player wearing a protector that conformed to ASTM F803 requirements. Similarly, there have been no reported significant eye injuries to any of the more than 1 million players wearing a full hockey face shield certified by HECC or CSA since the ASTM standard was first published in 1977 and HECC was founded in 1978.

Players of any sport assume some injury risk while participating, but players (and parents of minors) have the right to know the actual risk. The injury incidence should be documented by a prospective injury reporting system. The risk and the means of reducing it must be clearly articulated to players and players' parents. The vast majority of eye injuries can be prevented with existing protectors. The prudent school official will mandate eye protection for sports that use a stick or a ball or other projectile or that involve significant body contact. The team physician should insist that players of sports with an eye hazard wear certified protectors. Non-team physicians should include a sports history as part of the routine examination of all patients and recommend protective eyewear appropriate for the patient's activity.

References

1. Coroneo MT: An eye for cricket: ocular injuries in indoor cricketers. *Med J Aust* 1985;142(8):469-471.

2. Jaison SG, Silas SE, Daniel R, et al: A review of childhood admission with perforating ocular injuries in a hospital in northwest India. *Indian J Ophthalmol* 1994;42(4):199-201.

3. Pump-Schmidt C, Behrens-Baumann W: Changes in the epidemiology of ruptured globe eye injuries due to societal changes. *Ophthalmologica* 1999;213(6):380-386.

4. Drolsum L: Eye injuries in sports. *Scand J Med Sci Sports* 1999;9(1):53-56.

5. Lynch P, Rowan B: Eye injury and sport: sport-related eye injuries presenting to an eye casualty department throughout 1995. *Ir Med J* 1997;90(3):112-114.

6. Pikkel J, Gelfand Y, Miller B: Incidence of sports-related eye injuries (in Hebrew). *Harefuah* 1995;129(7-8):249-250, 294-295.

7. Lawson JS, Rotem T, Wilson SF: Catastrophic injuries to the eyes and testicles in footballers. *Med J Aust* 1995;163(5):242-244.

8. Ghosh F, Bauer B: Sports-related eye injuries. *Acta Ophthalmol Scand* 1995;73(4):353-354.

9.   Biasca N, Simmen HP, Bartolozzi AR, et al: Review of typical ice hockey injuries: survey of the North American NHL and Hockey Canada versus European leagues. *Unfallchirurg* 1995;98(5):283-288.

10. Pardhan S, Shacklock P, Weatherill J: Sport-related eye trauma: a survey of the presentation of eye injuries to a casualty clinic and the use of protective eye-wear. *Eye* 1995;9(pt 6 suppl):50-53.

11. Fong LP: Sports-related eye injuries. *Med J Aust* 1994;160(12): 743-747, 750.

12. Capoferri C, Martorina M, Menga M, et al: Eye injuries from traditional sports in Aosta Valley. *Ophthalmologica* 1994;208(1):15-16.

13. Jones NP: Eye injury in sport: incidence, biomechanics, clinical effects and prevention. *J R Coll Surg Edinb* 1993;38(3):127-133.

14. ten Napel JA: Eye injuries in sports (in Polish). *Klin Oczna* 1990;92(3-4):48-49.

15. Rapoport I, Romem M, Kinek M, et al: Eye injuries in children in Israel: a nationwide collaborative study. *Arch Ophthalmol* 1990;108(3):376-379.

16. Macewen CJ: Eye injuries: a prospective survey of 5671 cases. *Br J Ophthalmol* 1989;73(11):888-894.

17. Crowley PJ, Condon KC: Analysis of hurling and camogie injuries. *Br J Sports Med* 1989;23(3):183-185.

18. Pashby T: Eye injuries in sports. *J Ophthalmic Nurs Technol* 1989;8(3):99-101.

19. Jones NP: Eye injury in sport. *Sports Med* 1989;7(3):163-181.

20. Kelly SP: Serious eye injury in badminton players. *Br J Ophthalmol* 1987;71(10):746-747.

21. Prevent Blindness America (formerly National Society to Prevent Blindness): 1997 Sports and Recreational Eye Injuries. Schaumburg, IL, Prevent Blindness America, 1998.

22. Powell JW: National Athletic Injury/Illness Reporting System: eye injuries in college wrestling. *Int Ophthalmol Clin* 1981; 21(4):47-58.

23. Reif AE, Vinger PF, Easterbrook M: New developments in protection against eye injuries. *Squash News* 1981;4(6):10-14.

24. Genovese MT, Lenzo NP, Lim RK, et al: Eye injuries among pennant squash players and their attitudes towards protective eyewear. *Med J of Aust* 1990;153(11-12):655-658.

25. Soderstrom CA, Doxanas MT: Racquetball: a game with preventable injuries. *Am J Sports Med* 1982;10(3):180-183.

26. Rose CP, Morse JO: Racquetball injuries. *Phys Sportsmed* 1979;7(1):73-77.

27. Wilson K, Cram B, Rontal E, et al: Facial injuries in hockey players. *Minn Med* 1977;60(1):13-16.

28. Marton K, Wilson D, McKeag D: Ocular trauma in college varsity sports, abstracted. *Med Sci Sports Exerc* 1987;19(2 suppl):S53.

29. Schuster M: Baseball-Related Injuries Among Children: Statewide Comprehensive Injury Prevention Program. Boston, Bureau of Parent, Child and Adolescent Health, Massachusetts Department of Public Health, 1991.

30. Zagelbaum BM, Hersh PS, Donnenfeld ED, et al: Ocular trauma in major-league baseball players. *N Engl J Med* 1994;330(14):1021-1023.

31. Vinger PF: The eye and sports medicine, in Tasman W, Jaeger EA (eds): *Duane's Clinical Ophthalmology*. Philadelphia, JB Lippincott, 1994, pp 1-103.

32. Piltz W: Eye and facial injuries in women's lacrosse: a paper on women's lacrosse in Australia. Read before the Second International Symposium on Ocular Trauma. Geneva, Switzerland, April 2-5, 1992.

33. Zemper ED: Injury rates in a national sample of college football teams: a 2-year prospective study. *Phys Sportsmed* 1989;17(11):100-105.

34. Schein OD, Hibberd PL, Shingleton BJ, et al: The spectrum and burden of ocular injury. *Ophthalmology* 1988;95(3):300-305.

35. Jeffers JB: An ongoing tragedy: pediatric sports-related eye injuries. *Semin Ophthalmol* 1990;5(4):216-223.

36. Larrison WI, Hersh PS, Kunzweiler T, et al: Sport-related ocular trauma. *Ophthalmology* 1990;97(10):1265-1269.

37. Strahlman E, Sommer A: The epidemiology of sports-related ocular trauma. *Int Ophthalmol Clin* 1988;28(3):199-202.

38. American National Standards Institute: American National Standard Practice for Occupational and Educational Eye and Face Protection. Des Plaines, IL, American Society of Safety Engineers, 1998.

39. American Society for Testing and Materials: *1999 Annual Book of ASTM Standards: General Products, Chemical Specialties, and End Use Products*. West Conshocken, PA, American Society for Testing and Materials, 1999.

40. Federal Highway Administration: Manual on Uniform Traffic Control Devices for Streets and Highways. Washington, DC, US Department of Transportation, 1988.

41. Vinger PF, Parver L, Alfaro DV III, et al: Shatter resistance of spectacle lenses. *JAMA* 1997;277(2):142-144.

Dr. Vinger is a clinical professor of ophthalmology at Tufts University School of Medicine in Medford, Massachusetts. Address correspondence to Paul F. Vinger, MD, 297 Heath's Bridge Rd., Concord, MA 01742; e-mail to vingven@tiac.net.

Section 8.8

Eye Injuries

This information was provided by KidsHealth, one of the largest resources online for medically reviewed health information written for parents, kids, and teens. For more articles like this one, visit www.KidsHealth.org or www.TeensHealth.org. © 2001 The Nemours Center for Children's Health Media, a division of The Nemours Foundation.

You can treat many minor eye irritations by flushing the eye, but more serious injuries require medical attention. Injuries to the eye are the most common preventable cause of blindness, so when in doubt, err on the side of caution and call your child's doctor for help. Here's what to do:

Routine Irritations (Sand, Dirt, and Other Foreign Bodies on the Eye Surface)

- Do not try to remove any foreign body except by flushing because of the risk of scratching the surface of the eye, especially the cornea.

- Wash your hands thoroughly before touching the eyelids to examine or flush the eye.

- Do not touch, press, or rub the eye, and do whatever you can to keep the child from touching it (a baby can be swaddled as a preventive measure).

- Tilt the child's head over a basin with the affected eye down and gently pull down the lower lid, encouraging the child to open her eyes as wide as possible. For an infant or small child, it is helpful to have a second person hold the child's eyes open while you flush.

- Gently pour a steady stream of lukewarm water from a pitcher (do not heat the water) across the eye. Sterile saline solution can also be used.

83

- Flush for up to 15 minutes, checking the eye every 5 minutes to see if the foreign body has been flushed out.

- Since a particle can scratch the cornea and cause an infection, the eye should be examined by a doctor if there continues to be any irritation afterward.

- If a foreign body is not dislodged by flushing, it will probably be necessary for a trained medical practitioner to flush the eye.

Embedded Foreign Body (An Object Penetrates the Globe of the Eye)

- Call for emergency medical help.

- Cover the affected eye. If the object is small, use an eye patch or sterile dressing. If the object is large, cover the injured eye with a small cup taped in place. The point is to keep all pressure off of the globe of the eye.

- Keep your child (and yourself) as calm and comfortable as possible until help arrives.

Chemical Exposure

- Many chemicals, even those found around the house, can damage an eye. If your child gets a chemical in the eye and you know what it is, look on the product's container for an emergency number to call for instructions.

- Flush the eye (see above) with lukewarm water for 15 to 30 minutes. If both eyes are affected, do it in the shower.

- Call for emergency medical help.

- Call your local poison control center for specific instructions. Be prepared to give the exact name of the chemical, if you have it. However, do not delay flushing the eye first.

Black Eye, Blunt Injury, or Contusion

A black eye is often a minor injury, but it can also appear when there is significant eye injury or head trauma. A visit to your doctor or an eye specialist may be required to rule out serious injury, particularly if you're not certain of the cause of the black eye.

For a simple black eye:

- Apply cold compresses intermittently: 5 to 10 minutes on, 10 to 15 minutes off. If you are not at home when the injury occurs and there is no ice available, a cold soda will do to start. If you use ice, make sure it is covered with a towel or sock to protect the delicate skin on the eyelid.

- Use cold compresses for 24 to 48 hours, then switch to applying warm compresses intermittently. This will help the body reabsorb the leakage of blood and may help reduce discoloration.

- If the child is in pain, give acetaminophen (not aspirin or ibuprofen, which can increase bleeding). Prop the child's head with an extra pillow at night, and encourage her to sleep on the uninjured side of her face (pressure can increase swelling).

- Call your child's doctor, who may recommend an in-depth evaluation to rule out damage to the eye. Call immediately if any of the following symptoms are noted:

  1. increased redness
  2. drainage from the eye
  3. persistent eye pain
  4. any changes in vision
  5. any visible abnormality of the eyeball
  6. visible bleeding on the white part (sclera) of the eye, especially near the cornea

If the injury occurred during one of your child's routine activities such as a sport, follow up by investing in an ounce of prevention— protective goggles or unbreakable glasses are vitally important.

Note: All information on KidsHealth is for educational purposes only. For specific medical advice, diagnoses, and treatment, consult your doctor.

Part Two

Vision Correction and Refractive Surgery

Chapter 9

Vision Correction: Taking a Look at What's New

Vision correction has come a long way since the 13th century when the first pair of spectacles was made by riveting together the handles of two magnifying lenses. Today, surgical developments in vision correction, as well as advances in traditional eyeglasses and contact lenses, can potentially improve a person's vision to better than the optimal range of 20/20.

It's no surprise, then, that people dependent on glasses or contact lenses are visiting their eye-care specialists, hoping to find a quick fix for some age-old vision problems among the array of new techniques, products, and technologies. Learning about some of the common disorders that can threaten vision and how the eye sees can help you determine the best treatment to correct your vision. It's also important to understand the advantages, disadvantages, and limitations that come with vision correction procedures and aids.

How the Eye Sees

Having 20/20 vision means seeing at 20 feet what a person with normal vision sees at 20 feet. A person who has 20/40 vision can see at 20 feet what the person with normal vision sees at 40 feet. And so on.

"Vision Correction: Taking a Look at What's New," by Carol Lewis, *FDA Consumer*, U.S. Food and Drug Administration, October 2001; updated January 2002.

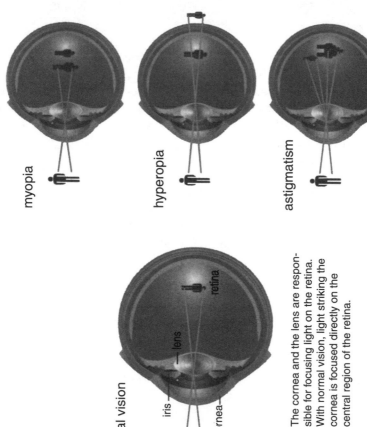

myopia

Myopia, or nearsightedness, occurs when the cornea is too thick and light is focused in front of the retina. Close objects appear clear and far objects are blurry.

hyperopia

Hyperopia, or farsightedness, occurs when the cornea is too thin and light is focused behind the retina. Distant objects appear clear and close objects appear blurry.

astigmatism

Astigmatism occurs when the surface of the cornea is oval-shaped, rather than round. Light rays have more than one focal point and can focus on different areas of the retina. Astigmatism creates double, distorted or blurry vision.

normal vision

iris

lens

retina

cornea

The cornea and the lens are responsible for focusing light on the retina. With normal vision, light striking the cornea is focused directly on the central region of the retina.

Infographic by Renée Gordon

The eye does not actually see objects. Instead, it sees the light that objects reflect. To see clearly, light striking the eye must be bent or refracted through the cornea—the clear window at the front of the eye that provides most of the focusing power. Light then travels through the lens, where it is fine-tuned to focus properly on the nerve layer that lines the back of the eye—the retina—and sent to the brain via the optic nerve. The retina acts like the film in a camera, and clear vision is achieved only if light from an object is precisely focused on it. If not, the image you see is blurred. This is called a refractive error.

Refractive errors usually occur in otherwise healthy eyes. They are caused mostly by an imperfectly shaped eyeball, cornea, or lens. There are four basic types of errors:

- Myopia or nearsightedness—Close objects appear sharp but those in the distance are blurred. The eyeball is longer than normal from front to back, so images focus in front of the retina instead of on it.

- Hyperopia or farsightedness—Distant objects can be seen clearly but objects up close are blurred. The eyeball is shorter than normal, so images focus behind the retina.

- Astigmatism—Objects are blurred at any distance. The cornea, lens, or both are shaped so that images aren't focused sharply on the retina.

- Presbyopia or aging eye—The eye loses its ability to change focus due to the natural aging process. This usually occurs between ages 40 and 50.

Glasses, contact lenses, and laser eye surgery attempt to reduce refractive errors by making light rays focus properly on the retina.

Laser Eye Surgery—A Popular Alternative

Laser eye surgery is intended for people who want to minimize their dependency on glasses or contact lenses. Laser surgery can provide vision correction similar to what would be obtained with glasses or contact lenses. People under the impression that surgery can improve their vision beyond what they can see with glasses or contact lenses, however, likely will be disappointed.

By far, the largest increase in laser eye surgery interest recently has been in a procedure called laser in situ keratomileusis, popularly known as LASIK.

Advertising for this technique appears prominently on broadcast outlets, including the Internet and in newspapers and magazines. Fortunately, says Terrence P. O'Brien, M.D., a spokesman for the American Academy of Ophthalmology (AAO), most surgeons and medical centers are doing a good job of educating the public about the risks and benefits of LASIK. "But patients need to be very well-informed in advance," he says.

LASIK permanently changes the shape of the cornea, and is performed for varying degrees of nearsightedness, farsightedness, and astigmatism. A surgical knife, called a microkeratome, is used to cut a flap in the cornea, leaving a hinge at one end of the flap. The flap is then folded back to reveal the middle layer of the cornea, called the stroma. Pulses from a computer-controlled excimer laser vaporize a portion of the stroma and the flap is then replaced. By removing this tissue, the shape of the central cornea is changed, and the refractive error is reduced.

O'Brien, who is also director of refractive surgery at the Wilmer Eye Institute at Johns Hopkins University in Baltimore, has performed over 10,000 eye surgeries. Still, he warns that people considering LASIK need to be wary of ads that make excessive promises.

"Price should not be the first factor" in considering to have delicate eye surgery, he says. "People fear blindness second only to cancer, and just as they wouldn't consider a discount open heart operation or budget brain surgery, they shouldn't take a chance with their eyes." The real struggle, he says, is in training doctors. "The most advanced technology and precise laser will give poor results if you don't have an experienced, capable surgeon."

This latest hype about LASIK's now-more-affordable advantage, coupled with some pretty appealing results, makes surgery one of the most exciting vision correction options available. Doctors say that LASIK gives a rapid visual recovery, with minimal pain, and little or no postoperative discomfort. In fact, most people who undergo LASIK, like Beth Polazzo—one of O'Brien's patients—can see well enough to drive immediately after surgery, and usually have excellent vision within a week.

"I had good vision immediately," says the 54-year-old Brooklyn, N.Y., resident, even though eventually one eye had to be retreated. "This is the best I've seen since I was seven years old." The laser does its work on each eye in less than a minute, and patients are typically back to work or normal activities within three days.

While most people are pleased with the results of their surgery, O'Brien says that, as with any medical procedure, there are risks involved. Some include: over- or under-treatment; the inability to wear contact lenses; permanent loss of vision; reduction in the quality of vision including the development of glare, halos, and starbursts; difficulty with night-driving; and reduced vision in dim lighting conditions. The risks are doubled when both eyes are treated at the same time.

Also, LASIK is not reversible. That's why in Polazzo's case, O'Brien intentionally undercorrected her distance eye. "We were aiming for modified monovision," he explains, which means that one eye would see close up while the other would be corrected to see distances. But Polazzo experienced some regression in her distance eye—that is, her distance vision began to worsen as she returned to nearsightedness—some weeks following surgery. However, because of the initial undercorrection, O'Brien was able to fix the problem.

A. Ralph Rosenthal, M.D., director of the Food and Drug Administration's division of ophthalmic and ear, nose and throat devices in the Center for Devices and Radiological Health, says that no one knows the long-term effects of laser eye surgery. "We just can't know that yet," he says, so when people call looking for a guarantee in years for the success of the procedure, "I can't give them one."

Before undergoing LASIK, Rosenthal says people should carefully weigh the risks and benefits based on what's important to them, and potential side effects, including the pros and cons of having one or both eyes done on the same day. It's also important to avoid being influenced by friends who have had LASIK surgery or doctors who encourage patients to do so.

A second laser procedure used today as an alternative to LASIK is photorefractive keratectomy, or PRK. Although O'Brien says that less than 5 percent of people undergo PRK, it is still the procedure of choice for certain eye conditions. This type of refractive surgery gently reshapes the cornea by removing microscopic amounts of tissue from the outer surface with a cool, computer-controlled ultraviolet beam of light. It does not, however, involve cutting. The procedure takes only a few minutes, and patients are typically back to daily routines in five to seven days.

Clinical studies indicate that about 5 percent of PRK recipients continued to need glasses for distance vision following the surgery, and up to 15 percent need glasses occasionally, such as when driving. In addition, many people experienced mild corneal haze following surgery, which is part of the normal healing process. The haze appeared to have little or no effect on final vision, and could only be seen by a doctor under a microscope. For about 5 percent of PRK patients, best-corrected vision without corrective lenses was slightly worse after surgery than before. These conditions, however, improved or disappeared in most people in six months.

Another new, less-invasive laser procedure—indicated for temporarily reducing hyperopia—is being aimed exclusively at people over 40. Laser thermal keratoplasty, or LTK, involves zapping 16 spots on the outer part of the cornea to shrink the tissue. People usually can leave 30 minutes after the procedure and resume normal activities the following day. The advantage of LTK is that it's a no touch procedure, meaning there's little chance of infection or loss of vision. The disadvantage is that the procedure is considered temporary since the treatment effect regresses—for many people, about half of the correction is gone within two years. Another drawback is that people may become nearsighted in the first six weeks, enough to require glasses for driving, and their vision can fluctuate for weeks after surgery.

Rosenthal wants people considering laser surgery to know and carefully weigh the pros and cons. "FDA mandated that manufacturers of all excimer lasers make available to people a patient information booklet," he says, that spells out this information. If the doctor fails to offer one, Rosenthal says that you should ask for it.

Experts say that the reliability of laser vision correction is quite good in mild to moderate levels of refractive errors. But people desperate for clear vision need to understand the dangers. The most satisfied laser surgery patient is one who has realistic expectations and a thorough understanding of the risks and possible complications of refractive surgery.

Contact Lenses—More Choices

Whether you're interested in wearing contact lenses for the first time, or are considering an upgrade for comfort and convenience, discussing the latest innovations with your eye-care practitioner will help make your choices easier and minimize the risks. Advances in materials for precision lenses have made soft and rigid gas permeable contacts—the two main contact lens groups—an option for more people. These medical devices are made of many different types of plastic, and offer numerous options. With daily wear or extended wear (overnight) lenses, the options include frequent- or planned-replacements, disposables, bifocals, UV-blocking contacts, and more. There are clear, tinted, opaque, spherical and rounded lenses. So where does someone start when deciding if contact lenses are the right choice for vision correction, and what to choose?

Hal Balyeat, M.D., professor of ophthalmology at the University of Oklahoma's Dean A. McGee Eye Institute, says people satisfied with their vision correction may not need to look very far. "If you are already a satisfied contact wearer," he says, "you may not consider other options worthwhile when you're wearing your contacts as well as you are." Satisfied wearers typically have no allergies and have not developed an intolerance to contact lenses. The bottom line: If contact lenses are working for you, Balyeat says, it's hard to justify other options, such as permanent laser alteration of otherwise healthy eyes.

Balyeat cites his wife, Marilyn, as an example. Although she was a good candidate for the LASIK surgery, she opted for monovision contacts—one lens focuses close up while the other lens corrects for distance vision. "At 60," she says, "I can still read without glasses." And that, says her husband, is the single most important factor: "If you like being able to take out your contacts and still see up close, surgery is not a worthwhile trade-off." Balyeat adds that many people don't realize that laser surgery, performed on people over 40, won't let you see up close without glasses or contacts unless you opt for monovision LASIK.

Contact lens quality continues to improve. Soft contacts contain from 25 percent to 79 percent water, are easy to adjust to, and are more comfortable than rigid gas permeable (RGP) lenses, thanks to their ability to conform to the eye and absorb water. Soft lenses aren't likely to pop out or capture foreign material such as dust underneath, as hard lenses are. Extra-thin soft lenses are available for very sensitive eyes.

While the ability to hold water increases oxygen permeability of soft lenses, it also makes them more fragile. And soft lenses are more likely to absorb chemicals and residues on the wearer's hands.

RGP lenses are more durable and resistant to deposit buildup, and they generally give clearer, crisper vision. They tend to be less expensive over the life of the lens, but the initial cost often is higher. RGP contacts last several years, while soft contacts, depending on the type, are meant to be replaced after periods ranging from a day to about a year. In addition, RGP lenses can be marked to show which lens is for which eye, and they're less likely to tear or rip, making them easier to handle. However, it often takes several weeks to get used to wearing rigid lenses, compared with several days for soft.

Many changes are occurring in the world of disposable (defined by the FDA as used once and discarded) and frequent- or planned-replacement contacts. The latest innovations include daily disposables, bifocals and toric contacts for astigmatism.

"It's healthier to replace lenses more often," says James Saviola, O.D., chief of the vitreoretinal and extraocular devices branch in the FDA. "And if you reuse your lenses, you need to do something more than store them in saline solution." The FDA approved in 2000 the first "no-rub" cleaning solution for contact lenses. The solution adds a safeguard for people who do not rub their lenses—but should—when cleaning. The no-rub directions for this first solution initially applied to lenses replaced within a month or less. Now, it has been expanded to include lenses that are replaced after a month or more. Other products also are available that have no-rub directions for lenses replaced within a month. But Saviola reminds people that in some cases, rubbing is still necessary to keep their lenses clean.

A new generation of lens materials is being studied. Lenses made of these materials provide a greater amount of oxygen permeability, says Saviola. Two types have received FDA approval, one for seven days of continuous wear, the other for 30 days. Others, such as the 30-day continuous wear contact, now are being considered.

The most serious safety concerns with any contact lens deal with overnight use, or extended-wear. Rigid or soft, wearing these types of contacts overnight increases the risk of corneal ulcers—infection-caused eruptions on the cornea that can lead to blindness. Symptoms include vision changes, eye redness, eye discomfort, and excessive tearing. Extended-wear rigid lenses also can cause unexpected, sometimes undesirable reshaping of the cornea. Saviola advises that keeping lenses clean, replacing them often, and wearing them as prescribed by your eye-care specialist increases the safety of wearing contacts.

People should not wear contact lenses longer than the time prescribed by their eye-care practitioner. But whatever he or she prescribes, be sure to ask for written instructions and follow them carefully. Patient package inserts usually accompany contact lenses, and Saviola emphasizes that people who are not offered this information by their doctors should ask for it.

For those who haven't been able to wear contacts, implantable lenses may be an option in the future.

Orthokeratology

Orthokeratology, or Ortho-K, is a procedure that uses RGP contact lenses to change the curvature of the cornea to improve its ability to refract light and successfully focus on objects. Unlike regular RGPs, Ortho-K RGPs have a design that can reshape the curvature of the cornea. This method, however, does not produce a permanent result.

With conventional Ortho-K, the lenses are worn about eight hours a day. After the cornea has achieved the best shape for optimal vision, the lenses are worn less frequently—perhaps for a few hours every two or three days. If someone starts and then discontinues Ortho-K, says Saviola, the corneas will eventually return to their natural state. People choose Ortho-K over refractive surgery because Ortho-K's effects are not permanent.

One disadvantage of Ortho-K is that clear vision may fluctuate during the day. Also, Ortho-K may take many months to change a person's vision. A more advanced technique known as accelerated Ortho-K takes less time, and may be recommended to achieve a rapid effect.

Since 1998, Saviola says the FDA has cleared a number of daily wear Ortho-K lenses, but overnight Ortho-K lenses have not been approved.

The best candidates for prescription Ortho-K are people of any age who have low amounts of nearsightedness or astigmatism. The goal is to bring the person's vision to at least 20/40. But for some, Ortho-K will provide 20/20 vision.

Corneal Ring Segments

In 1999, the FDA approved a non-laser surgical procedure for correcting small amounts of nearsightedness. Corneal ring segments are tiny, clear crescent-shaped pieces of plastic polymer that are implanted in the cornea. The ring segments reshape the cornea so that it becomes flatter, allowing it to focus light rays onto the retina and producing sharp vision. The procedure takes about 15 minutes and is done on an outpatient basis. Before surgery, anesthetizing drops are placed in the eyes.

Corneal rings are still being studied to treat mild hyperopia and astigmatism, although these uses have not been approved by the FDA. Several other intraocular and corneal implants, from several companies, also are in various stages of clinical study.

Eyeglasses—The Old Standby

In some cases, modern technology can provide the best vision correction option. In those cases in which it can't, eyeglasses can often help. Glasses correct refractive errors by adding or subtracting focusing power to the cornea and lens. The power needed to focus images directly on the retina is measured in diopters. This measurement is also your eyeglass prescription.

Like contact lenses, glasses come in all shapes and sizes, offering an array of choices for both function and fashion. Eyeglass frames, for example, are more durable and tout materials such as titanium and new memory metals. Lenses are thinner, stronger, and lighter. Lens options include antireflective coating, light-changing tints, progressive (line-free) bifocal lenses, and polycarbonate—the most impact-resistant lens material available.

Perhaps the greatest troubling aspect for eyeglass wearers is the constant feel of something sitting on the nose, despite such advances as featherweight glasses. Paul Trossevin of Falling Waters, W.Va., knows all too well the uncomfortable feeling of something permanently perched on his nose. Like a scar that never fades, Trossevin's glasses have been with him every day since he was 4 years old. Now 35, he says, "There was a time when I'd have done anything to get rid of my glasses." Or so he thought.

Although he could never wear contact lenses because of the severe flatness of his cornea, Trossevin was a candidate for laser eye surgery. But the one thing he was unable to obtain from any doctor was a guarantee that after surgery he wouldn't see starbursts and halos around lights—a big concern since he drives a good part of the day and plays baseball at night. "The guarantee was everything," he says. "When he couldn't give me that, suddenly my glasses took on new meaning—a guarantee of the good eyesight they have given me for over 30 years."

Looking Ahead

Among some of the more intriguing developments in the vision-correction pipeline is an alternative to LASIK, called LASEK, a new avenue for refractive surgeons that disturbs less corneal tissue than its sound-alike counterpart. There's also talk of investigational devices that could be placed inside the eye to correct refractive errors. Over the next decade, there are sure to be improvements in current techniques and technologies, in addition to new procedures.

Eye Tips

While you can't do anything about age or genetic makeup, you can eat a balanced diet, wear sunglasses that block ultraviolet light, and get regular eye exams to help maintain good vision. Regular eye exams are important because they can detect early signs of disease long before the disease leads to vision loss.

Doctors recommend that everyone have an eye exam shortly after birth, and at least every few years until age 40. After that, the eyes should be routinely checked every 2 or 3 years.

Buying Contact Lenses by Phone, Mail, or the Internet

If you buy contact lenses—an FDA-regulated product—on the Internet, over the phone, or by mail, the agency wants you to be well-informed. While such purchases are often a convenient and economical way to get your lenses, consumers need to exercise caution when using alternatives to a prescription from an eye-care specialist, or reputable pharmacy. The following information and tips can help:

Health-Related Information

- Get regular eye exams. You may have problems with your eyes that you are not aware of, and your contacts may not correct your vision properly. Some untreated infections can lead to blindness.

- Have an eye-care specialist check to make sure that your contact lenses fit properly and that the contact lens prescription was filled properly. Failure to do so could cause discomfort or damage to your eyes.

- Beware of attempts to substitute a different brand than what you normally wear. There are differences in water content and shape between brands. The choice of which lens is right for you should be made only based on examination by your eye-care specialist, not over the phone or the Internet.

- Request the manufacturer's written patient information for your contact lenses. It will give you important information, as well as instructions for use.

Prescription-Related Information

- The minimum elements contained on a valid contact lens prescription should include your name, doctor's name, contact lens brand name and material, expiration date (if mandated by your state), and lens measurements, including power, diameter and base curve.

- Make certain your contact lens prescription is current when ordering. The expiration date is currently set by each state. Some

99

states require one- or two-year expiration dates, while other states leave it to eye care-specialists to decide. Never order lenses using a prescription that has expired.

- Be sure the lenses the company sends matches your prescription exactly. Check that you have the brand and lens name you ordered, and that the numbers indicating power, sphere, cylinder and axis (if any), diameter, and base curve are the same as on your prescription. This information is required to appear on the contact lens package or container.

- If you think you have received an incorrect lens, check with your doctor. Don't accept substitutes for any contact lens unless your doctor approves.

- Some Internet sites ask for information about your doctor so that they can check the prescription. If they do check and receive a verbal OK, then they have complied with the Federal prescription device regulation. If the company does not check, they have not obtained a valid prescription. Some state laws require that a written prescription be presented.

- Order your contacts from a supplier you are familiar with and know is reliable.

- You won't break any laws if you buy lenses on the Internet, by phone, or through the mail without a prescription, but you should know that the company is selling you a prescription device as if it were an over-the-counter device. This violates federal regulation. Be wary when companies tell you they will check with your doctor to confirm the prescription. They don't always check.

Problems Relating to Purchases

- Report serious eye problems associated with your lenses to the FDA's MedWatch reporting program at www.fda.gov/medwatch. Also, contact your health professional for medical advice.

- Report problems involving contact lens sales by Web sites by sending an e-mail to webcomplaints@ora.fda.gov.

- If you do not get the exact lenses you ordered, you should report the problem directly to the company that supplied them.

Chapter 10

How to Read Your Eyeglasses Prescription

The numbers your Eye M.D. jots down during your eye exam describe what you're seeing, and what you're not seeing.

If you know how to read your prescription you can usually comparison shop for glasses over the phone, a good way to get a base price for the glasses of your choice. Don't forget that you will probably want lens enhancements, which will be an additional cost.

Whether your Eye M.D. writes your eye glass prescription on a preprinted form specifically for eye glasses or on a blank sheet of paper, the numbers will read the same. O.D. (oculus dextrus) is your right eye and O.S. (oculus sinister) is your left. You might see the abbreviations RE and LE, or possibly no designation at all. If that is the case, you can safely assume that the first set of numbers is for your right eye.

Table 10.1 reads, "Right eye, plus two point five zero, plus one point zero zero, axis 180. Left eye, plus one point seven five, plus one point five zero, axis one eighty. Plus two point zero zero add."

The sphere column indicates how nearsighted or farsighted you are. Cylinder refers to the measurable degree of astigmatism of your central cornea. The cylindrical number describes the dioptric difference between your cornea's steepest and lowest curves.

If you have astigmatism, your cornea is shaped like the back of a spoon, curved more on one side than the other. The orientation of the spoon shape can differ from person to person, for instance like a spoon standing on end or on its side. The axis column describes the orientation in degrees from horizontal. Most left and right eyes with astigmatism are symmetrical.

Table 10.1. Sample Prescription for Convex Lenses

	Sphere	Cylinder	Axis
O.D.	+2.50	+1.00	180
O.S.	+1.75	+1.50	180
		+2.00 add	

Table 10.2. Sample Prescription for Concave Lenses

	Sphere	Cylinder	Axis
O.D.	-1.25	-2.50	90
O.S.	-0.75	-2.25	90
		+1.50 add	

What Do the Numbers Mean?

Lens power is measured in units called diopters. Diopters are based on the extent light rays passing through the lens will be bent. As the power of the lens increases, so does the thickness of the lens. There are three different types of lenses:

• Convex lenses are thicker in the center than at the edges, like a magnifying glass. Light rays are gathered together toward a central point. Convex lenses are used in glasses for farsighted (hyperopic) eyes that can't bend light rays as much as they need to. Convex lenses are indicated with a plus (+) symbol on prescriptions.

- Concave lenses are thinner at the center than at the edges and spread light rays apart. These lenses are used for eyes that are nearsighted (myopic). Concave lenses are indicated with a minus (-) symbol.

- Cylindrical lenses are curved more in one direction than the other. To tell if your lenses are cylindrical, hold your glasses at arm's length and sight a straight line through the lens. Rotate the glasses clockwise and counterclockwise. If the line bends, it's a cylindrical lens. Cylindrical lenses, used for astigmatism, are usually part of a prescription for near- or farsightedness.

Table 10.2 reads, "Right eye, minus one point two five, minus two point five zero, axis ninety. Left eye, minus zero point seven five, minus two point two five, axis eighty-five."

This means the patient's right eye has 1¼ diopters of nearsightedness with 2½ diopters of astigmatism. The axis refers to the orientation of the cylindrical area of the lens. The axis can be anywhere from 1 to 180 degrees, with 90 being the vertical meridians. The left eye has ¾ diopters of nearsightedness, 2¼ diopters of astigmatism, axis 90.

Bifocal prescriptions are indicated with numbers such as the "+1.50 add" above. This number indicates the strength of the lens. This patient will need 1½ diopters of power for reading.

Chapter 11

Contact Lenses

Chapter Contents

Section 11.1

Keeping an Eye on Contact Lenses

"Keeping an Eye on Contact Lenses: Safety, Options Shape Contact
Lens Decisions," by Dixie Farley, *FDA Consumer*, U.S. Food and Drug
Administration, April 1998; updated August 1998.

Imagine wearing your contact lenses for a few hours and then, after you pop them out, still seeing clearly for a portion of the day. For
certain individuals with nearsightedness, that image can be reality,
thanks to a new lens the Food and Drug Administration recently
cleared for marketing.

The OK rigid gas-permeable contact lens, made by ConTEX,
Sherman Oaks, California, is the first lens designed to correct nearsightedness by temporarily reshaping the transparent tissue known
as the cornea that covers the iris and pupil. It is just one of many
choices for the 28 million Americans who wear contact lenses.

These medical devices, sold under more than 350 brand names,
offer numerous options, including rigid-lens handling ease, soft-lens
comfort, bifocal vision, a rainbow of colors, no-fuss disposables, and
even protective help against ultraviolet radiation.

Shaping up

The idea behind the OK lens is not new. Since the early 1960's, some
optometrists have used conventional daily-wear rigid lenses to reshape corneas. This procedure is called orthokeratology, or Ortho-K.
FDA considers such treatment of an individual patient to be the practice of medicine and therefore not subject to regulation. Selling contacts not cleared for Ortho-K to practitioners for this use is illegal
marketing, however, so the agency is helping manufacturers obtain
clearances specifically for Ortho-K.

Studies before FDA began regulating contact lenses, in 1976, show
that Ortho-K appears to be safe, says James Saviola, O.D., chief of the
vitreoretinal and extraocular devices branch at FDA's Center for Devices and Radiological Health. "The lower your amount of nearsightedness, the greater your probability of success with Ortho-K," he says.

Ortho-K reshaping involves the use of a series of lenses that apply pressure to the cornea. Once the desired result is achieved, use of daily-wear maintenance lenses is crucial to retain the reshaping. If you wear the maintenance lenses faithfully, Saviola says, "you may only need to wear the lenses for a portion of the day."

However, Ortho-K does not work for everyone. Some people do not experience any significant reduction in nearsightedness. "An individual's response is difficult to predict," Saviola says. "It may take weeks or months to have an effect."

Safety Concerns

The most serious safety concern with any contact lens is related to overnight use. Extended-wear (overnight) contact lenses—rigid or soft—increase the risk of corneal ulcers, infection-caused eruptions on the cornea that can lead to blindness. Symptoms include vision changes, eye redness, eye discomfort or pain, and excessive tearing.

The risk of corneal ulcers for people who keep extended-wear lenses in overnight is 10 to 15 times greater than for those who use daily-wear lenses only while awake, says James Saviola, O.D., chief of the vitreoretinal and extraocular devices branch at FDA's Center for Devices and Radiological Health.

When the eyes are open, he explains, tears carry adequate oxygen to the cornea to keep it healthy. But during sleep, the eye produces fewer tears, causing the cornea to swell. Under the binding down of a rigid contact lens during sleep, the flow of tears and oxygen to the cornea is further reduced. This lack of oxygen leaves the eye vulnerable to infection.

Extended-wear rigid lenses also can cause unexpected, sometimes undesirable, reshaping of the cornea.

Soft extended-wear lenses also bind down on the closed eye, but they are porous and allow some tears through during sleep. Because they have so little form, their binding has little effect on the shape of the eye.

FDA has approved extended-wear lenses for use up to seven days before removal for cleaning. Still, there are risks with use of extended-wear lenses, "even if it's just one night," Saviola says. Daily-wear lenses are removed daily for cleaning and are a safer choice, provided they aren't worn during sleep.

Another sight-threatening concern is the infection Acanthamoeba keratitis, caused by improper lens care. This difficult-to-treat parasitic infection's symptoms are similar to those of corneal ulcers.

The use of homemade saline from salt tablets is one of the biggest contributors to Acanthamoeba keratitis in contact lens wearers. "FDA no longer condones the use of salt tablets, and neither should a concerned pharmacist," writes Janet Engle, Pharm.D., in the 1996 *Handbook of Nonprescription Drugs*. Engle is associate dean for academic affairs and clinical associate professor of pharmacy practice at the University of Illinois in Chicago.

Microorganisms may also be present in distilled water, so always use commercial sterile saline solutions to dissolve enzyme tablets. Heat disinfection is the only method effective against Acanthamoeba, and it also kills organisms in and on the lens case.

The Options

Soft lenses are much more comfortable than rigid lenses, thanks to their ability to conform to the eye and absorb and hold water. You can get used to soft lenses within days, compared with several weeks for rigid. An added benefit is that soft lenses aren't as likely as rigid lenses to pop out or capture foreign material like dust underneath. Extra-thin soft lenses are available for very sensitive people.

While the ability to hold water increases oxygen permeability of soft lenses, it increases their fragility as well.

Rigid lenses generally give clearer vision. They can be marked to show which lens is for which eye. They don't rip or tear, so they're easy to handle.

Also, rigid lenses don't absorb chemicals, unlike soft lenses, which Saviola says are like sponges. "They'll suck up any residues on your hands—soap, lotion, whatever."

Both soft and rigid lenses offer bifocal correction. In some models, each lens corrects for near and distance vision. In others, one lens is for near vision, and the other is for distance. Middle-aged people who have good distance vision but need help for reading can get a monovision reading lens for one eye.

Soft lenses additionally come as disposable products (defined by FDA as used once and discarded) or as planned-replacement lenses.

With planned-replacement lenses, the practitioner works out a replacement schedule tailored to each patient's needs, says Byron Tart, director of promotion and advertising policy at FDA's devices center. "For patients who produce a higher level of protein in their eyes or don't take as good care of their lenses, it might be healthier to replace the lenses more frequently," he says.

Some practitioners prescribe disposables as planned-replacement lenses, which are removed, disinfected and reused before being discarded. Saviola cautions that lenses labeled disposable don't come with instructions for cleaning and disinfecting, while those labeled specifically for planned replacement do.

Whatever lenses your practitioner prescribes, be sure to ask for written instructions and follow them carefully.

In the U.S. contact lens marketplace, 82 percent wear soft lenses, 16 percent wear rigid gas-permeable, and 2 percent wear hard. Although very few people wear hard lenses, they are available for people who have adapted to them and want them. Hard lenses are not the same as rigid gas-permeable lenses, since they do not allow oxygen transmission through the lens.

Contacts Not for Everyone

People with inadequate tearing (dry eye syndrome) usually can't tolerate contacts, says Donna Lochner, chief of the intraocular and corneal implants branch of FDA's devices center. In addition, Lochner says, "Severe nearsightedness often can't be corrected effectively with contact lenses."

Saviola notes that certain working conditions, such as exposure to chemical fumes, may be undesirable for contact-lens wearers. Contacts may be ruled out by allergy to lens-care products or by corneal problems, such as a history of viral infection of the cornea. "Extra caution," he says, "should be exercised with diabetics, because they're susceptible to infection and have trouble healing."

Cosmetic use of contacts is limited in children. Adolescence is the youngest age as a rule to consider contact lenses, says Saviola, but some practitioners do fit 9- to 11-year-olds. "You may prescribe for a younger child who has the motor skills and responsibility to handle contact lenses."

For some people who haven't been able to wear contacts and want to, implantable lenses may be an option in the future.

Doctors are studying ring segments, "shaped like parentheses," Lochner says, which are implanted in the cornea. "They flatten out the cornea, changing the shape to give the correct optical power." Lenses that are implanted inside the eye are also being studied to correct refractive error, she says.

Correcting vision is not the only use for contact lenses.

Some soft contacts are used as bandage lenses after photorefractive keratectomy laser surgery for nearsightedness. The surgery removes the outer cell layer of the cornea, creating a large abrasion on the eye. "It's excruciatingly painful," Saviola says, "if you don't have a protective covering on the cornea after the anesthetic wears off."

Collagen eye shields are used as bandage lenses to relieve pain from other abrasions or sores on the cornea. They dissolve in a couple of days.

Comparison Shopping

Companies that sell contact lenses compete stiffly for business, offering discounts and premiums such as a second set free.

But a discount for the lenses might not save you money if the price doesn't include other needed products and services, such as a thorough eye examination, lens-care kit, and follow-up visits to make sure you're adapting. A moderate cost for a package that has everything you need may be the best deal.

Before you make an appointment, ask the practitioner these questions:

- Will you give me my prescription? (You may want the prescription if you decide to go to another practitioner or order lenses from an alternate source.)
- What tests are included in the eye examination?
- What do you charge for the examination, lenses, evaluation, fitting, lens-care kit, follow-up visits, and service agreements?
- What is your refund policy if I can't adapt to contact lenses?
- How many types and brands of contact lenses do you sell?
- How much do you charge for replacement lenses?

Asking questions about any new prescription treatment is always a good idea.

Like medicines, contact lenses provide benefits and pose risks. But even with the increased risk of corneal ulcers posed by extended-wear lenses, Saviola says this risk alone isn't enough to say the devices aren't safe and effective if properly used.

"If people are informed," he says, "then they're making a judgment based on available information. That's the thing we always struggle with, conveying enough information to people and having the practitioner convey enough information, so that the consumer can make an informed choice."

Buyer Beware

Sorting help from hype in any media—the World Wide Web, television, or print—can pose a problem. So remember: If a claim sounds too good to be true, it probably is.

Here are some recent examples of potential problems:

- Special effects contacts promoted on the Web with names like Vampire and Reptilian may sound fun to try, but they could be risky, says FDA's James Saviola, O.D. "We currently have no information that shows pigments in these lenses are safe in the eye." While FDA hasn't been strict about similar lenses used on a very limited basis by entertainers, Internet advertising takes them beyond isolated theatrical usage.

- Buying mail-order contacts with no prescription calls for caution, says Saviola. "If your current lens has a 14-millimeter (mm) diameter and 8.7 base curve, and the mail-order company switches to another brand lens with a 14.0-mm diameter and 8.8 curve, it seems like it's about the same size and shape and should fit well. Maybe it will. But the new brand is a different material. It may leave your eyes uncomfortable."

- A misleading print ad for Acuvue contacts was corrected last year after an FDA warning. The ad showed a man and woman half indoors and half outdoors on a sunny beach—no protective eyewear. "Open your eyes to the UV around you," it stated. "And you'll be glad Acuvue contact lenses are introducing UV protection." Writing to Vistakon Inc., of Johnson & Johnson Vision Products Inc., FDA warned: "The combination of this picture and the accompanying language implies that wearing the Acuvue UV-absorbing lens outside offers as much protection as one would naturally have indoors." Warnings in tiny print that the lenses were not substitutes for UV-absorbing eyewear did not "counteract the overall message" that the lenses provided full UV protection, the agency wrote. The company also corrected a similar TV ad.

- Misleading pricing a few years earlier prompted consumer lawsuits against Bausch & Lomb for selling the same lens under three different names, at three different prices.

- Charges of false claims were settled by the Federal Trade Commission last November against J. Mason Hurt, O.D., of Bartlett,

Tennessee. Hurt had touted his Precise Corneal Molding ortho-keratology treatment as a permanent cure for defective vision. A consent agreement prohibits Hurt from making further false claims and requires reliable scientific evidence for future claims.

Proper Care Gives Safer Wear

- Follow, and save, the directions that come with your lenses. If you didn't get a patient information booklet about your lenses, request it from your eye-care practitioner.

- Use only the types of lens-care enzyme cleaners and saline solutions your practitioner okays.

- Be exact in following the directions that come with each lens-care product. If you have questions, ask your practitioner or pharmacist.

- Wash and rinse your hands before handling lenses. Fragrance-free soap is best.

- Clean, rinse, and disinfect reusable lenses each time they're removed, even if this is several times a day.

- Clean, rinse, and disinfect again if storage lasts longer than allowed by your disinfecting solution.

- Clean, rinse and air-dry the lens case each time you remove the lenses. Then put in fresh solution. Replace the case every six months.

- Get your practitioner's okay before taking medicines or using topical eye products, even those you buy without a prescription.

- Remove your lenses and call your practitioner right away if you have vision changes, redness of the eye, eye discomfort or pain, or excessive tearing.

- Visit your practitioner every six months (more often if needed) to catch possible problems early.

Watch out

- Never use saliva to wet your lenses.

- Never use tap water, distilled water, or saline solution made at home with salt tablets for any part of your lens care. Use only commercial sterile saline solution.

- Never mix different brands of cleaner or solution.

- Never change your lens-care regimen or products without your practitioner's okay.

- Never let cosmetic lotions, creams or sprays touch your lenses.

- Never wear lenses when swimming or in a hot tub.

- Never wear daily-wear lenses during sleep, not even a nap.

- Never wear your lenses longer than prescribed by your eye-care practitioner.

Dixie Farley, who was on the staff of *FDA Consumer* for more than 13 years, retired from federal service in January 1998.

Section 11.2

Types of Contact Lenses

"Advantages and Disadvantages of Various Types of Contact Lenses,"
© 2001 American Optometric Association. Reprinted with permission.
For additional information, visit www.aoa.org.

Reasons to Consider Contact Lenses

- Contact lenses move with your eye, allow a natural field of view, have no frames to obstruct your vision, and greatly reduce distortions.

- They do not fog up, like glasses, nor do they get splattered by mud or rain.

- Contact lenses do not get in the way of your activities.

- Many people feel they look better in contact lenses.

Table 11.1. Advantages and Disadvantages of Various Types of Contact Lenses

Lens Types	Advantages	Disadvantages
Rigid gas-permeable (RGP) Made of slightly flexible plastics that allow oxygen to pass through to the eyes	Excellent vision, short adaptation period, comfortable to wear, correct most vision problems, easy to put on and to care for, durable with a relatively long life, available in tints (for handling purposes) and bifocals.	Require consistent wear to maintain adaptation, can slip off center of eye more easily than other types, debris can easily get under the lenses, requires office visits for follow-up care.
Daily-wear soft lenses Made of soft, flexible plastic that allows oxygen to pass through to the eyes.	Very short adaptation period, more comfortable and more difficult to dislodge than RGP lenses, available in tints and bifocals, great for active lifestyles.	Do not correct all vision problems, vision may not be as sharp as with RGP lenses, require regular office visits for follow-up care, lenses soil easily and must be replaced.
Extended-wear Available for overnight wear in soft or RGP lenses.	Can usually be worn up to seven days without removal.	Do not correct all vision problems, require regular office visits for follow-up care, increases risk of complication, requires regular monitoring and professional care.
Extended-wear disposable Soft lenses worn for an extended period of time, from one to six days and then discarded.	Require little or no cleaning, minimal risk of eye infection if wearing instructions are followed, available in tints and bifocals, spare lenses available.	Vision may not be as sharp as RGP lenses, do not correct all vision problems, handling may be more difficult.
Planned replacement Soft daily wear lenses that are replaced on a planned schedule, most often either every two weeks, monthly or quarterly.	Require simplified cleaning and disinfection, good for eye health, available in most prescriptions.	Vision may not be as sharp as RGP lenses, do not correct all vision problems, handling may be more difficult.

- Contact lenses, compared to eyeglasses, generally offer better sight.

Some Things to Remember about Contact Lenses

- Contact lenses, when compared with glasses, require a longer initial examination and more follow-up visits to maintain eye health and more time for lens care.

- If you are going to wear your lenses successfully, you will have to clean and store them properly; adhere to lens wearing schedules; and make appointments for follow-up care.

- If you are wearing disposable or planned replacement lenses, you will have to carefully follow the schedule for throwing away used lenses.

Section 11.3

Contact Lenses Dos and Don'ts

Get started off right with your contact lenses by going to a doctor who provides full-service care. This includes a thorough eye examination, an evaluation of your suitability for contact lens wear, the lenses, necessary lens care kits, individual instructions for wear and care, and unlimited follow-up visits over a specified time. The initial visit and examination can take an hour or longer. Here is a list of other specific dos and don'ts to lead you to successful wear.

Do

- Listen and watch closely as instructions are given and demonstrated.
- Practice the care routine in your optometrist's office.
- Follow lens care and wearing instructions/schedules to the letter.

- Schedule follow-up visits to your optometrist both during and after your adaptation period. This is important to maintaining good eye health and safe contact lens wear.

- Wash hands thoroughly before handling your lenses.

- Handle contact lenses over a clean towel. If your drop your lenses, they will stay clean and undamaged.

- Store your lenses in the case made for them and keep the case clean.

Don't

- Use cream soaps. They can leave a film on your hands that can transfer to the lenses.

- Put contact lenses in your mouth or moisten them with saliva, which is full of bacteria and a potential source of infection.

- Use homemade saline solutions. Improper use of homemade saline solutions has been linked with a potentially blinding condition among soft lens wearers.

Section 11.4

Buying Contact Lenses

"Buying Contact Lenses on the Internet, by Phone, or by Mail: Questions and Answers," Center for Devices and Radiological Health, U.S. Food and Drug Administration, May 2001.

The FDA wants you to be a wise consumer if you buy contact lenses, an FDA-regulated product, on the Internet, over the phone or by mail. While such purchases are often a convenient and economical way to get lenses, Internet, phone, or mail orders require consumers to exercise some caution. The following questions and answers should help you take simple precautions to make your Internet, phone, or mail purchase safe and effective for you.

What Do I Need to Consider When Buying Contact Lenses on the Internet, by Phone, or by Mail?

- Is my contact lens prescription current? You should always have a current, correct prescription when you order contact lenses.

- If you have not had a checkup in the last one to two years, you may have problems with your eyes that you are not aware of, or your contact lenses may not correct your vision well.

- The expiration date for your prescription is currently set by your state. Some require a one-year renewal, some a two-year renewal, while other states leave it to your doctor to decide.

- Never order lenses with a prescription that has expired.

What Does a Valid Contact Lens Prescription Include?

This depends on the state where your doctor practices. State laws often define a prescription's requirements. In states without a legal definition, the prescribing doctor includes some minimum elements.

The minimum elements usually include your name and the doctor's name along with the contact lens brand name and material. Also, lens measurements such as power, diameter, and base curve are included.

More detailed prescriptions will include directions for safe use such as wearing schedule, whether lenses are for daily or extended wear, the number of refills, whether lens material substitutions are allowed and an expiration date.

Some Internet sites ask for information about your doctor so that they may check the prescription with your doctor. If they do check with your doctor and receive a verbal okay, they comply with the Federal prescription device regulation. If the company does not check, then they have not obtained a valid prescription. Some state laws require that a written prescription be presented.

Will I Get in Legal Trouble If I Buy My Contact Lenses on the Internet, by Phone, or by Mail If I Don't Have a Copy of My Prescription?

You won't break any laws, but the company is selling you a prescription device as if it were an over-the-counter device. This is a violation of the Federal prescription device regulation. Often, the company will say that they will check back with your doctor to confirm the prescription. However, that may not always happen.

Some Internet sites will allow you to fill out a chart with the ordering information about your contact lenses and ask you to fill in your doctor's name and phone number. The site may not ask for an actual copy of your prescription.

Since individual states have different licensing requirements for optical dispensers, enforcement of prescription device sales has usually been left to the state in which the company selling the contact lenses is located.

What Harm Can Be Done If I Don't Have Regular Checkups with My Doctor or I Order Lenses without a Valid Prescription?

At your checkup, your eye doctor will re-evaluate the fit of your contact lenses and observe any changes in your cornea caused by your lenses. You will benefit by having a correct, current prescription and you may avoid serious problems, especially if you wear your lenses on an extended or overnight schedule.

Though infections of the cornea are rare, severe cases can cause loss of vision and even blindness. During regularly scheduled visits, your eye doctor looks for irregularities that, if left untreated, may lead to severe problems. These irregularities often have no symptoms and you may be totally unaware of them.

Contact lens wear causes many changes to cells and tissues of the eye, and sometimes wearing contact lenses can damage the cornea (the clear window of the eye). Even if you are currently experiencing no problems, the lenses may be causing damage to your eyes. Regular checkups will reduce the likelihood of damage going undetected.

Contact lenses that are not properly fitted by an eye doctor might not work well, or even worse, may harm your eyes.

Ask your eye doctor how often to have a checkup.

Will Regular Checkups Help Prevent Me from Having Problems with My Contact Lenses?

Anyone wearing contact lenses runs an increased risk of corneal infection. Regular checkups will help reduce your chances of having a problem. At your checkup, your doctor may find something that requires refitting with a new lens or requires modifying your wearing schedule.

What Can I Do to Avoid Serious Problems with My Contact Lenses?

- Ask your eye doctor how often you should have a checkup and see the doctor according to the recommended schedule.

- You run a greater risk of developing serious eye problems such as infection if you wear lenses overnight.

- Order your contact lenses from a supplier you are familiar with and know is reliable. Contact lenses are often more complex than they appear.

- Request the manufacturer's written patient information for your contact lenses. It will give you important risk/benefit information, as well as instructions for use.

- Beware of attempts to substitute a different brand than you presently have. While this may be acceptable in some situations, there are differences in the water content and shape between different brands. The correct choice of which lens is right for you should only be made based on examination by your doctor, not over the phone.

- Carefully check to make sure the company gives you: the exact brand; lens name; power; sphere; cylinder, if any; axis, if any; diameter; base curve; and peripheral curves, if any.

- If you think you have gotten an incorrect lens, check with your eye doctor. Don't accept a substitution unless your doctor approves it.

Where Can I Report Problems That I Have with My Contact Lenses?

You can report a serious eye problem associated with your contact lenses with FDA's MedWatch reporting form at: http://www.fda.gov/medwatch. Also, contact your health professional for medical advice.

You can report problems involving contact lens sales by Web sites by sending e-mail to webcomplaints@ora.fda.gov.

If you do not get the exact lenses that you ordered, you should report the problem directly to the company that supplied them.

Chapter 12

Vision Correction Procedures

If you're among the 68 million Americans who are nearsighted, you probably wear glasses or contact lenses to improve your distance vision. You also may hear a lot about radial keratotomy (RK) and photorefractive keratectomy (PRK)—surgical procedures that treat your vision problem—and orthokeratology (Ortho-K), a non-surgical procedure that claims to improve your vision by changing the shape of your cornea.

Don't throw away your glasses or contact lenses just yet. The Federal Trade Commission (FTC) cautions that RK, PRK, and Ortho-K are not always shortcuts to perfect vision, although some advertising and promotional materials for the procedures may suggest otherwise.

The RK and PRK Surgical Procedures

RK and PRK reduce nearsightedness by altering the shape of the cornea. In RK, the surgeon uses a diamond knife to make incisions in the cornea in a radial or spoke-like pattern. This causes the cornea's curvature to flatten, changing the way it focuses light on the retina. In PRK, the surgeon uses a computer-controlled excimer laser to sculpt the surface of the cornea, changing its shape and the way light is refracted to the retina.

RK and PRK are outpatient surgical procedures. They are not used to treat people who have trouble seeing near objects—those who are

Federal Trade Commission, November 1997; updated October 1999.

farsighted—or people who need reading glasses as a result of the aging process—those who are presbyopic.

Some surgeons who perform RK schedule two operations, allowing one eye to stabilize before operating on the second. The U.S. Food and Drug Administration (FDA) recommends a three-month waiting period between PRK operations. Many RK patients and a small percentage of PRK patients also need or want additional surgery—usually called an enhancement—to fine-tune the results of the initial operation. Neither RK nor PRK is considered medically necessary, because the operation is performed on a healthy organ. As a result, the surgery usually is not covered by health insurance.

The Ortho-K Non-Surgical Procedure

Ortho-K is defined as a procedure that involves fitting the patient with a series of rigid contact lenses in an attempt to reshape the cornea to improve vision. The last set of lenses become retainers that the patient wears for a limited time each day to maintain the new corneal shape. Some eye care providers use special names, such as precise corneal molding (PCM) or controlled kerato-reformation (CKR), to refer to their method of performing Ortho-K.

Published results of four controlled clinical studies conducted in the 1970's and 1980's showed that some contact lens wearers experienced changes in their nearsightedness after several months of contact lens wear. However, the studies show that any reduction in nearsightedness that may be achieved is temporary. In fact, the patient's nearsightedness returns to its original level when that patient stops wearing contact lenses. It also is not possible to predict who might respond positively to this procedure and by how much. Some practitioners claim that newer techniques achieve better results than what the four studies showed.

However, there is no scientific evidence to back this up. It is very important to know that the FDA, which regulates contact lenses as medical devices, has approved only one daily wear lens for orthokeratology. There are still no lenses that have FDA approval for overnight orthokeratology.

Seeing through Claims

Even with 20/20 vision, it can be difficult to read between the lines in promotional literature. If you or someone you care about is considering RK, PRK, or Ortho-K, here is some information to help you evaluate some of the claims about these procedures. Among the claims you may see or hear are:

No More Glasses or Contact Lenses

One claim about refractive surgery is that you'll never need glasses or contact lenses again. This claim is false for most people. The truth is that for a variety of reasons, you still may need corrective lenses after RK and PRK. Like any surgical procedure, refractive surgery is not 100 percent predictable. RK and PRK surgery may result in overcorrection, which renders you farsighted, or undercorrection, which leaves you nearsighted. And almost everyone who undergoes RK or PRK surgery eventually will need reading glasses.

What's more, studies have shown that a number of patients who undergo RK surgery to treat their nearsightedness may become farsighted and need corrective lenses for close vision because of a hyperopic shift—a gradual but continuing shift toward farsightedness. Some doctors deliberately undercorrect, leaving patients with residual nearsightedness after RK surgery to compensate for any slow drift toward farsightedness. In recent years, RK equipment and techniques have developed and surgical results have improved. Nevertheless, studies assessing RK surgery continue to document an ongoing need for corrective lenses after surgery for a significant number of patients.

The FDA recently approved two laser systems as safe and effective for performing PRK on adult patients with mild to moderate nearsightedness and mild astigmatism. In clinical studies that were submitted as part of the FDA approval process for one of the laser systems, about five percent of patients followed after surgery still needed corrective lenses often for distance vision, and up to 15 percent needed corrective lenses occasionally for distance vision. Those who wore reading glasses for near vision before the surgery still needed them afterward. In addition, there were indications that some patients who did not need reading glasses before surgery might need them afterward or earlier in life than they might have had they never had the surgery.

The claim that you won't need glasses or contact lenses following the Ortho-K procedure also is false. Even if Ortho-K helps reduce some of your nearsightedness, you must wear contact lenses at least part of the day to maintain the reduction. You might be told that you only have to wear retainer lenses at night, freeing you from contact lenses during the day. But no controlled study has been conducted to test the hypothesis that retainer lenses worn at night on a limited basis can stabilize the shape of the cornea. More importantly, overnight use of contact lenses is associated with greater risk of complications. The immediate and long-term health risks of Ortho-K performed in combination with overnight wear are unknown.[1]

Permanent, Stable, or Predictable Long-Term Results

Although research on RK surgery has identified a shift toward farsightedness in a significant number of patients, new RK techniques are being studied to determine whether they result in more stable vision. One technique, known as mini-RK, uses shorter and fewer incisions. It may provide more stable vision for people with a low degree of myopia only. Research on this technique continues.

One possible effect of PRK surgery may be a return to some degree of nearsightedness. Studies of the long-term effects of PRK are being conducted to determine whether vision remains stable over long periods of time.

Studies indicate that while Ortho-K can alter the corneal curvature, it is not possible to predict who will respond favorably to Ortho-K, by how much, and for how long. With lens removal, it is not possible to predict when unaided vision is at its best. The reason: unaided vision fluctuates.

Ninety-Five Percent of Patients Achieve 20/40 Vision or Better

You may have read or heard claims that a high percentage of PRK patients achieve unaided 20/40 vision or better. Although 20/40 vision may be enough to pass a driver's license eye test in most states, you still may need or choose to wear corrective lenses for distance vision, particularly at night. A 95 percent chance for unaided 20/40 vision or better does not mean that you have a 95 percent chance of never wearing glasses or contacts again.

In addition, you may have read testimonials from consumers who claim they've achieved unaided 20/20 or 20/40 vision with the Ortho-K procedure. These results are not typical or permanent. Ortho-K can reduce nearsightedness by a small amount, but most people who are nearsighted need more reduction to achieve unaided 20/20 or 20/40 vision.

You may read other claims about the safety and effectiveness of the surgical procedures as well. Keep in mind that no surgical procedure is risk-free. In rare instances, RK and PRK may result in serious complications, like loss of vision or infection. In addition, there are several potential side-effects. For example, after RK surgery, patients may experience fluctuating vision, a weakened cornea, halos around lights, increased sensitivity to light and glare, and temporary pain. Clinical studies submitted to the FDA by one laser manufacturer reported that those who have PRK surgery may experience pain 24 to 48 hours after surgery. In addition, other side-effects occurred within six months after surgery, including corneal haze, loss of best vision achieved with glasses, minor glare, and mild halos around images.

For More Information

For more information about possible benefits, limitations, side effects, and complications of vision correction options, consult your eye doctor. Remember to ask your eye doctor about his or her experience with these procedures.

Note

1. In June 2002, the U.S. Food and Drug Administration approved a corneal reshaping procedure in which special contact lenses are worn at night. The procedure, called Corneal Refractive Therapy (CRT), temporarily improves vision even after the contacts are removed. For more information about CRT, contact the U.S. Food and Drug Administration, Center for Devices in Radiological Health, http://www.fda.gov/cdrh.

Chapter 13

Laser Eye Surgery: Is It Worth Looking into?

For Jeri Goldstein everything was a blur. Without her contact lenses she couldn't distinguish people, the scenes on television, the stars at night, and, generally, the world at large. Then, in March 1998, the 49-year-old California resident had eye surgery, and all that changed.

"After wearing contact lenses for 35 years, you can't imagine the freedom I felt," says Goldstein.

Goldstein underwent refractive eye surgery, an elective procedure intended to correct common eye disorders, known as refractive errors, such as myopia (nearsightedness), hyperopia (farsightedness), and astigmatism (distorted vision). Although there are several types of surgical techniques being performed today to correct refractive errors, laser refractive correction is fast becoming the most technologically advanced method available, according to the American Academy of Ophthalmology in San Francisco. Doctors say it allows for an unparalleled degree of precision and predictability.

"Laser surgery is the most exciting advancement in ophthalmology," says James J. Salz, M.D., clinical professor of ophthalmology at the University of Southern California in Los Angeles and the doctor who performed Goldstein's surgery. But surprisingly, he says, despite its sudden popularity, "only 20 percent of ophthalmologists in the United States today are trained in its operation."

"Laser Eye Surgery: Is It Worth Looking Into?," by Carol Lewis, *FDA Consumer*, U.S. Food and Drug Administration, August 1998; updated April 1999.

The Food and Drug Administration first approved the excimer laser in October 1995 for correcting mild to moderate nearsightedness. With that approval, the agency also restricted use of the laser to practitioners trained both in laser refractive surgery and in the calibration and operation of the laser. Currently, the excimer laser has been approved for use in a procedure called photorefractive keratectomy (PRK), and, as of November 1998, for a procedure called laser in situ keratomileusis (LASIK).

Precision Surgery

PRK is an outpatient procedure generally performed with local anesthetic eye drops. This type of refractive surgery gently reshapes the cornea by removing microscopic amounts of tissue from the outer surface with a cool, computer-controlled ultraviolet beam of light. The beam is so precise it can cut notches in a strand of human hair without breaking it, and each pulse can remove 39 millionths of an inch of tissue in 12 billionths of a second. The procedure itself takes only a few minutes, and patients are typically back to daily routines in one to three days.

Before the procedure begins, the patient's eye is measured to determine the degree of visual problem, and a map of the eye's surface is constructed. The required corneal change is calculated based on this information, and then entered into the laser's computer.

Since 1995, a limited number of laser systems has been approved by FDA to treat various refractive errors, both with PRK and LASIK.

According to FDA's Center for Devices and Radiological Health, clinical studies showed that about 5 percent of patients continued to always need glasses following PRK for distance, and up to 15 percent needed glasses occasionally, such as when driving. In addition, many patients experienced mild corneal haze following surgery, which is part of the normal healing process. The haze appeared to have little or no effect on final vision, and could only be seen by a doctor with a microscope. Some patients experienced glare and halos around lights. These conditions, however, diminished or disappeared in most patients in six months. For about 5 percent of patients, however, best-corrected vision without corrective lenses was slightly worse after surgery than before. In view of these findings, FDA and the Federal Trade Commission (which oversees advertising) issued a letter to the eye-care community in May 1996 warning that unrealistic advertising claims, such as "throw away your eyeglasses," and unsubstantiated claims about success rates could be misleading to consumers.

LASIK

LASIK is a more complex procedure than PRK. It is performed for all degrees of nearsightedness. The surgeon uses a knife called a microkeratome to cut a flap of corneal tissue, removes the targeted tissue beneath it with the laser, and then replaces the flap.

"With LASIK, the skill of the surgeon is important because he'll be making an incision," says Stephen Crawford, O.D., an optometrist practicing in Virginia, "compared to the PRK method where the machine does more of the work." Crawford urges people to find qualified, experienced doctors to perform this surgery.

"You'll want someone who's done a number of LASIK procedures since this is a surgeon-dependent operation," he said.

According to Ken Taylor, O.D., vice president of Arthur D. Little, Inc., a technology and management consultant firm in Cambridge, Massachusetts, "Last year, across the country, 40 to 45 percent of refractive surgeries performed by physicians were LASIK, which equates to approximately 80,000 procedures."

Doctors not participating in clinical trials may choose to use the approved laser to perform LASIK procedures at their discretion, says Morris Waxler, Ph.D., chief of FDA's diagnostic and surgical devices section. But most uses are considered off label and are not regulated by FDA.

A. Ralph Rosenthal, M.D., director of FDA's division of ophthalmic devices, says, "The agency has ruled that individual physicians can perform LASIK under the general 'practice of medicine,' if it's in the patient's best interest."

Advantages of LASIK

Some doctors believe that LASIK is a suitable procedure for correcting the most severe refractive errors. They also say that there is generally a faster recovery time after LASIK than after PRK. In addition, LASIK patients can see well enough to drive immediately and have good vision within a week.

After studying the options, Goldstein first decided on the LASIK procedure, but was surprised to learn that her doctor advised against it.

"Initially, I wanted the quick recovery that LASIK offers," Goldstein says, "but the bottom line was, which surgery will give me the best results, and after considering everything, eventually we agreed on PRK."

James Salz is currently involved in an FDA-sanctioned clinical trial at Cedars-Sinai Medical Center in Los Angeles, which is now studying the laser system specifically for farsightedness (hyperopia) with astigmatism. Although routinely performing laser eye surgery, he still encourages a small percentage of his low to moderately nearsighted patients to undergo radial keratotomy, or RK, an earlier refractive correction procedure that does not require the excimer laser.

With RK, incisions are made in a radial pattern along the outer portion of the cornea using a hand-held blade. These incisions are designed to help flatten the curvature of the cornea, thereby allowing light rays entering the eye to properly focus on the retina. The number and length of the incisions determines the degree of correction attained.

"Typically, this is still a practiced procedure for select people with very small corrections of myopia," Salz says.

Conversely, Crawford says that although he will mention RK as an option to his patients considering eye surgery, he is not in favor of this method. He says studies indicate that incisions made during this procedure, which penetrate approximately 90 percent of the cornea, appear to weaken the structure of the eye. Also, once you've had RK done you can't repeat it or have PRK done.

"I think that patients should understand and consider all available options for correcting refractive errors," Crawford says, "but I would never recommend RK to anyone."

Is Laser Surgery for You?

For some, like Goldstein, laser surgery has been the ultimate freedom from the everyday hassles of contact lenses, and a second chance at having normal eyesight. But can everyone expect such dramatic results?

"The answer is no," says Rosenthal. "It's not a foolproof procedure and people need to know that some can end up with worse eyesight than before they went in."

Mary Ann Duke, M.D., a general ophthalmologist practicing in Potomac, Maryland, adds that there are other reasons why the expectations for laser surgery vary from person to person.

"People who are slow healers or who have ongoing medical conditions [such as glaucoma or diabetes] are not good candidates for laser surgery," she says. "That's why it's so important for patients to undergo a thorough examination with their doctor."

Poor candidates for this surgery also include those with uncontrolled vascular disease, autoimmune disease, or people with certain eye diseases involving the cornea or retina. Pregnant women should not have refractive surgery of any kind because the refraction of the eye may change during pregnancy.

Looking Ahead

At present, a number of other lasers for eye surgery are currently being tested in FDA-sanctioned studies to determine their safety and effectiveness.

Investigational Device Exemptions (IDEs) filed with FDA allow for clinical studies involving the excimer laser and the correction of far-sightedness. The IDE process is designed to investigate the safety and effectiveness of a device, or a new procedure with an already approved device, either to obtain information for publication or to generate the data needed to obtain marketing approval from FDA.

"If the refractive surgery center says the laser is approved by FDA, it probably is," Waxler concludes. "Still, it is wise for consumers to check that the device being used for their surgery is FDA-approved," he says, or that they make sure they are being treated with a laser that is under study in an FDA-sanctioned clinical trial.

During the first few weeks immediately following laser surgery, Goldstein says, "Every week I kept thinking, 'this is as good as it gets'?" Then, she discovered by the sixth week, as predicted by her surgeon, that her eyesight was noticeably better and eventually stabilized.

"I would tell others to be patient about their expected outcome," she advises. "Even though with LASIK you can expect quicker results, I'm happy with the choice of PRK."

Are You a Candidate for Laser Eye Surgery?

You may be a good candidate for laser eye surgery if you:

- are at least 21 years of age for a Summit laser or 18 years of age for a VISX laser, since the eyes are still growing to this point

- have healthy eyes that are free from retinal problems, corneal scars, and any eye disease (refractive errors are considered eye disorders, not diseases)

- have mild to moderate myopia (nearsightedness) within the range of treatment (see your doctor to determine your range)

- have a way to pay for the treatment since laser procedures are costly and probably not covered by health insurance policies

131

- are fully informed about the risks and benefits of laser surgery compared with other available treatments.

Frequently Asked Questions about Laser Eye Surgery

Is It Painful?

There is little if any discomfort during surgery because the cornea and eye are anesthetized by drops. Some patients experience a scratchy feeling. After the anesthetic wears off, the amount of discomfort varies with each individual, but any irritation is minor and usually disappears within a few hours. You may be sensitive to light for a few days.

When Will I Be Able to Return to Work?

Most people can return to work one to three days following surgery, but a rule of thumb is to wait until you feel up to it. Most return to normal activities as soon as the day after surgery.

What Are the Side Effects and Risks?

The most common side effects are a halo effect and some glare at night around lights.

How Long Does the Treatment Take?

Laser treatment itself takes only about 15 to 40 seconds, based on the degree of correction necessary. Recovery is minimal, and usually the patient is able to be driven home after about 30 minutes. Typically, you will notice improved sight in 3 to 5 days following treatment.

Is the Treatment Permanent?

According to the results of the U.S. clinical trials and results reported internationally, the treatment appears to be permanent. As people age, however, their eyes change and retreatment may be necessary.

Are There Any Activity Restrictions Following Surgery?

Following surgery, do not rub your eyes. Other than that, patients can do whatever they feel up to as long as they follow their doctors' instructions.

What If I Move My Head during Surgery?

This is the number one question that patients ask when undergoing laser treatment. The surgeon is skilled in the technique of removing his foot from the pedal that controls the ultraviolet beam as soon as a patient moves his or her head. This allows him to realign the beam with the corneal target and proceed with the surgery.

The Insight on Eyesight

In order to decide whether laser vision correction is a viable option for you, it is important to first understand how the eye works and why people need glasses or contact lenses to see well.

The eye works much like a camera; its primary function is to focus light. For the eye to see, light rays must be bent or refracted to meet at a single point through the cornea, the clear window at the front of the eye that provides most of the focusing power. Light then travels through the lens, where it is fine-tuned to focus properly on the retina, the nerve layer that lines the back of the eye and connects to the brain. The retina acts like the film in a camera, and clear vision is achieved only if light from an object is precisely focused onto it. If the light focuses either in front of or behind the retina, the image you see is blurred. A refractive error means that the shape of eye structures does not properly bend the light for focusing.

Having 20/20 vision means seeing at 20 feet what a normal person sees at 20 feet. However, if vision is measured at 20/40, it means a person has to walk up to 20 feet to see the same size letter that someone with 20/20 vision could see at 40 feet. And so on. People whose best-corrected visual acuity (what they see using glasses or contact lenses) is less than 20/200 in the better eye are considered legally blind, even though they still have enough vision to get around. Prior to laser surgery, Jeri Goldstein's visual acuity without her contact lenses was measured at 20/400 in her right eye and 20/200 in the left eye. Following surgery, her eyesight without contacts stands at 20/25 and 20/20, respectively.

What Are the Risks of Laser Surgery?

The risks outlined below apply to both PRK and LASIK procedures. The chances of having a serious vision-threatening complication are minimal, and there have been no reported cases of blindness following either PRK or LASIK, says James Salz, M.D., clinical professor of ophthalmology. However, FDA is aware of a few instances of severe eye injury requiring corneal transplant.

- **Infection and delayed healing**: There is about a 0.1 percent chance of the cornea becoming infected after PRK, and a somewhat smaller chance after LASIK. Generally, this means added discomfort and a delay in healing, with no long-term effects within a period of four years.

- **Undercorrection/Overcorrection**: It is not possible to predict perfectly how your eye will respond to laser surgery. As a result, you may still need corrective lenses after the procedure to obtain good vision. In some cases, a second procedure can be done to improve the result.

- **Decrease in Best-Corrected Vision**: After refractive surgery, some patients find that their best obtainable vision with corrective lenses is worse than it was before the surgery. This can occur as a result of irregular tissue removal or the development of corneal haze.

- **Excessive Corneal Haze**: Corneal haze occurs as part of the normal healing process after PRK. In most cases, it has little or no effect on the final vision and can only be seen by an eye doctor with a microscope. However, there are some cases of excessive haze that interferes with vision. As with undercorrections, this can often be dealt with by means of an additional laser treatment. The risk of significant haze is much less with LASIK than with PRK.

- **Regression**: In some patients the effect of refractive surgery is gradually lost over several months. This is like an undercorrection, and a retreatment is often feasible.

- **Halo Effect**: The halo effect is an optical effect that is noticed in dim light. As the pupil enlarges, a second faded image is produced by the untreated peripheral cornea. For some patients who have undergone PRK or LASIK, this effect can interfere with night driving.

- **Flap Damage or Loss (LASIK only)**: Instead of creating a hinged flap of tissue on the central cornea, the entire flap could come off. If this were to occur it could be replaced after the laser treatment. However, there is a risk that the flap could be damaged or lost.

- **Distorted Flap (LASIK only)**: Irregular healing of the corneal flap could create a distorted corneal shape, resulting in a decrease of best-corrected vision.

- **Incomplete Procedure**: Equipment malfunction may require the procedure to be stopped before completion. This is a more significant factor in LASIK, with its higher degree of complexity, than in PRK.

- **Problems with a Perfect Procedure:** Even when everything goes perfectly, there are effects that might cause some dissatisfaction. Older patients should be aware that they can't have both good distance vision and good near vision in the same eye without corrective lenses. Some myopic patients rely on their myopia (by taking off their glasses, or by wearing a weaker prescription) to allow them to read. Such a patient may need reading glasses after the myopia is surgically corrected. Another consideration is the delay between eye treatments. If one eye is being done at a time, then the eyes may not work well together during the time between treatments. If a contact lens is not tolerated on the unoperated eye, work and driving may be awkward or impossible until the second eye has been treated.

Carol Lewis is a staff writer for *FDA Consumer*.

Chapter 14

Laser-Assisted in Situ Keratomileusis (LASIK) Surgery

Chapter Contents

Section 14.1

What Is LASIK?

This section is excerpted from the Center for Devices and Radiological Health, U.S. Food and Drug Administration, 2000, updated May 2002.

LASIK is a surgical procedure intended to reduce a person's dependency on glasses or contact lenses. The goal of this chapter is to provide objective information to the public about LASIK surgery. See other sections to learn about what you should know before surgery, what will happen during the surgery, and what you should expect after surgery. There is a checklist of issues for you to consider, practices to follow, and questions to ask your doctor before undergoing LASIK surgery.

LASIK stands for laser-assisted in situ keratomileusis and is a procedure that permanently changes the shape of the cornea, the clear covering of the front of the eye, using an excimer laser. A knife, called a microkeratome, is used to cut a flap in the cornea. A hinge is left at one end of this flap. The flap is folded back revealing the stroma, the middle section of the cornea. Pulses from a computer-controlled laser vaporize a portion of the stroma and the flap is replaced.

The Eye and Vision Errors

The cornea is a part of the eye that helps focus light to create an image on the retina. It works in much the same way that the lens of a camera focuses light to create an image on film. The bending and focusing of light is also known as refraction. Usually the shape of the cornea and the eye are not perfect and the image on the retina is out-of-focus (blurred) or distorted. These imperfections in the focusing power of the eye are called refractive errors. There are three primary types of refractive errors: myopia, hyperopia and astigmatism. Persons with myopia, or nearsightedness, have more difficulty seeing distant objects as clearly as near objects. Persons with hyperopia, or farsightedness, have more difficulty seeing near objects as clearly as distant objects. Astigmatism is a distortion of the image on the retina caused by irregularities in the cornea or lens of the eye. Combinations of myopia and astigmatism or hyperopia and astigmatism are common. Glasses or contact lenses are designed to compensate for the eye's imperfections. Surgical procedures aimed at improving the focusing power of the eye are called refractive surgery. In LASIK surgery, precise and controlled removal of corneal tissue by a special laser reshapes the cornea changing its focusing power.

Other Types of Refractive Surgery

Radial keratotomy or RK and photorefractive keratectomy or PRK are other refractive surgeries used to reshape the cornea. In RK, a very sharp knife is used to cut slits in the cornea changing its shape. PRK was the first surgical procedure developed to reshape the cornea, by sculpting, using a laser. Later, LASIK was developed. The same type of laser is used for LASIK and PRK. Often the exact same laser is used for the two types of surgery. The major difference between the two surgeries is the way that the stroma, the middle layer of the cornea, is exposed before it is vaporized with the laser. In PRK, the top layer of the cornea, called the epithelium, is scraped away to expose the stromal layer underneath. In LASIK, a flap is cut in the stromal layer and the flap is folded back.

Another type of refractive surgery is thermokeratoplasty in which heat is used to reshape the cornea. The source of the heat can be a laser, but it is a different kind of laser than is used for LASIK and PRK. Other refractive devices include corneal ring segments that are inserted into the stroma and special contact lenses that temporarily reshape the cornea (orthokeratology).

What the FDA Regulates

In the United States, the Food and Drug Administration (FDA) regulates the sale of medical devices such as the lasers used for LASIK. Before a medical device can be legally sold in the United States, the person or company that wants to sell the device must seek approval from the FDA. To gain approval, they must present evidence that the device is reasonably safe and effective for a particular use— the indication. Once the FDA has approved a medical device, a doctor may decide to use that device for other indications if the doctor feels it is in the best interest of a patient. The use of an approved device for other than its FDA-approved indication is called "off-label use." The FDA does not regulate the practice of medicine.

The FDA does not have the authority to:

- Regulate a doctor's practice. In other words, FDA does not tell doctors what to do when running their business or what they can or cannot tell their patients.

- Set the amount a doctor can charge for LASIK eye surgery.

- Insist the patient information booklet from the laser manufacturer be provided to the potential patient.

- Make recommendations for individual doctors, clinics, or eye centers. FDA does not maintain nor have access to any such list of doctors performing LASIK eye surgery.

- Conduct or provide a rating system on any medical device it regulates.

The first refractive laser systems approved by FDA were excimer lasers for use in PRK to treat myopia and later to treat astigmatism. However, doctors began using these lasers for LASIK (not just PRK), and to treat other refractive errors (not just myopia). Over the last several years, LASIK has become the main surgery doctors use to treat myopia in the United States. More recently, some laser manufacturers have gained FDA approval for laser systems for LASIK to treat myopia, hyperopia, and astigmatism and for PRK to treat hyperopia and astigmatism.

Section 14.2

When Is LASIK Not for Me?

This section is excerpted from the Center for Devices and Radiological Health, U.S. Food and Drug Administration, 2000, updated May 2002.

You are probably **not** a good candidate for refractive surgery if:

*   You are not a risk taker. Certain complications are unavoidable in a percentage of patients, and there are no long-term data available for current procedures.

*   It will jeopardize your career. Some jobs prohibit certain refractive procedures. Be sure to check with your employer/professional society/military service before undergoing any procedure.

*   Cost is an issue. Most medical insurance will not pay for refractive surgery. Although the cost is coming down, it is still significant.

*   You required a change in your contact lens or glasses prescription in the past year. This is called refractive instability. Patients who are in their early 20s or younger, whose hormones are fluctuating due to disease such as diabetes, who are pregnant or breastfeeding, or who are taking medications that may cause fluctuations in vision are more likely to have refractive instability and should discuss the possible additional risks with their doctor.

*   You have a disease or are on medications that may affect wound healing. Certain conditions, such as autoimmune diseases (e.g., lupus, rheumatoid arthritis), immunodeficiency states (e.g., HIV) and diabetes, and some medications (e.g., retinoic acid and steroids) may prevent proper healing after a refractive procedure.

*   You actively participate in contact sports. You participate in boxing, wrestling, martial arts or other activities in which blows to the face and eyes are a normal occurrence.

141

- You are not an adult. Currently, no lasers are approved for LASIK on persons under the age of 18.

Precautions

The safety and effectiveness of refractive procedures has not been determined in patients with some diseases. Do **not** have LASIK surgery if you have a history of any of the following:

- Herpes simplex or Herpes zoster (shingles) involving the eye area

- Glaucoma, glaucoma suspect, or ocular hypertension

- Eye diseases, such as uveitis/iritis (inflammations of the eye) and blepharitis (inflammation of the eyelids with crusting of the eyelashes)

- Eye injuries or previous eye surgeries

- Keratoconus

Other Risk Factors

Your doctor should screen you for the following conditions or indicators of risk:

- Large pupils: Make sure this evaluation is done in a dark room. Younger patients and patients on certain medications may be prone to having large pupils under dim lighting conditions. This can cause symptoms such as glare, halos, starbursts, and ghost images (double vision) after surgery. In some patients these symptoms may be debilitating. For example, a patient may no longer be able to drive a car at night or in certain weather conditions, such as fog.

- Thin corneas: The cornea is the thin clear covering of the eye that is over the iris, the colored part of the eye. Most refractive procedures change the eye's focusing power by reshaping the cornea (for example, by removing tissue). Performing a refractive procedure on a cornea that is too thin may result in blinding complications.

- Previous refractive surgery (e.g., RK, PRK, LASIK): Additional refractive surgery may not be recommended. The decision to have additional refractive surgery must be made in consultation with your doctor after careful consideration of your unique situation.

- Dry eyes: LASIK surgery tends to aggravate this condition.

Section 14.3

What Are the Risks and How Can I Find the Right Doctor for Me?

This section is excerpted from the Center for Devices and Radiological Health, U.S. Food and Drug Administration, 2000, updated May 2002.

Most patients are very pleased with the results of their refractive surgery. However, like any other medical procedure, there are risks involved. That's why it is important for you to understand the limitations and possible complications of refractive surgery.

Before undergoing a refractive procedure, you should carefully weigh the risks and benefits based on your own personal value system, and try to avoid being influenced by friends that have had the procedure or doctors encouraging you to do so.

What Are the Risks?

You may be undertreated or overtreated. Only a certain percent of patients achieve 20/20 vision without glasses or contacts. You may require additional treatment, but additional treatment may not be possible. You may still need glasses or contact lenses after surgery. This may be true even if you only required a very weak prescription before surgery. If you used reading glasses before surgery, you may still need reading glasses after surgery.

Results are generally not as good in patients with very large refractive errors of any type. You should discuss your expectations with your doctor and realize that you may still require glasses or contacts after the surgery.

Results may not be lasting. The level of improved vision you experience after surgery may be temporary, especially if you are farsighted or currently need reading glasses. It is especially important for farsighted individuals to have a cycloplegic refraction (a vision exam with lenses after dilating drops) as part of the screening process.

Patients whose manifest refraction (a vision exam with lenses before dilating drops) is very different from their cycloplegic refraction are more likely to have temporary results.

Some patients lose vision. Some patients lose lines of vision on the vision chart that cannot be corrected with glasses, contact lenses, or surgery as a result of treatment. Even with good vision on the vision chart, some patients do not see as well in situations of low contrast, such as at night or in fog, after treatment as compared to before treatment. Some patients experience glare, halos, and double vision that can seriously affect nighttime vision. It is important for you to know that not all eye centers test contrast sensitivity, and that when it is tested, it should be done in a dark room.

Some patients may develop severe dry eye syndrome. As a result of surgery, your eye may not be able to produce enough tears to keep the eye moist and comfortable. This condition may be permanent. Intensive drop therapy and the use of plugs or other procedures may be required.

Additional Risks If You Are Considering the Following

Monovision

Monovision is one clinical technique used to deal with the correction of presbyopia, the gradual loss of the ability of the eye to change focus for close-up tasks that progresses with age. The intent of monovision is for the presbyopic patient to use one eye for distance viewing and one eye for near viewing. This practice was first applied to fit contact lens wearers and more recently to LASIK and other refractive surgeries. With contact lenses, a presbyopic patient has one eye fit with a contact lens to correct distance vision, and the other eye fit with a contact lens to correct near vision. In the same way, with LASIK, a presbyopic patient has one eye operated on to correct the distance vision, and the other operated on to correct the near vision. In other words, the goal of the surgery is for one eye to have vision worse than 20/20, the commonly referred to goal for LASIK surgical correction of distance vision. Since one eye is corrected for distance viewing and the other eye is corrected for near viewing, the two eyes no longer work together. This results in poorer quality vision and a decrease in depth perception. These effects of monovision are most noticeable in low lighting conditions and when performing tasks requiring very sharp vision. Therefore, you may need to wear glasses or contact lenses to fully correct both eyes for distance or near when performing visually demanding tasks, such as driving at night, operating dangerous equipment, or performing occupational tasks requiring very sharp close vision (e.g., reading small print for long periods of time).

Many patients cannot get used to having one eye blurred at all times. Therefore, if you are considering monovision with LASIK, make sure you go through a trial period with contact lenses to see if you can tolerate monovision, before having the surgery performed on your eyes. Find out if you pass your state's driver's license requirements with monovision.

In addition, you should consider how much your presbyopia is expected to increase in the future. Ask your doctor when you should expect the results of your monovision surgery to no longer be enough for you to see near-by objects clearly without the aid of glasses or contacts, or when a second surgery might be required to further correct your near vision.

Bilateral Simultaneous Treatment

You may choose to have LASIK surgery on both eyes at the same time or to have surgery on one eye at a time. Although the convenience of having surgery on both eyes on the same day is attractive, this practice is riskier than having two separate surgeries. The second eye may have a higher risk of developing an inflammation if surgery is done on the same day than if surgery is performed on separate days. If a malfunction of the laser or microkeratome occurs causing a complication with the first eye, the second eye is more likely to also experience the same complication if the surgery is performed on the same day rather than on separate days.

If you decide to have one eye done at a time, you and your doctor will decide how long to wait before having surgery on the other eye. If both eyes are treated at the same time or before one eye has a chance to fully heal, you and your doctor do not have the advantage of being able to see how the first eye responds to surgery before the second eye is treated.

Another disadvantage to having surgery on both eyes at the same time is that the vision in both eyes may be blurred after surgery until the initial healing process is over, rather than being able to rely on clear vision in at least one eye at all times.

Finding the Right Doctor

If you are considering refractive surgery, make sure you:

- Compare. The levels of risk and benefit vary slightly not only from procedure to procedure, but from device to device depending on the manufacturer, and from surgeon to surgeon depending on their level of experience with a particular procedure.

- Don't base your decision simply on cost and don't settle for the first eye center, doctor, or procedure you investigate. Remember that the decisions you make about your eyes and refractive surgery will affect you for the rest of your life.

- Be wary of eye centers that advertise 20/20 vision or your money back or package deals. There are never any guarantees in medicine.

- Read. It is important for you to read the patient handbook provided to your doctor by the manufacturer of the device used to perform the refractive procedure. Your doctor should provide you with this handbook and be willing to discuss his/her outcomes (successes as well as complications) compared to the results of studies outlined in the handbook.

Even the best screened patients under the care of most skilled surgeons can experience serious complications.

- During surgery. Malfunction of a device or other error, such as cutting a flap of cornea through and through instead of making a hinge during LASIK surgery, may lead to discontinuation of the procedure or irreversible damage to the eye.

- After surgery. Some complications, such as migration of the flap, inflammation, or infection, may require another procedure and/ or intensive treatment with drops. Even with aggressive therapy, such complications may lead to temporary loss of vision or even irreversible blindness.

Under the care of an experienced doctor, carefully screened candidates with reasonable expectations and a clear understanding of the risks and alternatives are likely to be happy with the results of their refractive procedure.

Advertising

.   Be cautious about slick advertising and/or deals that sound too good to be true. Remember, they usually are. There is a lot of competition resulting in a great deal of advertising and bidding for your business. Do your homework.

Section 14.4

What Should I Expect before, during, and after Surgery?

This section is excerpted from the Center for Devices and Radiological Health, U.S. Food and Drug Administration, 2000, updated May 2002.

What to expect before, during, and after surgery will vary from doctor to doctor and patient to patient. This chapter is a compilation of patient information developed by manufacturers and healthcare professionals, but cannot replace the dialogue you should have with your doctor. Read this information carefully and with the checklist, discuss your expectations with your doctor.

Before Surgery

If you decide to go ahead with LASIK surgery, you will need an initial or baseline evaluation by your eye doctor to determine if you are a good candidate. This is what you need to know to prepare for the exam and what you should expect:

If you wear contact lenses, it is a good idea to stop wearing them before your baseline evaluation and switch to wearing your glasses full-time. Contact lenses change the shape of your cornea for up to several weeks after you have stopped using them depending on the

147

type of contact lenses you wear. Not leaving your contact lenses out long enough for your cornea to assume its natural shape before surgery can have negative consequences. These consequences include inaccurate measurements and a poor surgical plan, resulting in poor vision after surgery. These measurements, which determine how much corneal tissue to remove, may need to be repeated at least a week after your initial evaluation and before surgery to make sure they have not changed, especially if you wear RGP or hard lenses. If you wear:

- soft contact lenses, you should stop wearing them for 2 weeks before your initial evaluation.

- toric soft lenses or rigid gas permeable (RGP) lenses, you should stop wearing them for at least 3 weeks before your initial evaluation.

- hard lenses, you should stop wearing them for at least 4 weeks before your initial evaluation.

You should tell your doctor:

- about your past and present medical and eye conditions

- about all the medications you are taking, including over-the-counter medications and any medications you may be allergic to

Your doctor should perform a thorough eye exam and discuss:

- whether you are a good candidate

- what the risks, benefits, and alternatives of the surgery are

- what you should expect before, during, and after surgery

- what your responsibilities will be before, during, and after surgery

You should have the opportunity to ask your doctor questions during this discussion. Give yourself plenty of time to think about the risk/benefit discussion, to review any informational literature provided by your doctor, and to have any additional questions answered by your doctor before deciding to go through with surgery and before signing the informed consent form.

You should not feel pressured by your doctor, family, friends, or anyone else to make a decision about having surgery. Carefully consider the pros and cons.

The day before surgery, you should stop using:

- creams
- lotions
- makeup
- perfumes

These products as well as debris along the eyelashes may increase the risk of infection during and after surgery. Your doctor may ask you to scrub your eyelashes for a period of time before surgery to get rid of residues and debris along the lashes.

Also before surgery, arrange for transportation to and from your surgery and your first follow-up visit. On the day of surgery, your doctor may give you some medicine to make you relax. Because this medicine impairs your ability to drive and because your vision may be blurry, even if you don't drive make sure someone can bring you home after surgery.

During Surgery

The surgery should take less than 30 minutes. You will lie on your back in a reclining chair in an exam room containing the laser system. The laser system includes a large machine with a microscope attached to it and a computer screen.

A numbing drop will be placed in your eye, the area around your eye will be cleaned, and an instrument called a lid speculum will be used to hold your eyelids open. A ring will be placed on your eye and very high pressures will be applied to create suction to the cornea. Your vision will dim while the suction ring is on and you may feel the pressure and experience some discomfort during this part of the procedure. The microkeratome, a cutting instrument, is attached to the suction ring. Your doctor will use the blade of the microkeratome to cut a flap in your cornea.

The microkeratome and the suction ring are then removed. You will be able to see, but you will experience fluctuating degrees of blurred vision during the rest of the procedure. The doctor will then lift the flap and fold it back on its hinge, and dry the exposed tissue.

The laser will be positioned over your eye and you will be asked to stare at a light. This is not the laser used to remove tissue from the cornea. This light is to help you keep your eye fixed on one spot once the laser comes on. NOTE: If you cannot stare at a fixed object for at least 60 seconds, you may not be a good candidate for this surgery.

When your eye is in the correct position, your doctor will start the laser. At this point in the surgery, you may become aware of new sounds and smells. The pulse of the laser makes a ticking sound. As the laser removes corneal tissue, some people have reported a smell similar to burning hair. A computer controls the amount of laser delivered to your eye. Before the start of surgery, your doctor will have programmed the computer to vaporize a particular amount of tissue based on the measurements taken at your initial evaluation. After the pulses of laser energy vaporize the corneal tissue, the flap is put back into position.

A shield should be placed over your eye at the end of the procedure as protection, since no stitches are used to hold the flap in place. It is important for you to wear this shield to prevent you from rubbing your eye and putting pressure on your eye while you sleep, and to protect your eye from accidentally being hit or poked until the flap has healed.

After Surgery

Immediately after the procedure, your eye may burn, itch, or feel like there is something in it. You may experience some discomfort, or in some cases, mild pain and your doctor may suggest you take a mild pain reliever. Both your eyes may tear or water. Your vision will probably be hazy or blurry. You will instinctively want to rub your eye, but don't! Rubbing your eye could dislodge the flap, requiring further treatment. In addition, you may experience sensitivity to light, glare, starbursts or haloes around lights, or the whites of your eye may look red or bloodshot. These symptoms should improve considerably within the first few days after surgery. You should plan on taking a few days off from work until these symptoms subside. You should contact your doctor immediately and not wait for your scheduled visit, if you experience severe pain, or if your vision or other symptoms get worse instead of better.

You should see your doctor within the first 24 to 48 hours after surgery and at regular intervals after that for at least the first six months. At the first postoperative visit, your doctor will remove the eye shield, test your vision, and examine your eye. Your doctor may give you one or more types of eye drops to take at home to help prevent infection and/or inflammation. You may also be advised to use artificial tears to help lubricate the eye. Do not resume wearing a contact lens in the operated eye, even if your vision is blurry.

You should wait one to three days following surgery before beginning any non-contact sports, depending on the amount of activity required, how you feel, and your doctor's instructions.

To help prevent infection, you may need to wait for up to two weeks after surgery or until your doctor advises you otherwise before using lotions, creams, or make-up around the eye. Your doctor may advise you to continue scrubbing your eyelashes for a period of time after surgery. You should also avoid swimming and using hot tubs or whirlpools for 1 to 2 months.

Strenuous contact sports such as boxing, football, karate, etc. should not be attempted for at least four weeks after surgery. It is important to protect your eyes from anything that might get in them and from being hit or bumped.

During the first few months after surgery, your vision may fluctuate.

- It may take up to three to six months for your vision to stabilize after surgery.

- Glare, haloes, difficulty driving at night, and other visual symptoms may also persist during this stabilization period. If further correction or enhancement is necessary, you should wait until your eye measurements are consistent for two consecutive visits at least 3 months apart before re-operation.

- It is important to realize that although distance vision may improve after re-operation, it is unlikely that other visual symptoms such as glare or haloes will improve.

- It is also important to note that no laser company has presented enough evidence for the FDA to make conclusions about the safety or effectiveness of enhancement surgery.

Contact your eye doctor immediately, if you develop any new, unusual or worsening symptoms at any point after surgery. Such symptoms could signal a problem that, if not treated early enough, may lead to a loss of vision.

Section 14.5

LASIK Surgery Checklist

This section is excerpted from the Center for Devices and Radiological Health, U.S. Food and Drug Administration, 2000, updated May 2002.

Know What Makes You a Poor Candidate

- Career impact—does your job prohibit refractive surgery?

- Cost—can you really afford this procedure?

- Medical conditions—e.g., do you have an autoimmune disease or other major illness? Do you have a chronic illness that might slow or alter healing?

- Eye conditions—do you have or have you ever had any problems with your eyes other than needing glasses or contacts?

- Medications—do you take steroids or other drugs that might prevent healing?

- Stable refraction—has your prescription changed in the last year?

- High or low refractive error—do you use glasses/contacts only some of the time? Do you need an unusually strong prescription?

- Pupil size—are your pupils extra large in dim conditions?

- Corneal thickness—do you have thin corneas?

Know All the Risks and Procedure Limitations

- Overtreatment or undertreatment—are you willing and able to have more than one surgery to get the desired result?

- May still need reading glasses—do you have presbyopia?

- Results may not be lasting—do you think this is the last correction you will ever need? Do you realize that long-term results are not known?

- May permanently lose vision—do you know some patients may lose some vision or experience blindness?

- Development of visual symptoms—do you know about glare, halos, starbursts, etc. and that night driving might be difficult?

- Contrast sensitivity—do you know your vision could be significantly reduced in dim light conditions?

- Bilateral treatment—do you know the additional risks of having both eyes treated at the same time?

- Patient information—have you read the patient information booklet about the laser being used for your procedure?

Know How to Find the Right Doctor

- Experienced—how many eyes has your doctor performed LASIK surgery on with the same laser?

- Equipment—does your doctor use an FDA-approved laser for the procedure you need?

- Informative—is your doctor willing to spend the time to answer all your questions?

- Long-term care—does your doctor encourage follow-up and management of you as a patient? Your preop and postop care may be provided by a doctor other than the surgeon.

- Be comfortable—do you feel you know your doctor and are comfortable with an equal exchange of information?

Know Preoperative, Operative, and Postoperative Expectations

- No contact lenses prior to evaluation and surgery—can you go for an extended period of time without wearing contact lenses?

- Have a thorough exam—have you arranged not to drive or work after the exam?

- Read and understand the informed consent—has your doctor given you an informed consent form to take home and answered all your questions?

- No makeup before surgery—can you go 24 to 36 hours without makeup prior to surgery?

- Arrange for transportation—can someone drive you home after surgery?

- Plan to take a few days to recover—can you take time off to take it easy for a couple of days if necessary?

- Expect not to see clearly for a few days—do you know you will not see clearly immediately?

- Know sights, smells, sounds of surgery—has your doctor made you feel comfortable with the actual steps of the procedure?

- Be prepared to take drops/medications—are you willing and able to put drops in your eyes at regular intervals?

- Be prepared to wear an eye shield—do you know you need to protect the eye for a period of time after surgery to avoid injury?

- Expect some pain/discomfort—do you know how much pain to expect?

- Know when to seek help—do you understand what problems could occur and when to seek medical intervention?

- Know when to expect your vision to stop changing—are you aware that final results could take months?

- Make sure your refraction is stable before any further surgery—if you don't get the desired result, do you know not to have an enhancement until the prescription stops changing?

Section 14.6

FDA-Approved Lasers

This section is excerpted from the Center for Devices and Radiological Health, U.S. Food and Drug Administration, 2000, updated May 2002.

Information about FDA-approved lasers for LASIK eye surgery is given in Tables 14.1 and 14.2. The tables list lasers by company and model and provide facts about the approval date and indications. Table 14.1 includes lasers approved for LASIK eye surgery; Table 14.2 provides information about lasers approved for PRK and other eye surgeries.

Table 14.1. LASIK Eye Surgery: FDA-Approved Lasers (continued on page 156)

Company and model	Approval number and date	Approved indications (D = diopters)
Autonomous Technology —LADARVision	P970043/S5 (5/9/00)	Myopia less than -9.0D with or without astigmatism from -0.5 to -3.0D
Bausch & Lomb Surgical —Technolas 217a	P990027 (2/23/00)	Myopia from -1.0 to -7.0D with or without astigmatism less than -3.0D
Bausch & Lomb Surgical —Technolas 217a	P990027/S2 (5/15/02)	Myopia less than -11D with or without astigmatism less than -3.0D
Dishler	P970049 (12/16/99)	Myopia from -0.5 to -13.0D with or without astigmatism between -0.5 to -4.0D
Kremer	P970005 (7/30/98)	Myopia from -1.0 to -15.0D with or without astigmatism up to -5.0D

Table 14.1. LASIK Eye Surgery: FDA-Approved Lasers (continued from page 155)

Company and model	Approval number and date	Approved indications (D = diopters)
LaserSight —LaserScan LSX	P980008/S5 (9/28/01)	Myopia from -0.5 to -6.0D with or without astigmatism up to 4.5D
Nidek—EC5000	P970053/S2 (4/14/00)	Myopia from -1.0 to -14.0D with or without astigmatism less than 4.0D
Summit—Apex Plus	P930034/S13 (10/21/99)	Myopia less than -14.0D with or without astigmatism from 0.5 to 5.0D
Summit Autonomous —LADARVision	P970043/S7 (9/22/00)	Hyperopia less than 6.0D with or without astigmatism less than -6.0D
VISX—Star S2 & S3	P930016/S12 (4/27/01)	Hyperopia between +0.5 and +5.0D with or without astigmatism up to +3.0D
VISX—Star S2 & S3	P930016/S14 (11/16/01)	Mixed astigmatism up to 6.0D; cylinder is greater than sphere and of opposite sign
VISX—Star S2	P990010 (11/19/99)	Myopia less than -14.0D with or without astigmatism between -0.5 and -5.0D
VISX—Star S3 (EyeTracker)	P990010/S1 (4/20/00)	Same as S2, except with eye tracker

Table 14.2. FDA-Approved Lasers for PRK and Other Refractive Surgeries (continued on page 158)

Company and model	Approval number and date	Approved indications (D = diopters)
Autonomous Technology —LADARVision	P970043 (11/2/98)	PRK; Myopia from -1.0 to -10.0D with or with out astigmatism less than -4.0D
Bausch & Lomb Surgical —KERACOR 116	P970056 (9/28/99)	PRK; Myopia from -1.5 to -7.0D with or without astigmatism less than -4.5D
LaserSight— LaserScan LSX	P980008 (11/12/99)	PRK; Myopia from -1.0 to -6.0D with or without astigmatism less than 1.0D
Nidek—EC5000	P970053 (12/17/98)	PRK; Myopia from -0.75 to -13.0D
Nidek—EC5000	P970053/S1 (9/29/99)	PRK; Myopia from -1.0 to -8.0D with or without astigmatism from -0.5 to -4.0D
Summit—Apex & Apex Plus	P930034 (10/25/95)	PRK; Myopia from -1.5 to -7.0D
Summit—Apex Plus	P930034/S9 (3/11/98)	PRK; Myopia from -1.0 to -6.0D with or without astigmatism from -1.0 to -4.0D
Summit—Apex Plus	P930034/S12 (10/21/99)	PRK; Hyperopia from +1.5 to +4.0D with or without astigmatism less than -1.0D
Summit Autonomous —LADARVision	P970043/S8 (7/11/00)	Name Change Only

Table 14.2. FDA-Approved Lasers for PRK and Other Refractive Surgeries (continued from page 157)

Company and model	Approval number and date	Approved indications (D = diopters)
Sunrise—Hyperion	P990078 (6/30/00)	Laser Thermokerato-plasty (LTK); Hyperopia from +0.75 to +2.5D with or without astigmatism less than 0.75D
VISX—Model B & C (Star & Star S2)	P930016 (3/27/96)	PRK; Myopia from 0 to -6.0D
VISX—Model B & C (Star & Star S2)	P930016/S3 (4/24/97)	PRK; Myopia from 0 to -6.0D with or without astigmatism from -0.75 to -4.0D
VISX—Model B & C (Star & Star S2)	P930016/S5 (1/29/98)	PRK; Myopia from 0 to -12.0D with or without astigmatism from 0 to -4.0D
VISX—Star S2	P930016/S7 (11/2/98)	PRK; Hyperopia from +1.0 to +6.0D
VISX—Star S2 & S3	P930016/S10 (10/18/00)	PRK; Hyperopia from +0.5 to +5.0D with or without astigmatism +0.5 to +4.0D
VISX—Star S2 & S3	P930016/S13 (3/19/01)	Add myopia blend zone; increase overall ablation zone from 6.5 to 8.0mm

Chapter 15

Laser Epithelial Keratomileusis (LASEK) Surgery

A slight variation on the traditional LASIK procedure is becoming available, LASEK [laser epithelial keratomileusis]. This procedure may be an option for patients who are not good candidates for the traditional procedure.

LASEK is a relatively new surgery that utilizes a trephine to create an epithelial flap (as opposed to a deeper stromal flap with LASIK) and an alcohol solution to preserve the epithelial cells. Once the epithelial flap is created and lifted, the treatment proceeds as for traditional PRK, with light smoothing at its conclusion. Then, the epithelial flap is repositioned with a small spatula.

LASEK preserves more corneal tissue, on average, than a typical LASIK procedure. Therefore, for patients who have thin corneas, LASEK may offer a safer alternative than LASIK.

Several small peer-reviewed studies have recently been published about the LASEK procedure.[1-5] All have concluded that this technique has the potential for use within the clinical practice, noting patients achieved results similar to those achieved with LASIK or PRK. All also noted that additional long-term studies were needed to confirm these early results. As more ophthalmologists are trained in the procedure and offer this technique as an alternative to patients, we expect to see more studies collaborating these initial results.

The FDA [U.S. Food and Drug Administration] approves drugs and devices, not specific surgeries. However, the FDA evaluates the safety and efficacy of a device within the context of studies that have been done on a particular procedure, like PRK or LASIK.

On those lasers that have earned approval based on PRK or LASIK data, LASEK is permitted as a practice of medicine. The use of devices during a procedure deemed a practice-of-medicine is called an off label use of these devices. Because the approved lasers and trephines have proven safe and effective in other procedures, ophthalmologists may use them off-label if they feel it is in their patients' best interest to do so.

We have listed below a few more questions for your doctor that will be of assistance if you are considering LASEK.

- What training have you received on this particular surgical procedure?

- What should my expectations be for healing at one day? one week? one month?

- Are there any quality of vision issues I need to understand? (risk of glare/halos, decreased contrast sensitivity, etc.)

- What complications are associated with this procedure? How are they different from those of LASIK or PRK?

- What about my eyes makes me a good candidate for LASEK?

- What is the advantage of this procedure over LASIK for me?

As always, there are no right or wrong answers to these questions; however, the answers should be of assistance in your evaluation.

The US FDA LASIK website provides a checklist for prospective refractive surgery patients. You should carefully review those questions. We suggest you review that list and ask yourself the following:

- Are the risks associated with the surgery worth the potential benefit derived from the surgery?

- Am I generally a risk taker?

- Do I generally adopt new technology early on, before others, or do I wait until it is more mainstream?

In sum, LASEK may offer patients with thin corneas a viable option to preserve more corneal tissue. However, the LASEK procedure is relatively new and is an off-label use of the excimer laser. Patients should be sure to discuss this option fully with their ophthalmologist.

References

1. Claringbold TV 2nd. Laser-assisted subepithelial keratectomy for the correction of myopia. *J Cataract Refract Surg* 2002 Jan;28(1):18-22.

2. Azar DT, Ang RT, Lee JB, Kato T, Chen CC, Jain S, Gabison E, Abad JC. Laser subepithelial keratomileusis: electron microscopy and visual outcomes of flap photorefractive keratectomy. *Curr Opin Ophthalmol* 2001 Aug;12(4):323-8.

3. Kornilovsky IM. Clinical results after subepithelial photorefractive keratectomy (LASEK). *J Refract Surg 2001* Mar-Apr;17(2 Suppl):S222-3.

4. Scerrati E. Laser in situ keratomileusis vs. laser epithelial keratomileusis (LASIK vs. LASEK). *J Refract Surg* 2001 Mar-Apr;17(2 Suppl):S219-21.

5. Lee JB, Seong GJ, Lee JH, Seo KY, Lee YG, Kim EK. Comparison of laser epithelial keratomileusis and photorefractive keratectomy for low to moderate myopia. *J Cataract Refract Surg* 2001 Apr;27(4):565-70.

Chapter 16

Photorefractive Keratectomy (PRK) Surgery

The PRK laser is computer-controlled and programmed by an Eye M.D. to specifically address a patient's own unique corneal shape and refractive error.

The laser produces a highly concentrated beam of light which flattens the front surface of the cornea by removing micro-thin layers of tissue.

What Is PRK?

Photorefractive keratectomy is an outpatient corneal surgery that can reduce or correct mild to moderate myopia. This is done by use of a laser that precisely reshapes the cornea. The goal of PRK is to reduce or eliminate dependency on glasses or contact lenses.

Most of the people who have had PRK report they no longer need to wear glasses or contacts. In a large clinical trial, two thirds of the patients who had PRK can see 20/20 or better without corrective lenses. Ninety-five percent can see at least 20/40, well enough to pass a driver's test.

Risks

Although unlikely, there is a chance that complications may arise as a result of having PRK. Anyone considering the surgery should weigh the potential risks against the benefits of PRK.

- Undercorrection: It's possible that the PRK treatment could result in undercorrection and some degrees of nearsightedness may remain. Retreatments often correct this problem.

- Overcorrection: It's possible that overcorrection could occur; meaning patients may need to wear glasses or contact lenses after PRK. Overcorrections are generally not retreated.

- Night vision difficulties: Some PRK patients report difficulty with night vision. For instance, tasks performed without visual difficulty during the day are more difficult in low light or at night.

- Loss of best corrected vision: A small percentage of PRK patients experience a decrease in best corrected vision. This means if they could see images with a certain clarity wearing glasses before PRK, they might not be able to see as well, even with glasses, after PRK.

Other Risks

As with all surgeries, there is the rare possibility of infection or drug reaction that could cause loss of vision. Some people find they need reading glasses at an earlier age after PRK even though they did not need them before. Whether they've had PRK or not, most people need to wear reading glasses after the age of 40.

How to Make an Informed Decision about PRK

PRK is an elective procedure, so be sure to make an informed decision. The most satisfied patient is one who has realistic expectations and a thorough understanding of the risks and possible complications of refractive surgery. If you are considering the surgery, be certain to talk with your Eye M.D.

The following are questions your Eye M.D. will be able to address to help you make an informed decision.

- Am I a good candidate for PRK?
- What are the benefits of the surgery?
- What are the alternatives to PRK, both surgical and non-surgical?
- What are the possible complications and side effects of the surgery?
- Will I need additional surgery after the initial procedure?

- Will I still have to wear glasses after PRK?
- Will I need reading glasses as I age?

  Questions to ask yourself before you make a decision:

- Will I be satisfied with PRK if I still need to wear eyeglasses all or part of the time?
- Can I tolerate the temporary discomfort and inconvenience that may follow the PRK operation?

Consult Your Eye M.D.

Anyone considering PRK should make an informed decision. This chapter can't provide all the information a person should have. Discuss PRK with your Eye M.D. and study all the literature provided. Carefully review the consent form before making a decision.

Guidelines for Appropriate Referral of Persons with Possible Eye Diseases or Injuries Policy

The American Academy of Ophthalmology supports the concept of prompt appropriate referral of persons to a doctor of medicine or osteopathy (M.D. or D.O.), preferably to an Eye M.D., when certain signs are observed and/or certain symptoms are reported of possible eye disease or injury.

Background

Many eye diseases, systemic diseases, and injuries that affect the eyes may begin with subtle signs and either minimal or barely detectable symptoms. Most of these diseases and injuries require prompt and appropriate medical treatment in order to minimize risks of impaired vision or even blindness.

Eye M.D.'s are medical specialists qualified by education, training, and clinical experience to provide total eye care, which includes a vision examination (refraction), a medical eye examination, and necessary medical and surgical care and treatment.

Guidelines

A person exhibiting any of the following signs or symptoms should be referred promptly to an M.D. or D.O., preferably to an Eye M.D., for definitive diagnosis and necessary medical treatment:

165

- failure to achieve normal visual acuity in either eye unless the cause of the impairment has been medically confirmed by prior examination and visual acuity is stabilized (in preschool children, different levels of screening visual acuity for different ages have been established, which reflect the maturity of the child);

- significant eye injury or eye pain;

- symptoms of flashes of light, recent onset of floaters, halos, transient dimming or distortion of vision, obscured vision, loss of vision or pain in the eye, lids or orbits, double vision, or excessive tearing in the eye;

- transient or sustained loss of any part of the visual field or clinical suspicion or documentation of such field loss;

- abnormalities or opacities in the normally transparent media of the eye, or abnormalities of the ocular fundus or the optic nerve head;

- tumor or swelling of the eyelids or orbit or protrusion of one or both eyes;

- inflammation of the lids, conjunctiva or globe, with or without discharge;

- strabismus or diplopia;

- intraocular pressure at abnormal level;

- diabetes mellitus;

- eye and orbital abnormalities associated with thyroid disease (Graves' disease);

- HIV-positive patients with ocular symptoms and all patients with AIDS;

- newborn babies at risk, by prematurity, family history of retinoblastoma, or serious ocular symptoms; other history, symptoms, or signs that indicate need for ophthalmologist-performed eye examination or treatment.

Chapter 17

Use of Laser Surgery in Ophthalmology

The art and science of surgery have evolved remarkably over the past centuries. While the knife traditionally has been regarded as the quintessential surgical tool, the advent of sophisticated medical devices has extended the armamentarium and precision of surgical techniques.

The newest surgical devices utilized by surgeons are lasers. Lasers use extremely high energy light waves in order to cut through tissue in a very accurate manner, and to coagulate and remove tissue. Lasers have produced dramatic surgical effects that have improved the quality of care for patients. Lasers are used for many surgical applications. For example, lasers are employed to prevent visual loss in patients with diabetes, to reduce intraocular pressure in patients with glaucoma, to remove cancerous lesions inside the body, to cut away plaques in the blood vessels of the heart, and to treat skin cancer. As with any surgical procedure, the key to a successful outcome is a knowledgeable, experienced and skillful surgeon. The surgeon who uses lasers should understand the technology being employed, be well trained in its use and be capable of managing potential complications and meet the high standards of his or her medical peers.

This statement is in keeping with the policies for use of lasers developed by other physician medical and surgical specialty societies.

These policies stress medical training and experience in laser surgery and patient care, as well as expert knowledge of alternative medical and surgical techniques for the treatment of these conditions.

The following sections describe laser surgery applications in ophthalmology in greater detail. Ophthalmology has been acknowledged as a pioneer and innovator in laser surgery. The clinical experience of ophthalmologists with lasers dates back to the early 1960's, prior to that of any other medical specialty. Almost all types of lasers have found application in ophthalmology, and innovation in laser techniques continues at a rapid pace. The major areas of clinical application described here are treatment of glaucoma, management of patients who have had cataracts, retinal surgery, and corneal surgery. In each case, the significant risks and potential complications are described.

Laser Surgery in the Treatment of Glaucoma

The treatment of glaucoma is aimed primarily at reducing the level of intraocular pressure, because pressure is the major risk factor in the development of optic nerve damage from glaucoma. In most cases, treatment is limited to the use of topical and systemic medications. However, in some instances, surgery is indicated in order to reduce the intraocular pressure. Surgical techniques include manual incisional or laser incisional methods. The laser surgical techniques of laser trabeculoplasty, laser iridotomy, and laser photocoagulation are described below.

Argon Laser Trabeculoplasty

The concept of using the argon laser to treat the trabecular meshwork in patients with glaucoma was developed and refined in the 1970s. The trabecular meshwork is the mesh-like structure within the eye that filters aqueous fluid and controls its flow. Since 1980, argon laser surgery has proven to be a very effective surgical modality in improving the outflow of aqueous humor from the anterior chamber, thereby reducing intraocular pressure.

During argon laser trabeculoplasty, the surgeon applies a special mirrored contact lens to the patient's cornea. This device allows direct observation of the angle of the anterior chamber of the eye. The surgeon then directs the aiming beam of the argon laser at the trabecular meshwork. Thorough knowledge of the spectrum of anatomy and physiology of the trabecular meshwork region by the surgeon is crucial to the accuracy of laser application.

Laser applications are made to specific areas of the trabecular meshwork in order to create a very subtle but definite burn of tissue in the trabecular meshwork. Studies have shown that the facility of outflow is improved after such treatment and intraocular pressure is reduced in approximately three quarters of the cases treated. However, because the argon laser has also been used in experimental situations to create glaucoma, it is imperative that the surgeon be aware of the histopathological processes which take place following the application of laser energy to tissues, and that the margin of error is quite narrow.

In certain instances, the trabecular meshwork is obscured by iris tissue which is bowed forward. Under these conditions, the surgeon may determine that the procedure of laser peripheral iridoplasty is necessary in order to flatten the iris near the base of the filtration angle. This allows a better direct view of the trabecular meshwork to allow argon laser trabeculoplasty to be performed.

Argon or Neodymium:YAG (Nd:YAG) Laser Iridotomy

Although most patients with glaucoma have open-angle glaucoma, a significant number have anatomically narrow anterior chamber angles, which restrict the egress of aqueous fluid. Some patients have acute angle-closure glaucoma in which the pathways for drainage of aqueous fluid are completely blocked. When the ophthalmologist diagnoses acute angle-closure glaucoma and/or a critical narrow anterior chamber angle, then the ophthalmologist will recommend creating a surgical opening in the iris. Such an opening can either be created with the use of conventional surgical instruments or with the use of a surgical laser.

During laser iridotomy, the ophthalmologist will apply a special contact lens to the patient's cornea, which helps to focus the laser, allowing the creation of an opening. Again, the surgeon's knowledge of the range of variability of the anatomy and physiology of the iris is essential in iris surgery, and particularly so in laser surgery, because the iris is often found in close proximity to the easily damaged corneal endothelium, or the undersurface of the cornea.

Inappropriate use of the surgical laser can result in permanent damage to the cornea as well as to the lens of the eye and to an intraocular lens. In addition, bleeding from the iris can occur when an Nd:YAG laser application penetrates a blood vessel. In laser surgical iridotomy, a significant risk is the elevation of intraocular pressure following the procedure. Knowledge of the medical treatment for such adverse effects is necessary to safeguard the patient's vision.

Trans-scleral Laser Cyclophotocoagulation

Trans-scleral Nd:YAG thermal laser surgical cyclophotocoagulation can be utilized when other surgical modalities have failed to halt the advancement of glaucoma. Surgical laser energy is applied through the sclera, or the outer layer of the eye, to the ciliary body. The ciliary body produces aqueous fluid, which maintains the intraocular pressure. The selective destruction of the ciliary processes reduces aqueous production and lowers intraocular pressure. Because this procedure can be painful, a retrobulbar anesthetic is administered prior to the performance of trans-scleral cyclophotocoagulation. In addition, trans-scleral Nd:YAG laser surgery may be used to produce filtration via trans-scleral sclerostomy.

Laser Surgery in the Management of Patients after a Cataract Operation

Lasers are not utilized in the surgical removal of cataracts. However, the use of laser surgery may be indicated in the post-operative management of a patient who already has had a cataract extracted.

The most common surgical treatment of cataracts is the operation called extracapsular cataract extraction. In this procedure, the clear posterior lens capsule is left in place, in order to stabilize the artificial lens implant. However, 20 to 30% of patients will develop clouding of the posterior capsule within two years following extra-capsular cataract surgery. In these cases, a clear window can be created in the cloudy membrane with the Nd: YAG laser.

In this surgical procedure, the laser is used as a photodisruptor, which applies tiny but powerful shock waves to make minute tears in the membrane. The surgeon performs a series of carefully focused laser applications in order to restore clarity to the optical path of the eye. The complication rate with this procedure is low and is primarily that of elevated intraocular pressure, although other adverse events, such as retinal disorders and intra-ocular bleeding, may also occur.

Laser Surgery in the Treatment of Retinal Diseases

Diabetic retinopathy, a condition characterized by blood vessel changes in the retina of patients with diabetes, is the leading cause of blindness in working-age Americans. Diabetes is one of the most serious, generalized blood vessel, or vascular, disorders in modern medicine. The blood vessel changes in the retina are just one component of the serious complications of diabetes throughout the body. High blood pressure, itself a common complication of diabetes, elevated blood sugar levels, kidney disease, and pregnancy are each associated with an increased risk of developing retinopathy. A thorough medical understanding of the systemic diabetic disease process is therefore required to manage diabetic retinopathy optimally.

Laser Photocoagulation

In the condition known as proliferative diabetic retinopathy, abnormal new blood vessels develop from the optic nerve area or elsewhere in the retina and frequently lead to severe visual loss from hemorrhage and other complications. The National Eye Institute-sponsored Diabetic Retinopathy Study proved the beneficial role of laser surgery for proliferative diabetic retinopathy. Laser photocoagulation is applied extensively from near the optic nerve margin to the periphery of the retina while sparing the central macular area, which is functionally important for reading.

The extensive laser applications required to treat proliferative diabetic retinopathy produce side effects in the majority of patients, including a reduction in peripheral vision and in the ability to adapt to changes in light level. Some other potential complications are burns and scarring of the cornea, glaucoma, cataracts, thermal damage to the optic nerve, rupture of blood vessels, vitreous hemorrhage, and macular edema, which requires treatment as described below for spontaneously occurring diabetic macular edema.

Because such laser surgery can be uncomfortable and patients may find it difficult to cooperate, there is also a need in some patients for injection of an anesthetic agent around or behind the eyeball, which may be associated with serious complications. A medical decision must then be made for the type of anesthesia, which includes peribulbar, epibulbar, and retrobulbar injection of anesthetic agents.

The list of potential complications of anesthesia injection includes hemorrhage behind the eye, closure of the central artery nourishing the retina, and perforation of the eyeball or optic nerve from the needle, all of which can lead to blindness, if not immediately recognized and treated by appropriate emergency measures. General or systemic complications of anesthesia injections include a significant drop in blood pressure with a severe loss of consciousness, respiratory and possible cardiac arrest, and grand mal seizures.

Laser Surgery for Diabetic Macular Edema

In diabetic macular edema, microaneurysms, or local balloon-like swellings of the capillaries in the retina, and weakened capillaries in the macular area allow fluid leakage or edema that can seriously impair reading vision. A National Eye Institute-sponsored, multi-center study demonstrated a highly beneficial effect of laser surgery for diabetic macular edema. In this procedure, the surgeon applies the laser to the microaneurysms and leaking retinal capillaries. These vessels are identified by fluorescein angiography. Fluorescein angiography involves the injection of a dye, fluorescein, which can be photographed as it is carried through the eye's blood vessels.

The complication rate for laser surgery treatment of macular edema is low in an experienced surgeon's hands. But experience is critical because of the potential for damage to the macula. Even with appropriate treatment, some patients will develop a slight permanent reduction of reading vision. Occasionally, the treatment of patients with macular edema will require the injection of anesthesia behind the eyeball with the same serious risks noted above.

Laser Surgery for Age-Related Macular Degeneration

Age-related macular degeneration involves the central area of the retina used for straight ahead vision as in reading. This condition is usually slowly progressive, but about 15 percent of patients develop abnormal blood vessels beneath the retina. These vessels can bleed and impair vision. Delicate laser surgery can be effective in closing these vessels.

High quality fluorescein angiography is required and the surgeon must be skilled in the interpretation of the findings. When laser applications must be placed within or near the macula, some patients require retrobulbar anesthesia. This helps stabilize the eyeball in order to minimize the risk of inadvertent laser burns close to the center of the macula.

Laser Surgery in Treatment of Corneal Disease and Refractive Errors

Excimer laser surgery is capable of removing corneal tissue with an accuracy and precision that has never before been available. Possible applications of this new surgical technique include the treatment of refractive errors by modifying the surface of the cornea (photo-refractive keratectomy) and the removal of corneal opacities (photo-therapeutic keratectomy).

Patients who undergo excimer laser corneal surgery face the same complications as those who undergo conventional corneal surgery, including inadvertent damage to other ocular structures, corneal scarring, infection, lack of healing and regression of the intended refractive effects. Thus, a physician who performs excimer laser corneal surgery should be trained, licensed, and prepared to provide local and systemic therapy with antibiotics, corticosteroids, and other prescription drugs. He should be able to perform corneal transplants or other surgical procedures that may be indicated and should also be able to offer surgical alternatives to laser surgery. The physician should be sufficiently trained to assess the risks and benefits of all available treatment alternatives and to discuss these with the patient before proceeding.

Because of the large number of individuals who now wear glasses and would be candidates for photo-refractive keratectomy, public safety concerns have been raised over these procedures. The safety and efficacy of both photo-refractive keratectomy and photo-therapeutic keratectomy must be established by clinical trials before FDA approval can be obtained for these uses of the excimer laser. These trials are currently underway.

Summary

Laser surgery provides an alternative to older, more invasive surgical techniques, resulting in more rapid healing and a reduction of complications. However, laser surgery is neither simple nor without associated serious risks, including edema, elevation of intraocular pressure, penetration of a blood vessel with bleeding, tissue necrosis, etc. As exemplified by the descriptions above, the optimal use of lasers demands much more than just technical expertise; a comprehensive knowledge and experience related to pathologic disease processes and their treatment is also required.

Lasers have proven to be safe and effective instruments in ophthalmology, when used by surgeons possessing a broad base of knowledge, training, and clinical experience. Continued success in existing and new laser surgical applications will depend on many interrelated aspects of the physician's expertise and judgment: a comprehensive eye examination and an astute medical diagnosis; a weighing of risks, benefits, and available recourse to alternative surgical and medical treatments; precise timing and selection of the laser technique to fit the individual patient's circumstances; a technical proficiency in controlling and manipulating lasers; a familiarity with associated adverse events and a readiness to respond as warranted; and a personal responsibility for the post-operative management of patients undergoing laser surgery.

Note: This article was written for physicians. Patients should talk to their Eye M.D. if they have questions about the content.

Chapter 18

Acupuncture for Ocular Conditions and Headaches

Summary

Introduction to the Topic

Acupuncture refers broadly to a group of procedures that stimulate the skin. The most common technique uses thin, solid metallic needles, which are manipulated either manually or by electrical stimulation.

Conclusions

Based on available evidence in the peer-reviewed scientific literature, the Task Force on Complementary Therapies believes that scientific evidence has not been found to demonstrate the safety or effectiveness of acupuncture for treatment of various ocular conditions when compared to standard therapies.

Also, the quality of the scientific evidence, as reviewed by the National Institutes of Health (NIH) Consensus Development Panel, is not sufficient at this time to provide a determination of efficacy on the use of acupuncture for headaches. However, acupuncture may be useful as an adjunct treatment or as an acceptable alternative to standard therapies or be included in a comprehensive management program for headaches.

175

Benefits

Ocular Conditions

Acupuncture use has been reported for treating and alleviating a variety of ocular conditions. One randomized controlled double-blind study was found that examined the use of acupuncture for dry eye. Statistically significant differences were found between the needle acupuncture group and the control group (P<0.01). Longer-term studies with larger samples of patients and adequate sham control groups to compare with needle acupuncture are needed to validate the results of this one study.

Headaches

Sixteen controlled studies of the use of acupuncture for tension and migraine headaches were reviewed. In eight of the nine studies, acupuncture was found to be more effective than the control, reaching significance in three studies. In seven of the studies that compared acupuncture to standard therapy, acupuncture was found to be as effective as standard therapy. However, these studies are not considered methodologically rigorous.

Risks

Overall, the rate of general adverse effects from acupuncture has been reported to be low. They result from improper needling, organ puncture injuries, and the risk of infection related to use of unsterilized needles. Specific risks with use of acupuncture in ocular conditions have not been described.

Report

Description of the Technology

Acupuncture has been a part of the health care system in China for several thousand years. It refers broadly to a group of procedures that stimulate the skin using a variety of techniques, and they are usually performed in an office setting. The most common technique involves inserting thin, solid metallic needles no more than three inches into the surface of the skin to the deep tissue. They are manipulated either manually or by electrical stimulation. This assessment focuses on the application of acupuncture for eye conditions and for tension and migraine headaches. Other techniques, such as moxibustion that applies heat to an acupuncture point, have too few studies to evaluate.

Mechanism of Action

The rationale behind acupuncture is that there is an energy flow (Qi) along specific channels throughout the body. According to this theory, disease occurs when there is too little or too much Qi or when the flow is blocked or interrupted. Stimulation of acupuncture points corrects the imbalance of energy flow. Studies in animals and humans have demonstrated that biological responses occur as a result of acupuncture.[1-2] These responses include the release of opioid peptides, which can account for the analgesic effects of acupuncture. There are also studies that have shown that acupuncture can alter immune functions, the secretion of neurotransmitters and neurohormones, and the regulation of blood flow. However, there is much that remains unknown about the anatomy and physiology of acupuncture points and the scientific basis for the theory of circulating energy flow. Further research is important.

Definition of the Problems

Ocular Conditions

Acupuncture use has been reported for treating and alleviating a variety of ocular conditions, including myopia,[3-4] high myopia,[5] paralytic strabismus,[6] retinitis pigmentosa,[7] optic atrophy, retrobulbar neuritis, maculopathy,[8] iritis, conjunctivitis, cataracts, and dry eye.[9] Acupuncture has also been used for anesthesia during extraocular muscle surgery.

Headaches

Headache is a common complaint that patients present with when visiting an ophthalmologist. It is reported that up to 14 percent of all males and 28 percent of all females in the United States complain of relatively frequent headaches.[10] Headaches secondary to ocular causes are rare. Migraine headaches are characterized by repetitive bouts of headaches, and they occur more commonly in women and can have associated visual symptoms. Tension headaches are precipitated by stress, and are chronic in nature; they are characterized by aching pain. Treatment of headaches is guided by the type of headache and

177

symptoms. It can include eliminating contributory factors and using analgesics such as ergotamines, serotonergic agents, nonsteroidal anti-inflammatory and other medications.

FDA Status

In 1996, the U.S. Food and Drug Administration removed acupuncture needles from the category of Class 3 experimental medical devices and now regulates them as Class 2 devices, subjecting them to good manufacturing practices and single-use standards of sterility.

Summary of Evidence

Statistical Issues and Study Design

There are inherent difficulties and complexities in designing studies of acupuncture, mainly in using appropriate controls, such as placebos and sham acupuncture groups. This is complicated by the fact that many of the published studies involve issues of methodology, including insufficient sample size, questions about the effectiveness of randomization, lack of use of standardized outcome measures, short follow-up intervals, and inadequate placebo treatments for control groups.[11] The NIH Consensus Development Panel on Acupuncture concluded that "according to contemporary research standards, there is a paucity of high-quality research assessing efficacy of acupuncture compared with placebo or sham acupuncture. The vast majority of studies on acupuncture in the biomedical literature consist of case reports, case series, or intervention studies with designs inadequate to assess efficacy."[1]

Search Methods and Study Selection

Ocular conditions: In March 1999, the American Academy of Ophthalmology searched through MEDLINE in the English language for articles from January 1970 to March 1999 relating to acupuncture and ocular conditions. A total of 12 articles were identified; a total of 7 were defined as relevant and were reviewed for study design and implementation.

Headaches: In November 1997, a 12-member panel representing the fields of acupuncture, pain, psychology, psychiatry, physical medicine and rehabilitation, drug abuse, family practice, internal medicine, health policy, epidemiology, statistics, physiology, and biophysics were assembled as the NIH Consensus Development Panel on Acupuncture.

The panel developed conclusions based on scientific literature and evidence presented by experts. The evidence presented in this assessment is based on the reports and data presented at this conference. The NIH Consensus Development Panel searched through MEDLINE, Allied and Alternative Medicine, EMBASE, MANTIS, and journals not indexed by the National Library of Medicine for the period from January 1970 to October 1997. An extensive bibliography of 2,302 references was assembled.

Benefits

Ocular Conditions

Of the seven articles reviewed, only one was a randomized controlled, double-blind study. The rest of the articles were reports of case-series (4 articles) or comparative studies without adequate control groups. The one randomized double-blind study of dry eye used soft laser devices to deliver the point stimulation treatment similar to needle acupuncture, one emitting infrared light (32 cases) and one without any function (30 cases) as a placebo.[9] These patients were compared with a group of 30 patients treated with needle acupuncture and 22 patients treated with artificial tears. Outcomes were defined as results of the Schirmer II test, break-up time, and frequency of use of artificial tears. The multiple Tukey-Kramers test was used for statistical analysis. Statistically significant differences were found between the two lasers that were used (the functional laser group showing improved outcomes), and between the needle acupuncture group and the control group (the needle acupuncture group showing improved outcomes) ($P<0.01$). There was no statistically significant difference between the functional laser group and the needle acupuncture group. Longer-term studies with larger samples of patients and adequate sham control groups compared with needle acupuncture are needed to validate the results of this one small study.

Headaches

Sixteen controlled studies for acupuncture of tension and migraine headaches were reviewed. In nine of the studies, acupuncture was compared to a control group receiving needling treatment or some form of placebo treatment. In eight of these studies, acupuncture was found to be more effective than the control, reaching significance in three studies. In seven other studies, acupuncture was compared to standard treatment such as medication or physiotherapy. In all of these studies acupuncture was found to be as effective as standard therapy. However, most of these studies were not adequately designed, with insufficient sample size, outcome measures, problems with the control group, or inadequate use of acupuncture.[10] Thus, the weight of evidence seems positive, with a need for larger, well-designed studies for replication of previous results.[11] The NIH Consensus Development Panel concluded that although research evidence is not sufficient to provide firm evidence of efficacy at this time, acupuncture may be useful as an adjunct treatment or as an acceptable alternative that could be included in a comprehensive management program for headaches.

Risks

The overall rate of general adverse effects from acupuncture has been reported to be low. There have been rare events of potentially life-threatening events such as pneumothorax caused by improper needling or other organ puncture injuries. Fainting, local infection, and increased pain are more common adverse effects. It has been reported that 126 cases of hepatitis B have been linked to practitioners using unsterilized needles. Technical problems that can occur include bent or broken needles. Risks have not been described with use of acupuncture in ocular conditions.

Questions for Scientific Inquiry

If further scientific investigation is desired, the following questions are posed:

Ocular Conditions

- What is the biological basis for acupuncture for treating various eye conditions, i.e., dry eye, myopia, optic nerve atrophy?

- Is acupuncture effective treatment for ocular conditions using randomized controlled clinical trials in larger, well-designed studies with adequate statistical analyses?

- How effective is acupuncture compared to standard therapies for these ocular conditions?

Headaches

- What is the biological basis for using acupuncture to treat headaches?

- Is acupuncture effective treatment for headaches in a randomized controlled clinical trial, with larger, well-designed studies?

- How effective is acupuncture compared to conventional therapies for headache?

Information for Patients

Physicians can advise their patients who are contemplating acupuncture treatment to ask the following questions:

- Does the provider have state licensure and credentialing? (A majority of states provide licensure or registration.)

- What other treatment options are available?

- What are the expected prognosis and risks associated with the use of acupuncture?

- What safety protocols are in place to minimize the risks of acupuncture?

- Does the provider follow FDA regulations for acupuncture needles, including using sterile, single-use needles?

Summary and Conclusions

Ocular Conditions

Based on available evidence in the peer-reviewed scientific literature, the Task Force on Complementary Therapies believes that scientific evidence has not been found to demonstrate the safety or effectiveness of acupuncture to treat various ocular conditions compared to standard therapies. These conditions include myopia, high myopia, paralytic strabismus, retinitis pigmentosa, optic atrophy, retrobulbar neuritis, maculopathy, iritis, conjunctivitis, cataracts, and dry eye.

Headaches

As reviewed by the NIH Consensus Development, the quality of the scientific evidence is not sufficient to provide a determination of efficacy at this time on the use of acupuncture for headaches. Acupuncture could be useful for headaches as part of a comprehensive management program or as an alternative for patients who have not had satisfactory results with conventional therapies. The clinician relies on clinical experience, scientific evidence regarding conventional therapies, weighing the benefits and risks, and information about patient characteristics and preferences to make these decisions.

Development of Complementary Therapy Assessments

Complementary, or alternative therapies, are a growing part of health care in America. Americans spend an estimated $14 billion a year on alternative treatments. Mainstream medicine is recognizing a need to learn more about alternative therapies and determine their true value. About 37 U.S. medical schools are beginning to devote a small part of training to alternative therapies. The editors of the *Journal of the American Medical Association* announced that publishing research on alternative therapies will be one of its priorities. The NIH National Center for Complementary and Alternative Medicine has broadly defined complementary and alternative medicine as those treatments and health care practices that are not taught widely in medical schools, not generally used in hospitals, and not usually reimbursed by medical insurance companies. More scrutiny and scientific objectivity is being applied to determine whether evidence supporting their effectiveness exists.

In the fall of 1998, the Board of Trustees appointed a Task Force on Complementary Therapy to evaluate complementary therapies in eye care and develop an opinion on their safety and effectiveness, based on available scientific evidence, in order to inform ophthalmologists and their patients. A scientifically grounded analysis of the data will help ophthalmologists and patients evaluate the research and thus make more rational decisions on appropriate treatment choices.

The Academy believes that complementary therapies should be evaluated similarly to traditional medicine: evidence of safety, efficacy, and effectiveness should be demonstrated.[12] Many therapies used in conventional medical practice also have not been as rigorously tested as they should be. But given the large numbers of patients affected and the health care expenditures involved, it is important that data and scientific information be used to base all treatment recommendations. In this way, we can encourage high-quality, rigorous research on complementary therapies, such as the gold standard for clinical research, and the randomized controlled clinical trial.[13]

Ideally, a study of efficacy compares a treatment to a placebo or another treatment, using a double-blind controlled trial and well-defined protocol. Reports should describe enrollment procedures, eligibility criteria, clinical characteristics of the patients, methods for diagnosis, randomization of treatment, control conditions, and length of treatment. They should also use standardized outcomes and appropriate statistical analyses.

The goal of these assessments is to provide objective information about complementary therapies and to provide a scientific basis for physicians to advise their patients, when asked.

To accomplish these goals, the assessments, in general, are intended to do the following:

- Describe the scientific rationale or mechanism for action for the complementary therapy.

- Describe the methods and basis for collecting evidence.

- Describe the relevant evidence.

- Summarize the benefits and risks of the complementary therapy.

- Pose questions for future research inquiry.

- Summarize the evidence on safety and effectiveness.

References

1. NIH consensus conference. Acupuncture. *JAMA* 1998; 280:1518-24. [Also available at http://consensus.nih.gov]

2. Leake R, Broderick JE. Treatment efficacy of acupuncture: a review of the research literature. *Integrative Medicine* 1998; 1:107-15.

3. Liu H, Lu Y, Dong Q, Zhong X. Treatment of adolescent myopia by pressure plaster of semen impatientis on otoacupoints. *J Tradit Chin Med* 1994; 14:283-6.

4. Yang C, Hu L, Zhu F, Li L. 268 cases of myopia treated with injection and pellet pressure at auriculoacupoints. *J Tradit Chin Med* 1993; 196-8.

5. Wong S, Ching R. The use of acupuncture in ophthalmology. *Am J Chin Med* 1980; 8:104-53.

6. Liu C, Wang Y. 81 cases of paralytic strabismus treated with acupuncture. *J Tradit Chin Med* 1993; 13:101-2.

7. Dabov S, Goutoranov G, Ivanova R, Petkova N. Clinical application of acupuncture in ophthalmology. *Acupunct Electrother Res* 1985; 10:79-93.

8. Omura Y. Non-invasive circulatory evaluation and electro-acupuncture and TES treatment of diseases difficult to treat in western medicine. *Acupunct Electrother Res* 1983; 8:177-256.

9. Hepp J, Wedrich A, Akramian J et al. Dry eye treatment with acupuncture; a prospective, randomized, double-masked study. In: Sullivan DA, Dartt DA, Meneray MA, eds. *Lacrimal gland, tear film and dry eye syndromes* 2. New York: Plenum Press, 1998.

10. Birch S. Overview of the efficacy of acupuncture in the treatment of headache and face and neck pain. NIH Consensus Development Conference on Acupuncture, Bethesda, MD, 1997. [Available at http://consensus.nih.gov]

11. Berman BM. Overview of clinical trials on acupuncture on pain. NIH Consensus Development Conference on Acupuncture, Bethesda, MD, 1997. [Available at http://consensus.nih.gov]

12. Fontanaros PB, Lundberg GD. Alternative medicine meets science [editorial]. *JAMA* 1998; 280: 1618-9.

13. Margolin A, Avants SK, Kleber HD. Investigating alternative medicine therapies in randomized controlled trials. *JAMA* 1998; 280:1626-8.

Prepared by the American Academy of Ophthalmology Complementary Therapy Task Force: Ivan R. Schwab, M.D., Chair; Harold P. Koller, M.D.; Roger Husted, M.D.; Sayoko E. Moroi, M.D., Ph.D.; Jeffrey Todd Liegner, M.D.; Denise Satterfield, M.D.; and Peter R. Holyk, M.D., Consultant.

Chapter 19

Vision Therapy

Introduction

Society places a premium on efficient vision. Schools and most occupations require increasing amounts of printed and computer information to be handled accurately and in shorter periods of time. Vision is also a major factor in sports, crafts, and other pastimes. The efficiency of our visual system influences how we collect and process information. Repetitive demands on the visual system tend to create problems in susceptible individuals. Inefficient vision may cause an individual to slow down, be less accurate, experience excessive fatigue, or make errors. When these types of signs and symptoms appear, the individual's conscious attention to the visual process is required. This, in turn, may interfere with speed, accuracy, and comprehension of visual tasks. Many of these visual dysfunctions are effectively treated with vision therapy.

Pertinent Issues

Vision is a product of our inherited potentials, our past experiences, and current information. Efficient visual functioning enables us to understand the world around us better and to guide our actions accurately and quickly. Age is not a deterrent to the achievement of successful vision therapy outcomes.

Vision is the dominant sense and is composed of three areas of function:

- Visual pathway integrity including eye health, visual acuity, and refractive status.

- Visual skills including accommodation (eye focusing), binocular vision (eye teaming), and eye movements (eye tracking).

- Visual information processing including identification, discrimination, spatial awareness, and integration with other senses.

Learning to read and reading for information require efficient visual abilities. The eyes must team precisely, focus clearly, and track quickly and accurately across the page. These processes must be coordinated with the perceptual and memory aspects of vision, which in turn must combine with linguistic processing for comprehension. To provide reliable information, this must occur with precise timing. Inefficient or poorly developed vision requires individuals to divide their attention between the task and the involved visual abilities. Some individuals have symptoms such as headaches, fatigue, eyestrain, errors, loss of place, and difficulty sustaining attention. Others may have an absence of symptoms due to the avoidance of visually demanding tasks.

Vision Therapy

The human visual system is complex. The problems that can develop in our visual system require a variety of treatment options. Many visual conditions can be treated effectively with spectacles or contact lenses alone; however, some are most effectively treated with vision therapy.

Vision therapy is a sequence of activities individually prescribed and monitored by the doctor to develop efficient visual skills and processing. It is prescribed after a comprehensive eye examination has been performed and has indicated that vision therapy is an appropriate treatment option. The vision therapy program is based on the results of standardized tests, the needs of the patient, and the patient's signs and symptoms. The use of lenses, prisms, filters, occluders, specialized instruments, and computer programs is an integral part of vision therapy.

Vision therapy is administered in the office under the guidance of the doctor. It requires a number of office visits and depending on the severity of the diagnosed conditions, the length of the program typically ranges from several weeks to several months. Activities paralleling in-office techniques are typically taught to the patient to be practiced at home to reinforce the developing visual skills.

Research has demonstrated vision therapy can be an effective treatment option for:

- Ocular motility dysfunctions (eye movement disorders)

- Non-strabismic binocular disorders (inefficient eye teaming)

- Strabismus (misalignment of the eyes)

- Amblyopia (poorly developed vision)

- Accommodative disorders (focusing problems)

- Visual information processing disorders, including visual-motor integration and integration with other sensory modalities

Summary

Vision therapy is prescribed to treat diagnosed conditions of the visual system. Effective therapy requires visual skills to be developed until they are integrated with other systems and become automatic, enabling individuals to achieve their full potential. The goals of a prescribed vision therapy treatment regimen are to achieve desired visual outcomes, alleviate the signs and symptoms, meet the patient's needs, and improve the patient's quality of life.

This Policy Statement was formulated by a working group representing the American Academy of Optometry, American Optometric Association, the College of Optometrists in Vision Development, and the Optometric Extension Program Foundation. The following individuals are acknowledged for their contributions: Gary J. Williams, OD; Chair; Susan A. Cotter, OD; Kelly A. Frantz, OD; Louis G. Hoffman, OD, MS; Glen T. Steele, OD; Stephen C. Miller, OD; Jeffrey L. Weaver, OD, MS.

Approved by: American Academy of Optometry, April 27, 1999; American Optometric Association, June 22, 1999; College of Optometrists in Vision Development, June 25, 1999; Optometric Extension Program Foundation, June 25, 1999.

Bibliography

1. American Optometric Association. Position statement on vision therapy. *J Am Optom Assoc* 1985;56:782-3.

2. Caloroso EE, Rouse MW, Cotter SA. *Clinical management of strabismus*. Boston: Butterworth-Heinemann, 1993.

3. Ciuffreda KJ, Levi DM, Selenow A. *Amblyopia: basic and clinical aspects*. Boston: Butterworth-Heinemann, 1991.

4. Coffey B, Wick B, Cotter S, et al. Treatment options in intermittent exotropia: a critical appraisal. *Optom Vis Sci* 1992;69:386-404.

5. Cooper J, Medow N. Intermittent exotropia: basic and divergence excess type. *Binoc Vis Eye Muscle Surg Q* 1993;8:185-216.

6. Cooper J, Selenow A, Ciuffreda KJ, et al. Reduction of asthenopia in patients with convergence insufficiency after fusional vergence training. *Am J Optom Physiol Opt* 1983;60:982-9.

7. Daum KM. The course and effect of visual training on the vergence system. *Am J Optom Physiol Opt* 1982;59:223-7.

8. Flax N, Duckman RH. Orthoptic treatment of strabismus. *J Am Optom Assoc* 1978;49:1353-61.

9. Garzia RP. Efficacy of vision therapy in amblyopia: a literature review. *Am J Optom Physiol Opt* 1987;64:393-404.

10. Griffin JR. Efficacy of vision therapy for nonstrabismic vergence anomalies. *Am J Optom Physiol Opt* 1987;64:411-4.

11. Grisham JD, Bowman MC, Owyang LA, Chan CL. Vergence orthoptics: validity and persistence of the training effect. *Optom Vis Sci* 1991;68:441-51.

12. Liu JS, Lee M, Jang J, et al. Objective assessment of accommodation orthoptics. I. Dynamic insufficiency. *Am J Optom Physiol Opt* 197956:285-94.

13. The 1986/87 Future of Visual Development/Performance Task Force. The efficacy of optometric vision therapy. *J Am Optom Assoc* 1988;59:95-105.

14. *Optometric clinical practice guideline: care of the patient with accommodative and vergence dysfunction*. St. Louis: American Optometric Association, 1998.

15. Press LJ. *Applied concepts in vision therapy*. St. Louis: Mosby, 1997.

16. Rouse MW. Management of binocular anomalies: efficacy of vision therapy in the treatment of accommodative deficiencies. *Am J Optom Physiol Opt* 1987;64:415-20.

17. Scheiman M, Wick B. *Clinical management of binocular vision: heterophoric, accommodative, and eye movement disorders*. Philadelphia: Lippincott, 1994.

18. Suchoff IB, Petito GT. The efficacy of visual therapy: accommodative disorders and non-strabismic anomalies of binocular vision. *J Am Optom Assoc* 1986;57:119-25.

19. Wick BW. Accommodative esotropia: efficacy of therapy. *J Am Optom Assoc* 1987;58:562-6.

20. Wick B, Wingard M, Cotter S, Scheiman M. Anisometropic amblyopia: is the patient ever too old to treat? *Optom Vis Sci* 1992;69:866-78.

Chapter 20

Eye-Related Quackery

Since ancient times, many people have held the mistaken belief that poor eyesight can be cured by special eye exercises. This belief was brought to its highest state of fruition by a one-time reputable physician, William Horatio Bates, M.D., who in 1920 published *The Cure of Imperfect Eyesight by Treatment Without Glasses*.

In 1917, Bates teamed up with Bernarr Macfadden, a well known food faddist who published the magazine *Physical Culture*. Together they offered a course in the Bates System of Eye Exercises for a fee that included a subscription to the magazine. This venture met with considerable success and led many people to believe in the Bates System. However, the big impact of Bates' work materialized after publication of his book. This book attracted large numbers of charlatans, quacks, and gullible followers who then published scores of unscientific books and articles of their own on the subject of vision. Extolling the Bates System, these authors urged readers to throw away their glasses. Some of these writers even established schools.

Contrary to scientific fact, Bates taught that errors of refraction are due, not to the basic shape of the eyeball or the structure of the lens, but to a functional and therefore curable derangement in the action of the muscles on the outside of the eyeball. All defects in vision, he said, were caused by eyestrain and nervous tension; and perfect vision could be achieved by relaxing the eyes completely. Bates

From "Eye-Related Quackery," by Russell S. Worrall, O.D., Jacob Nevyas, Ph.D., and Stephen Barrett, M.D., © 2002 Quackwatch, Inc. Reprinted with permission.

warned that eyeglasses cause the vision to deteriorate; he also deplored the use of sunglasses. Bates claimed his exercises could correct nearsightedness, farsightedness, astigmatism, and presbyopia (the inability of older people to focus their eyes on nearby objects). They could also cure such diseases as cataracts, eye infections, glaucoma, and macular degeneration. His exercises included palming (covering the eyes and attempting to see blackness) and shifting or swinging the gaze from object to object.

It should be obvious that these exercises cannot influence eyesight disorders as Bates claimed. Nearsightedness, farsightedness, astigmatism, and presbyopia result from inborn and acquired characteristics of the lens and the eyeball—which no exercise can change. As for eye diseases, the only thing the exercises can do is delay proper medical or surgical treatment and result in permanent impairment of vision. The claims Bates made in advertising his book were so dubious that in 1929 the Federal Trade Commission issued a complaint against him for advertising "falsely or misleadingly."

After Bates died in 1931, his office and teaching practices were taken over very successfully by his wife Emily with the help of Dr. Harold M. Peppard. Mrs. Bates had worked with her husband for a number of years, and Peppard was an ardent advocate of the Bates System. An edited version of Dr. Bates' book was published in 1940 as *Better Eyesight Without Glasses*. This version was revised several times and is still in print. Its recommendations include sun treatment in which the sun is permitted to shine on closed eyes and then on the sclera (white portion of the eye) while looking downward. The book states: "One cannot get too much sun treatment."

Other dubious promoters followed Bates' path. One of the best known was Gaylord Hauser, popular food faddist and Hollywood favorite, who in 1932 published *Keener Sight Without Glasses*. By combining eye exercise and diet theories, Hauser furthered the sale of his own dietary products.

In the mid-1950s, Philip Pollack, O.D., a prominent optometrist in New York City, wrote a blistering critique of the Bates System[1]; and the vast majority of optometrists and ophthalmologists regard Bates' notions as wrong. Yet Bates still has advocates today. Some cling to traditional Bates techniques, while others use expensive computerized biofeedback machines. Their promotion is not limited to books and magazine articles but includes direct-mail campaigns with glossy brochures and toll-free numbers, pitching similar programs with new gadgets and mail-order videos. Beware of "Institutes" using well-known college towns in their names or "doctors" with dubious credentials, such as one we encountered with a degree from the "University in California" (not the University *of* California).

Vision Therapy

Like Bates, vision therapists claim to strengthen eyesight through a series of exercises. In contrast to Bates' use of relaxation, vision therapists promote active exercises. They emphasize exercising focusing, eye pointing, and eye movement skills. Exercises may include eye-hand coordination drills, watching a series of blinking lights, staring at colored lights (Syntonics), bouncing on a trampoline, and even sleeping in a certain position. Often they prescribe bifocal and prism glasses to prevent or cure nearsightedness. In addition to promising to eliminate glasses, they claim that these methods can also improve school and athletic performance, increase IQ, help overcome learning problems and attention disorders, and even prevent juvenile delinquency. However, no scientific evidence supports such claims.[2-4]

There is a proven segment of vision therapy known as orthoptics, which can help with symptoms of visual strain or fatigue in individuals with mild eye coordination or focus problems, double vision, or even strabismus (crossed or turned eyes) and amblyopia (lazy eye).[5-6] Many optometrists, ophthalmologists, and Certified Orthoptists offer orthoptic diagnostic and treatment services.

Vision therapists who refer to themselves as "developmental" or "behavioral" optometrists assert that most vision disorders are the result of learned or environmental factors and can be corrected through eye training. For example, they may suggest biofeedback training to reverse nearsightedness or recommend low-power glasses (learning lenses) to children with reading problems. The initials C.O.V.D. after a practitioner's name refer to the College of Optometrists in Vision Development, which is a national organization that provides training, promotional, and referral services for its members. Another proponent group is the Optometric Extension Program (O.E.P.), which began as the Oklahoma Extension Program in the 1920s. O.E.P. has contributed greatly to advancing the optometric profession by providing optometrists with postgraduate continuing education. In recent years, however, its programs have emphasized 'behavioral optometry" and vision therapy. Even though there is no scientific evidence that vision therapy can improve academic performance, the public relations activities of these two organizations have persuaded many teachers and counselors to refer children with dyslexia to a behavioral or developmental optometrist.

Dyslexia, a term that is often misunderstood, simply refers to severe reading problems in an otherwise normal person. Reading experts have identified many causes of dyslexia, with the majority related to the brain's ability to interpret the sound of spoken words or to process language information rapidly.[7-11] Because reading involves sight, teachers and parents often incorrectly assume that vision problems are the cause of reading problems. Vision and eye-coordination problems, however, are not the cause of dyslexia. Glasses can help if a child has trouble focusing on words, but they are often prescribed unnecessarily. Muscle-strengthening exercises (orthoptics) may help relieve fatigue symptoms if a mild eye coordination or focusing problem exists, but exercises to improve coordination are not helpful for dyslexia. The preponderance of studies have found that vision-related training has no effect or even a negative effect on learning to read.[2-4]

Parents often abandon common sense in their quest to help their struggling children and are easy prey for therapists promising a cure.[12] A few years ago, a vision training program was promoted in supermarkets with tear-off advertisements targeted to unsuspecting parents. The practitioner, boasting that vision training is a low-cost, high-profit specialty, claimed that he generated close to $950,000 in new billings during the first twelve months of the supermarket campaign.[13]

Promises of dramatically improved reading speed are often made by vision therapists and speed- reading courses. If you can read but have symptoms of fatigue or read slowly, these programs may help. However, they are unlikely to double or triple your speed, as is typically claimed. Studies have shown that many people can gain 20 to 50% in speed and experience more comfort while reading with the proper glasses and vision therapy if needed.[6,14,15]

Many self-help books are aimed at people who want to improve their eyes naturally without glasses. They include *Dr. Friedman's Vision Training Program*, *Lisette Scholl's Visionetics: The Holistic Way to Better Eyesight*, *Taber's Eye-Robics*, and *Dr. Salov's Hidden Secrets for Better Vision*. Similar claims are made on the website of the American Vision Institute (AVI), which markets the See Clearly Method "to help you eliminate or reduce" nearsightedness, farsightedness, astigmatism, presbyopia, and eyestrain. The program is based on Bates and other vision training methods. The See Clearly claims are peppered with "may" and "it depends" and supported by testimonials preceded by the disclaimer "Results not typical; individual results will vary." The first sentence of the See Clearly research page states that "No formal research studies have been done yet on the See Clearly

Method." This is despite the fact that AVI, founded in 1979, describes itself as "dedicated to research." All of these programs are long on claims and short on evidence that any of them will actually improve the user's vision.

Dubious Diagnosis

Iridology is based on the notion that each area of the body is represented by a corresponding area in the iris of the eye (the colored area surrounding the pupil). Iridologists claim that states of health and disease can be diagnosed according to the color, texture, and location of various pigment flecks in the eye. Iridology practitioners purport to diagnose imbalances and treat them with vitamins, minerals, herbs, and similar products. They may also claim that the eye markings can reveal a complete history of past illnesses as well as previous treatment.

Most iridology practitioners are chiropractors and naturopaths, but laypersons who do nutrition counseling also are involved. Bernard Jensen, D.C., the leading American iridologist, states that "Nature has provided us with a miniature television screen showing the most remote portions of the body by way of nerve reflex responses." He also claims that iridology analyses are more reliable and "offer much more information about the state of the body than do the examinations of Western medicine." However, in two large studies, Jensen and seven other prominent iridologists could not distinguish between patients who had kidney or gallbladder disease and those who were healthy. Nor did they agree with each other about which was which.[16,17] This is not surprising, because there is no known way that body organs could be represented at specific locations in the iris.

Other Unproved Method

Pressing on the eyes or surrounding bones has been a perennial favorite for all manner of eye disease. John Quincy Adams once wrote a paper claiming this method could return the "convexity of youth" and eliminate the need for reading glasses. Small eye-stones placed under the lids were popular until the early 1900s. Chiropractors who use "craniopathy" or "neural organization technique" claim that vision and eye coordination can be improved by manipulating (adjusting) the eyes and skull. Current devices include the Natural Eye Normalizer for massaging the eyelids, and a pneumatic bag for placement over the head to cure all visual problems.

The use of color to treat various ailments, including those affecting the eye, has been promoted for many years. Edwin Babbit popularized the use of colored light with his book *The Principles of Light and Color: The Healing Power of Color* published in 1878. Today's practice of syntonics—also called photoretinology—evolved from these theories. Its practitioners use expensive machines to direct various pulsating colored lights into the eyes, claiming to cure optical errors, eye coordination problems, and even general health problems! There is no scientific evidence to support these claims.

Another approach involving color has been popularized by Helen Irlen, a marriage, family, and child counselor, who has appeared on CBS-TV's *60 Minutes* and franchised more than 2,000 individuals and clinics nationwide since 1983. She claims that scotopic sensitivity syndrome is a leading cause of learning problems and affects 65% of those with reading problems (dyslexia), and can be remedied with colored eyeglasses. Her recommended diagnosis and treatment can cost more than $500. I do not believe that Irlen's theory or claimed success rates have been scientifically substantiated. Although more than 50 studies of her methods have been reported, many have methodologic flaws such as lack of a control group and the results do not give a clear consensus.[18,19] One study finds that "lens color was not a critical diagnostic factor" just a reduction in contrast was important.[20] Poor test-retest reliability has been reported raising questions about diagnostic methods.[21] Another study reports an increase in comprehension but not reading rate, but a control group with symptoms was not included.[22] Another reports modest gains in both (12% in rate and 7% in comprehension),[23] and yet another well designed study produced no change in rate, accuracy or comprehension.[24] Several studies suggest that inexpensive blue tinted overlays may be beneficial.[23,25] Some studies question the prevalence of scotopic sensitivity syndrome when other factors are ruled out.[26,27]

Overall, these studies indicate that fewer than 5% of readers who experience discomfort benefit from a change in contrast, brightness, or color on the page beyond what would be expected from a placebo treatment alone. Remember that even if a treatment makes the print more comfortable to look at, proper reading instruction is still needed to improve reading skills.

Several entrepreneurs have marketed pyramid or pinhole glasses consisting of opaque material with multiple slits or perforations. The technology involved has been known for centuries and was used before glass lenses were invented. Light passing through a small hole (or holes) is restricted to rays coming straight from the viewed object;

these rays do not need focusing to bring them to a point. Modern promoters claim their products are better than conventional lenses. Actually, both reduce the focus effort needed to read, but pinhole glasses are much less useful because they restrict contrast, brightness, and the field of view.[28] Worn as sunglasses, they can even be harmful because the holes allow damaging ultraviolet rays to reach the eye.

Regulatory Actions

In 1992, the Missouri Attorney General obtained a consent injunction and penalties totaling $20,000 against a New York company that sold aerobic glasses. These glasses, which sold for $19.95 plus postage and handling, had black plastic lenses with tiny holes. The company's ads had falsely claimed that its "Aerobic Training Eyeglass System exercises and relaxes the eye muscles through use of scientifically designed and spaced 'pin dot' openings that change the way light enters the eye." The company had also advertised that continued wear and exercises should enable eyeglass wearers to change to weaker prescription lenses and reduce the need for bifocals or trifocals.

In 1997, the FTC obtained a consent agreement banning misleading claims optometrists were making for orthokeratology devices and Precise Corneal Molding (PCM) services, which involved the use of a series of contact lenses purportedly to reshape the cornea gradually for the treatment of nearsightedness, farsightedness, and astigmatism. No such device can permanently reshape the cornea.

In 1997, Richard C. Davis, Jr., M.D., opened RheoTherapyCenters of Tampa Bay, Florida (a subsidiary of OccuLogix Corporation) which offered a "revolutionary" treatment for age-related macular degeneration (AMD) of the eye. AMD is a disease in which pathologic changes in the macula result in loss or reduction of central vision. It is a leading cause of vision loss in the elderly. Laser coagulation may slow progression of the disease, but there is no known cure. Occulogix advertised that rheotherapy "removes toxic proteins and fatty substances" from the blood, thereby allowing increased blood flow to the macula; and a clinic videotape stated that rheotherapy had been shown to be effective in the vast majority of patients with macular degeneration who had undergone the treatment. A few months later, the Florida Board of Medicine concluded that (a) these claims were unsubstantiated, (b) the procedure was "experimental," and (c) Davis's practice constituted "an immediate and serious danger to the health, safety and welfare of the public."[26] However, while the Board continued to investigate, Davis was permitted to continue offering the treatment so long as patients were informed that it was experimental. In 1999, RheoTherapy Centers was closed and Davis signed a consent agreement with the Board under which he agreed to: (a) pay an administrative fine of $10,000, (b) perform 50 hours of community service, and (c) not to provide apheresis or any other clinical services for AMD (except within the context of an FDA-approved clinical trial) unless and until such treatment is cleared by the FDA.[27] OccuLogix Corporation has abandoned the term rheotherapy and is sponsoring an FDA-approved clinical trial of a plasma filtration process it calls Rheopheresis, which differs from the procedure Davis used.

Stick with Proven Treatment

There is one rational method of eye training and eye exercises—orthoptics—carried out under competent optometric and medical supervision to correct coordination or binocular vision problems such as crossed eyes and amblyopic (lazy) eyes. If the muscles that control eye movements are out of balance, the function of one eye may be suppressed to avoid double vision. (The suppressed eye is called an amblyopic eye.) Covering the good eye can often stimulate the amblyopic eye to work again to provide binocular vision for the patient. Orthoptics, surgery, or a combination of the two often can improve problems in pointing and focusing the eyes due to poor eye-muscle control.

Remember: no type of eye exercise can improve a refractive error or cure any ailment within the eyeball or in any remote part of the body. If you are considering a vision training program, request a written report detailing the problem, the proposed treatment plan, an estimate of the time and costs involved, and the prognosis. If the plan is not targeted toward a specific visual problem (such as amblyopia), or if it includes a broad promise such as improving IQ, forget about it. If you are not sure what to do, invest in a second opinion, preferably from a university-affiliated practitioner.

References

1. Pollack P. *The Truth about Eye Exercises*. Philadelphia: Chilton Co., 1956, Chapter 3.

2. Kavale K, Mattson P.D. "One Jumped Off The Balance Beam": Meta-analysis of Perceptual-motor Training. *Journal of Learning Disabilities* 16:165-174, 1983.

3. Keogh BK and Pelland, M. Vision training revisited. *Journal of Learning Disabilities* 18:228-235, 1985.

4. Koller H. Is vision therapy quackery. *Review of Ophthalmology* March:38-49, 1998.

5. Solan HA. In support of vision therapy. *Review of Ophthalmology* March:44-45, 1998.

6. Keech RV. Symposium: Near Vision and Reading Disorders. *American Orthoptic Journal* 49:1-47, 1999

7. Adams MJ. *Beginning to Read: Thinking and Learning about Print*. Cambridge: MIT Press, 1994.

8. McGuinness D. *A Scientific Revolution in Reading: Why Our Children Can't Read*. New York: Simon & Schuster, 1999.

9. Shaywitz SE. Dyslexia. *Scientific American* Nov: 98-104, 1996.

10. Richardson SO. Historical perspectives on dyslexia. *Journal of Learning Disabilities* 25:40-47, 1992.

11. Worrall RS. Reading disability: a discussion of visual, auditory and linguistic factors. *Journal of the American Optometric Association* 57:60-64, 1986.

12. Worrall RS. Detecting health fraud in the field of learning disabilities. *Journal of Learning Disabilities* 23:207-212, 1990.

13. Berstein AL. Could you succeed in this specialty? *Review of Optometry*, March: 23-24, 1988.

14. Calef T and others. Comparisons of eye movements before and after a speed-reading course. *Journal of the American Optometric Association* 70:60-64, 1999.

15. Peters, HB. The influence of orthoptic training on reading ability. *Archives of the American Academy of Optometry* 19:95-176, 1942.

16. Simon A and others. An evaluation of iridology. *JAMA* 242:1385-1387, 1979.

17. Knipschild P. Looking for gall bladder disease in the patient's iris. *British Medical Journal* 297:1578-1581, 1988.

18. Robinson GL. Coloured Lenses and Reading: A Review of Research into Reading Achievement, Reading Strategies and Causal Mechanisms. *Australian Journal of Special Education* 18(1):3-14, 1994.

19. Cardinal DN, Griffin JR, Christenson,GN. Do Tinted Lenses Really Help Students with Reading Disabilities? *Intervention in School and Clinic* 28:275-279, 1993.

20. Spafford CS and others. Contrast sensitivity differences between proficient and disabled readers using colored filters. *Journal of Learning Disabilities* 28:240-252, 1995.

21. Woerz M, Maples, WC. Test-retest reliability of colored filter testing. *Journal of Learning Disabilities* 30:214-221, 1997.

22. Robinson GL, Foreman, PJ. Scotopic Sensitivity/Irlen Syndrome and the use of coloured filters: A long-term placebo controlled and masked study of reading achievement and perception ability. *Perceptual Motor Skills*, 89:83-113, 1999.

23. Solan HA and others. Eye movement efficiency in normal and reading disabled elementary school children: effects of varying luminance and wavelength. *Journal of the American Optometric Association* 69:455-464, 1998.

24. Gole, GA and others.Tinted lenses and dyslexia—A controlled study. *Australian and New Zealand Journal of Ophthalmology* 17:137-141, 1989.

25. Williams MC, LeCluyse K, Rock-Faucheux A. Effective intervention for reading disability. *Journal of the American Optometric Association* 63:411-417, 1992.

26. McNamara, R. Detecting children who will benefit from treatment in an orthoptic clinic for specific learning difficulties. *British Orthoptic Journal* 56:22-30, 1999.

27. Scheiman, M and others. Vision characteristics of individuals identified as Irlen Filter candidates. *Journal of the American Optometric Association* 61:600-605, 1990.

28. Wittenberg S. Pinhole eyewear systems: A special report. *Journal of the American Optometric Association* 64:112-116, 1993.

29.   State of Florida Department of Health. In re: Emergency restriction of the license of Richard Clair Davis, Jr., M.D., Case No. 97-13662, filed Jan 27, 1998.

30.   Consent agreement. Florida Department v. Richard Clair Davis, Jr., M.D. Signed July 1, 1999.

This article was updated from a corresponding chapter in *The Health Robbers: A Close Look at Quackery in America*. Dr. Worrall, who practices optometry in Colfax, California, is assistant clinical professor at the School of Optometry, University of California, Berkeley, and is a board member of the National Council Against Health Fraud. Dr. Nevyas, now deceased, taught biochemistry at the Pennsylvania College of Optometry and edited scientific publications. The sections on iridology and regulatory actions were added by Dr. Barrett.

Part Three

Age-Related Eye Problems

Chapter 21

Trends in Vision in Older Americans

Overview

For the elderly, sensory impairments increase vulnerability and limit the quality of life. Dimming eyesight and failing hearing can reduce physical, functional, emotional, and social well-being. Visual and hearing impairments decrease independence in performing the activities of daily living, getting from place to place, or communicating with others. Isolation, depression, and poorer social relationships often accompany sight and hearing loss.[1-3]

Older persons are disproportionately affected by sensory impairments. Although those 65 and over make up only 12.8 percent of the U.S. population, they account for roughly 37 percent of all hearing-impaired individuals and 30 percent of all visually-impaired individuals. Moreover, nearly 37 percent of all visits to physicians' offices for eye care are made by persons 65 years of age and older.

This chapter explores the levels of vision and hearing impairments among the elderly, the changes in those levels over the last decade, common devices and procedures used to reduce the impact of these impairments, and the potential for future reductions.

Older Americans can expect to live longer than ever before. Under existing conditions, women who live to age 65 can expect to live

"Trends in Vision and Hearing among Older Americans," By Mayur Desai, Ph.D., Laura A. Pratt, Ph.D., Harold Lentzner, Ph.D., Kristen N. Robinson, Ph.D., National Center for Health Statistics, Centers for Disease Control and Prevention, *Aging Trends*, No. 2, March 2001.

about 19 years longer, men about 16 years longer. Whether the added years at the end of the life cycle are healthy, enjoyable, and productive depends, in part, upon preventing and controlling a number of chronic diseases and conditions.

This chapter is one of a series undertaken by the National Center for Health Statistics, with support from the National Institute on Aging, to help meet the challenge of extending and improving life. By monitoring the health of the elderly, using information compiled from a variety of sources, we hope to help focus research on the most effective ways to use resources and craft health policy.

Visual Impairment Limits the Elderly

Visual impairment is an important cause of activity limitation and disability among the elderly. Approximately 1.8 million non-institutionalized elderly report some difficulty with basic activities such as bathing, dressing, and walking around the house, in part because they are visually impaired. Visual impairment increases the risk of falls and fractures, making it more likely that an older person will be admitted to a hospital or nursing home, be disabled, or die prematurely.[4-5]

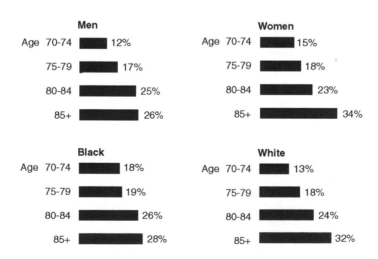

Figure 21.1. Percent of elderly who reported being visually impaired by age, sex, and race, 1995.

Visual Impairment, Defined as Vision Loss That Cannot Be Corrected by Glasses or Contact Lenses Alone, Increased with Age

Prescription lenses were almost universal among older persons. Ninety-two percent of persons 70 years of age and older wore glasses. Eighteen percent also used a magnifying glass for reading and close work. Trouble seeing even when wearing glasses increased steadily, from 14 percent among persons 70 to 74 years of age to 32 percent for those 85 years of age and older. Fewer than 2 percent of persons 70 years of age and older with a visual impairment reported using other equipment to help them overcome their disability such as telescopic lenses, braille, readers, canes, or computer equipment.

The prevalence of blindness also increased with age, reaching its peak at 85 years of age and older. In 1995, the prevalence of blindness in both eyes was about 1 percent among persons 70 to 74 years of age compared with 2.4 percent among those 85 years of age and older. The prevalence of blindness in the population 70 years of age and older changed little between 1984 and 1995. At both points in time, there were no differences in rates of blindness between men and women or between black and white elderly.

Visual Impairment and Blindness Have Four Main Causes: Cataracts, Age-Related Macular Degeneration, Glaucoma, and Diabetic Retinopathy

Cataracts, a clouding of the lens of the eye, are a leading cause of visual impairment in the elderly. According to the National Eye Institute, over half of all Americans aged 65 years and older have cataracts. In the early stages, they do not seriously impair vision. Then as vision begins to worsen, corrective lenses can often be used to improve vision. If vision becomes too impaired, cataract removal surgery is performed. Cataract surgery is one of the most common surgeries performed in America, approximately 1.5 million surgeries per year. Cataract surgery is generally an outpatient procedure and is very successful; 90% of patients have improved vision after recovering from their surgery.

Approximately one-fourth of the noninstitutionalized population 70 years of age and older reported currently having cataracts in 1995. Cataracts were more common among women than men. The number of persons reporting currently having cataracts was similar in 1984 and 1995, 23% and 26% respectively.

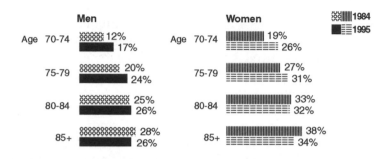

Figure 21.2. *Percent of elderly men and women who reported currently having cataracts, 1984 and 1995.*

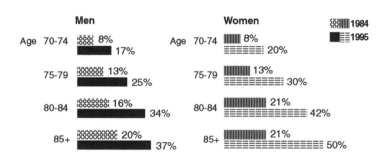

Figure 21.3. *Percent of elderly men and women who reported ever having cataract operations, 1984 and 1995.*

Cataract surgery to reverse the impairment more than doubled between 1984 and 1995. Among the youngest (70 to 74 years of age), the percent who had ever had cataract surgery increased from about 8 percent in 1984 to 18 percent in 1995. In 1995, almost half of those 85 years of age and older reported ever having had cataract surgery, up from about one-fifth a decade earlier. In 1984, the rate of cataract operations was similar for men and women. By 1995, however, women were more likely than men to report having had operations for cataracts.

Age-related macular degeneration (AMD) was the leading cause of irreversible visual impairment in the elderly. More common than either glaucoma or diabetic retinopathy (which will be discussed in the following sections), early or late stage AMD affected roughly one-quarter of persons 70 years of age and older or approximately 3.6 million elderly persons.

As with cataracts, the early stages of the disease may not greatly impair vision. The rate of AMD increased sharply with age, from 18 percent among persons 70 to 74 years of age to 47 percent among persons 85 and older. In the adult population (18 years and older) the prevalence of AMD was similar for black and white persons and for both sexes. For the group 70 years and older, however, AMD was more common in women than in men and in white than in black older persons. Unlike cataracts, the most common potential cause of visual impairment, there is currently no treatment to save the sight of a person with AMD.

Glaucoma was twice as common among black elderly as it was among white elderly. Glaucoma is irreversible damage to the optic nerve caused by increased pressure in the eye. It is an insidious, slow-progressing disease that if left untreated can cause irreversible blindness. In 1984, about 5 percent of the noninstitutionalized elderly population reported having glaucoma. In 1995, the rate had risen to approximately 8 percent. The National Eye Institute (NEI) estimates that half the people who have glaucoma are unaware of their condition.

Older blacks were twice as likely to have glaucoma as older whites (15 percent versus 7 percent). This racial differential, which characterized both men and women, has widened considerably since 1984 when the prevalence rates were 7.5 percent for blacks and 5 percent for whites. The prevalence of glaucoma among elderly black persons doubled in the decade between 1984 and 1995.

Diabetic retinopathy, a complication of diabetes, causes visual impairment and can result in blindness. In contrast to cataracts and

AMD, diabetic retinopathy is not clearly related to advanced age. Almost half of those with AMD were 70 years of age and older, but only 25 percent of persons with diabetic retinopathy were over 70 years of age. Approximately 4 percent of men and 6 percent of women 70 years of age and older had diabetic retinopathy. The prevalence among black elderly 70 years of age and older was 7 percent, while among white elderly of the same age it was 5 percent.

References

1. Keller BK, Morton JL, Thomas VS, Potter JF. The effect of visual and hearing impairments on functional status. *J Am Geriatr Soc*. 47:1319-1325, 1999.

2. Rovner BW, Ganguli M. Depression and disability associated with impaired vision: the MoVIES Project. *J Am Geriatr Soc*. 46:617-619, 1998.

3. Tinetti ME, Inouye SK, Gill TM, Doucette JT. Shared risk factors for falls, incontinence, and functional dependence: unifying the approach to geriatric syndromes. *JAMA*. 273:1348-1353, 1995.

4. Ding YY, Choo P. Epidemiology of falls among the elderly community dwellers in Singapore. *Singapore Med J*. 38:427-431, 1997.

5. Ivers RQ, Cumming RG, Mitchell P, Attebo K. Visual impairment and falls in older adults: the Blue Mountains Eye Study. *J Am Geriatr Soc*. 46:58-64, 1998.

Chapter 22

Saving Your Sight: Early Detection Is Critical

Sometimes eye diseases occur with the natural aging process. Other times, they run in families, in the same way that cancer or heart disease might. Diseases and conditions such as diabetes and high blood pressure also increase the risk for eye problems. The leading causes of irreversible blindness—glaucoma, diabetic retinopathy, and macular degeneration—tend to come on silently, without pain or other symptoms in the earliest stages. The later an eye problem is diagnosed, the harder it becomes to treat. In some cases, any vision that has slipped away may be gone forever.

Experts say that skipping regular and thorough eye exams is chief among the barriers to early detection. It's important to have your eyes regularly checked through dilated pupils so doctors can get a good three-dimensional view of the optic nerve and retina. For a dilated exam, an eye specialist places drops in the eye to enlarge the pupils. "Without dilating the eye, it's like looking inside a room through a keyhole instead of an open door," according to George Blankenship, M.D., immediate past president of the American Academy of Ophthalmology (AAO).

Also problematic is the tendency to ignore symptoms when they do present themselves, says Lee R. Duffner, M.D., an ophthalmologist in Hollywood, Florida. "It's not uncommon to see patients who say they've been having eye problems for a whole year before coming in

"Saving Your Sight—Early Detection Is Critical," by Michelle Meadows, *FDA Consumer*, U.S. Food and Drug Administration, April 2002.

to get checked—usually because of a spouse or other relative who encouraged them to come in."

Here's a look at four eye diseases you can't afford to miss.

Glaucoma

The Problem

It's not known why, but people with glaucoma typically experience an imbalance in eye fluid production and drainage. Fluid that normally flows in and out of the eye drains too slowly. As that fluid builds up, pressure in the eyeball increases and becomes abnormally high, a condition that can damage the optic nerve, the retina, or other parts of the eye.

It's important to note that there are also patients with glaucoma who actually have what would be considered normal eye pressure, says Sheryl Berman, M.D., a medical officer in the Food and Drug Administration's division of ophthalmic and ear, nose, and throat devices. "This is why it is so critical to have dilated examinations, since routine pressure screening would miss the diagnosis of glaucoma in these eyes." For these people, there are other factors at play that may lead to optic nerve damage.

If glaucoma is left untreated, blindness is likely. The most common form of glaucoma is primary open-angle glaucoma, also known as chronic glaucoma. Nearly 3 million Americans have glaucoma, according to the National Eye Institute (NEI), and about half do not know it. That's because glaucoma is a silent stealer of sight; there are usually no symptoms in the early stages. As the disease progresses, people with glaucoma may notice their side (peripheral) vision failing. But by this time, the disease is usually quite advanced and the damage is irreversible. Once vision is lost, it can't be restored. Glaucoma usually affects both eyes, one shortly after the other.

Ida Miggins, 52, a computer specialist from Takoma Park, Maryland, says she learned she had glaucoma three years ago by chance. She hadn't had an eye exam since childhood and hadn't noticed any vision problems. "I was actually taking my mother to her eye appointment, and the doctor suggested that I be checked too," says Miggins. The doctor diagnosed glaucoma in both eyes.

Risk Factors

Early detection is the best way to control glaucoma and prevent major vision loss. Elevated pressure in the eye is the major risk factor for glaucoma. Other risk factors associated with the disease include having high blood pressure, diabetes, and certain diseases that affect blood vessels. A family history of the disease, aging, and African ancestry also increase your risk for glaucoma.

Studies have shown that for unknown reasons, glaucoma presents at an earlier age in blacks, is five times more likely to occur in blacks than in whites, and is about four times more likely to cause blindness in blacks than whites.

Miggins, who is black, says she had heard of glaucoma. "But I didn't have a clue what it was, nor did I think I was at risk for it because it doesn't run in my family."

If you are in any of the high-risk groups for glaucoma—everyone over age 60, those with a family history of the disease, and blacks over age 40—you should get a complete eye exam at least every two years.

Treatment

Though glaucoma is not curable, there are treatments that successfully lower pressure in the eye. The first line of treatment is drugs, and whether you're prescribed eye drops or pills, taking your drugs as prescribed is critical.

The development of several classes of medications to reduce pressure in the eye has allowed for more effective treatment over time, says Wiley Chambers, M.D., deputy director of the FDA's division of anti-inflammatory, analgesic and ophthalmic drug products. For now, glaucoma medications only tackle eye pressure, says Chambers. "We're looking for treatments that can also protect the optic nerve."

Miggins says the first medication she took caused bleeding gums and eye pain. Some side effects may lessen over time, but be sure to report them to your doctor because it could be that the drug or dose needs to be changed.

In March 2001, the FDA approved two new drugs to treat elevated eye pressure, Lumigan (bimatoprost ophthalmic solution), marketed by Allergan Inc. of Irvine, Calif., and Travatan (travoprost ophthalmic solution), marketed by Alcon Laboratories Inc. of Fort Worth, Texas. These medications provide alternatives for people who are intolerant or unresponsive to other drugs and who otherwise may need surgery. Potential side effects of these two drugs include gradual darkening of eye color and darkening of eyelid skin.

When glaucoma can't be controlled with medication, doctors may turn to laser surgery in which a focused beam of light creates openings in the part of the eye where fluid drains to make draining easier.

The next line of treatment is a surgical procedure called trabeculectomy, in which a small opening is made in the front chamber of the eye to make a new pathway from which fluid can drain. Even with surgery, many patients who have glaucoma still need medication.

For those with very advanced disease, or when conventional medical and surgical treatments have failed to control the disease, glaucoma may be treated with a drainage device, a little plastic tube. These devices are surgically implanted to create a new drainage pathway. In July 2001, the FDA approved the AquaFlow Collagen Glaucoma Drainage Device from STAAR Surgical Company in Monrovia, Calif., to manage open-angle glaucoma. A small cylinder made of collagen is implanted in the eye to absorb excess fluid. The device is designed to maintain a space under the white part of the eye, and it slowly dissolves in the eye until it's completely absorbed within nine months, leaving behind a drainage route for the fluid.

Age-Related Macular Degeneration (AMD)

The Problem

The cause is unknown, but AMD occurs when light-sensing cells in the macula break down. The macula is the central part of the retina and is responsible for clear, sharp vision.

About 90 percent of people with AMD have what's known as the dry type, and the remaining 10 percent have the wet type. The wet type of AMD is more severe and causes the most vision loss. In the dry type, the light-sensitive vision cells deteriorate but there is no bleeding. In the wet type of AMD, new blood vessels grow and leak blood and fluid under the macula. For some people with the disease, vision is affected very slowly. But for others, the disease progresses rapidly over the course of weeks to months.

"Macular degeneration rarely leads to complete blindness, but often causes severe and irreversible loss of central vision," says Stuart L. Fine, M.D., chairman of the department of ophthalmology at the University of Pennsylvania. Side vision remains, but the center of vision, which is needed for daily tasks like reading and driving, is destroyed.

About 1.7 million Americans have some form of AMD, according to the National Eye Institute (NEI). It's the leading cause of vision loss among Americans ages 65 and over. The disease is painless, and common symptoms include blurry vision, distorted vision, such as seeing straight lines as crooked or wavy, or a dark, empty area appearing in the center of vision.

Dorothy Borne, 66, a retired food technician from Hahnville, Louisiana, was diagnosed with wet AMD and experienced blurriness in her left eye about three years ago. It presented abruptly because a large quantity of fluid leaked into the macula from abnormal blood vessels.

"When I got to work that morning, I noticed that everything looked blurry," she says. "I didn't know what was wrong."

Risk Factors

Age and a family history of AMD are the biggest risk factors. People over age 60 are at the highest risk, and should get an eye exam at least every two years.

Fine says, "Other risk factors may include smoking, low lifetime intake of dark green leafy vegetables, high blood pressure, and cardiovascular disease. Some epidemiological studies have identified farsightedness and light eye color as risk factors."

According to NEI, women tend to be at greater risk for AMD than men, and whites are much more likely to lose vision from AMD than blacks.

Those at risk should get in the habit of checking their central vision in each eye separately by covering one eye while evaluating the other eye, Fine suggests. It is recommended that some patients keep an Amsler Grid on their refrigerator as a reminder to check their eyes at home. You look at the dot in the center of the grid to see if lines around it appear wavy or distorted, which could be a sign of AMD. Once you have AMD in one eye, there is a roughly 50 percent chance that it could occur in the other eye, so it's important to report any vision changes to your doctor and routinely test the other eye.

Studies have suggested that a diet rich in dark green, leafy vegetables such as spinach and collard or mustard greens lowers the risk of AMD. These foods are a source of nutrients such as vitamin A, vitamin C, and vitamin E. But experts say it's important to recognize that a balanced diet is generally important for eye health, the same way it is for the rest of the body.

Recent NEI research has shown that nutritional supplements—vitamin E, vitamin C, beta carotene, and zinc—may benefit some people who have advanced AMD. The American Academy of Ophthalmology recommends that if you have intermediate or advanced AMD in one eye only, you should talk with your physician about whether nutritional supplements may help you and how to take them safely. Not everybody needs supplements. For example, in large quantities, zinc can be toxic. Beta-carotene can increase the risk of lung cancer in smokers. High-dose nutrients can also interfere with medications and decrease the absorption of other nutrients into the body.

Treatment

"For the dry form of AMD there is no specific treatment other than low vision rehabilitation, which shouldn't be underestimated," says Fine.

The biggest advance in AMD treatment so far was the approval in April 2000 of Visudyne (verteporfin for injection) for treatment of the classic type of wet AMD. About half of those with wet AMD have the classic type. Visudyne is manufactured by QLT Photo Therapeutics Inc., Seattle, and marketed by Novartis Ophthalmics, Duluth, Georgia.

Visudyne can't restore vision that's been lost, but it can slow the loss of vision from AMD. It's injected into the patient's arm and it travels to the abnormal blood vessels in the eye. Then a laser is aimed at the patient's eye for a little over a minute to activate the drug. The drug works to stop or slow blood leakage. Common side effects include light sensitivity and reactions at the injection site.

Some cases of wet AMD can be treated with laser surgery. Again, lost vision usually can't be restored, but the laser aims a light beam onto new blood vessels to destroy them to preserve what central vision remains. Borne had laser surgery immediately and ended up having several more surgeries in the span of a few months, which left her with some scarring in the eye. "She needed the surgeries because some of the blood vessels around the macula continued to bleed," says Monica L. Monica, M.D., Borne's doctor and an ophthalmologist in New Orleans.

In the end, the laser surgeries stopped the bleeding. "If the hemorrhage isn't stopped, there could be even more extensive loss of vision than just central vision," Monica says.

Borne has lost central vision in her left eye, but still has side vision in that eye and can grossly see large objects like cars.

Borne, who can still see clearly out of her right eye, says, "I can read, just not for very long. After a while, words start jumbling together." She knows that if her right eye bothers her, day or night, she should call her doctor right away. "I just hope my right eye will stay OK," she says.

Cataracts

The Problem

Cataracts are areas that distort light as it passes through the lens of the eye (opacities). The most common type of cataract is age-related.

As we get older, protein in the lens of our eyes can clump together and cloud the lens, which is located behind the iris and the pupil. The lens is responsible for focusing light and producing sharp images.

Cataracts form slowly and typically cause no pain. In late 2000, David Guillot, 65, a retired aerospace engineer from Covington, Louisiana, noticed blurry vision. "I couldn't make out road signs even with my glasses on," he says. Shortly after, he was diagnosed with cataracts in both eyes. In addition to blurriness, common symptoms of cataracts are reduced night vision, problems with glare, frequent eyeglass prescription changes, impaired depth perception, and color distortion. Cataracts usually occur in both eyes.

Risk Factors

Anyone can get cataracts, but it's for those over 60 that cataracts are most likely to interfere with vision. Cataracts can result from natural aging of the lens, but also can occur as a result of eye injury. An eye exam at least every two years is recommended for those over 60.

Some studies suggest that exposure to bright sunlight over several years may lead to cataracts, while other studies refute this, says Walter J. Stark, M.D., professor of ophthalmology at The Johns Hopkins University School of Medicine in Baltimore and director of the corneal and cataract services at the Wilmer Eye Institute. "The recommendation is that if one is outside a lot, say because of occupation, it may help to wear sunglasses that block ultraviolet rays," Stark says. "It won't hurt." Your sunglasses should offer 100 percent or nearly total UV protection. Wide-brimmed hats can also help block sunlight.

People with diabetes are at higher risk for cataracts, and smoking is a suspected risk factor. "It appears that smoking generally makes things worse when it comes to the eyes," Stark says. Taking corticosteroids for other medical conditions also can cause cataracts.

It had been believed that certain vitamins, such as vitamin C, might affect cataracts, but recent research has shown that nutritional supplements do not appear to prevent cataracts or keep them from getting worse.

Treatment

For some people with cataracts, a stronger eyeglass prescription may be all that's needed. Keep up with regular eye appointments and talk with your doctor about how the cataracts affect your ability to work, read, and take part in other routine activities.

When cataracts interfere with daily activities, surgery may be recommended to remove the clouded lens and replace it with a new, artificial one. Monica says it's probably the most satisfying operation for an eye doctor and patient. Cataract surgery has an overall success rate of about 98 percent. According to NEI, it's the most frequently performed surgery in the United States, with over 1.5 million cataract surgeries performed each year.

Like any eye surgery, there are risks such as eye infection and swelling. "Cystoid macular edema is an uncommon complication of cataract surgery that causes swelling and blurry vision," says FDA's Berman.

The most common complication is formation of a secondary opacification (known as posterior capsular opacification) behind the new lens implant, Berman says. "This is treated with a laser that creates an opening through which clear vision is regained."

Just 10 years ago, cataract surgery required a hospital stay of several days. Now, the surgery can sometimes be done in less than 30 minutes on an outpatient basis. Guillot says his surgery took about 20 minutes and he went home that day. He had a cataract removed from one eye in June 2001, and had eye surgery on the second eye about three weeks later. His doctor broke up his cataracts with a high-frequency ultrasound. "I can see much better," Guillot says. "I can read the newspaper, watch TV, and I notice a big difference when I'm on the Internet. Sometimes I don't even need my glasses."

Advances in lens technology have improved cataract surgery over the last several years. "New lens materials, such as soft silicone, acrylic, and hydrogels, are more flexible and foldable," Berman says. "They permit surgery through smaller incisions and some appear to have lower rates of secondary opacification formation." And multifocal lens designs have been approved that provide both distance and near vision, so that reading glasses may not always be necessary. "Future advances might come," Berman says, "as a result of research on lens materials able to form a new lens within the eye itself."

Diabetic Retinopathy

The Problem

When diabetes is uncontrolled, chronic high blood sugar levels can damage the blood vessels that feed the retina of the eye. In nonproliferative diabetic retinopathy (NPDR), an early stage of diabetic eye disease, the blood vessels may leak fluid. This may cause the retina to swell and vision to blur, a condition called diabetic macular edema. In what's known as advanced or proliferative diabetic retinopathy (PDR), abnormal new blood vessels grow on the surface of the retina. The abnormal blood vessels don't supply the retina with normal blood flow, and in addition may eventually pull on the retina and cause detachment.

Diabetic retinopathy is the leading cause of new cases of blindness, accounting for about 8,000 cases each year. It's the most common and serious threat to vision that people with diabetes face. Nearly half of all people with diabetes eventually develop some degree of diabetic retinopathy. It usually occurs in both eyes. There may be no early signs of the disease. More advanced cases may be signaled by floaters, blurred vision, eye pain, or gradual vision loss.

Experts say the rate of diabetic retinopathy is likely to get worse because the number of people with diabetes is increasing. About 16 million people have diabetes and many don't know it. In one recent National Institutes of Health study of Mexican-Americans over age 40, 23 percent of those who didn't know they had diabetes also had early to moderate diabetic retinopathy.

Risk Factors

Uncontrolled diabetes is the prime risk factor for retinopathy. Diabetic retinopathy can usually be managed with a combination of tight blood sugar control, appropriate exercise and diet, and early detection. People who are diagnosed with diabetes before age 30 should begin having dilated exams every year beginning five years after diagnosis. All others with diabetes should have an eye exam every year. A recent study in the AAO's journal *Ophthalmology* showed that more than one-third of Americans with diabetes don't get a yearly dilated exam as recommended, putting them at risk for vision loss.

Treatment

Some cases of diabetic retinopathy can be treated with laser surgery that aims a strong beam of light onto the retina to shrink or seal leaking or abnormal vessels. But it can't restore vision already lost, which is why early detection is important. In some advanced cases of PDR, a vitrectomy is recommended, in which the surgeon removes the vitreous portion of the eye and replaces it with a clear solution.

Josephine Grant, 54, a former cafeteria worker from Gaithersburg, Maryland, says she had diabetes for several years and then experienced major vision loss seven years ago because of diabetic retinopathy. She is blind in her right eye, and can see a little bit with the left eye. Unfortunately, Grant came to treatment with an advanced form of the disease, which made her prognosis poor, says T. S. Melki, M.D., the Maryland ophthalmologist who performed Grant's surgeries.

If laser surgery is done in time, he says, the disease can be stopped or slowed. Melki says hundreds of patients with diabetes come see him regularly, sometimes as frequently as every four to five months, so that the level of diabetic retinopathy can be followed closely. "If a patient has minimal disease then the follow-up is less frequent," Melki says. "There are some patients we refer to as 'The Golden Club,' who have had diabetes for over 20 years with no effect on the eye," he says. "So it can be done."

Free and Low-Cost Eye Screenings

EyeCare America-National Eye Care Project is a program of the American Academy of Ophthalmology to provide free or low-cost eye exams. Those who are eligible are people who are 65 or older, U.S. citizens, not in a health maintenance organization, not receiving care through the armed forces or Department of Veterans Affairs, and who haven't seen an ophthalmologist in the last three years. Call (800) 222-EYES [(800) 222-3937].

Volunteers in Service in Our Nation (VISION) USA is a program to give free eye care to uninsured, low-income workers and their families, sponsored by the American Optometric Association. Eligibility requirements may vary by state. But generally, participants must have a job or live in a household where there is one working member, have no vision insurance, have income below an established level, and have not had an eye exam in the last two years. The deadline to enroll for free services in 2002 just passed. In January 2003, you can call (800) 766-4466. The toll-free line is only operational during January of each year.

Chapter 23

Cataract

Chapter Contents

Section 23.1

Facts about Cataract

"Facts about Cataract," National Eye Institute, available online at
http://www.nei.nih.gov, October 2001.

A cataract is a clouding of the eye's lens that can cause vision problems. The most common type is related to aging. More than half of all Americans age 65 and older have a cataract. In the early stages, stronger lighting and eyeglasses may lessen vision problems caused by cataracts. At a certain point, however, surgery may be needed to improve vision. Today, cataract surgery is safe and very effective.

What Is the Lens?

The lens is the part of the eye that helps focus light on the retina. The retina is the eye's light-sensitive layer that sends visual signals to the brain. In a normal eye, light passes through the lens and gets focused on the retina. To help produce a sharp image, the lens must remain clear.

What Is a Cataract?

The lens is made mostly of water and protein. The protein is arranged to let light pass through and focus on the retina. Sometimes some of the protein clumps together. This can start to cloud small areas of the lens, blocking some light from reaching the retina and interfering with vision. This is a cataract.

In its early stages, a cataract may not cause a problem. The cloudiness may affect only a small part of the lens. However, over time, the cataract may grow larger and cloud more of the lens, making it harder to see. Because less light reaches the retina, your vision may become dull and blurry. A cataract won't spread from one eye to the other, although many people develop cataracts in both eyes.

Although researchers are learning more about cataracts, no one knows for sure what causes them. Scientists think there may be several causes, including smoking, diabetes, and excessive exposure to sunlight.

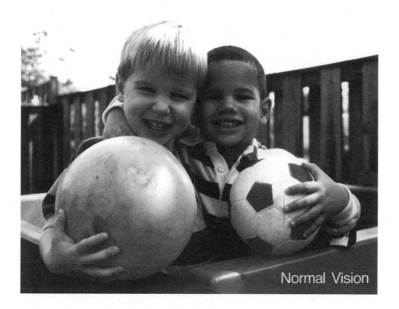

Figure 23.1. *View of boys by person with normal vision.*

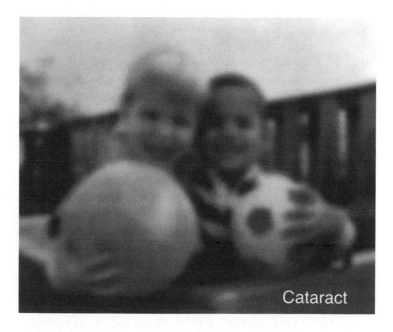

Figure 23.2. *View of boys by person with cataracts.*

What Are the Symptoms?

The most common symptoms of a cataract are:

- Cloudy or blurry vision.

- Problems with light. These can include headlights that seem too bright at night; glare from lamps or very bright sunlight; or a halo around lights.

- Colors that seem faded.

- Poor night vision.

- Double or multiple vision (this symptom often goes away as the cataract grows).

- Frequent changes in your eyeglasses or contact lenses.

These symptoms can also be a sign of other eye problems. If you have any of these symptoms, check with your eye care professional.

When a cataract is small, you may not notice any changes in your vision. Cataracts tend to grow slowly, so vision gets worse gradually. Some people with a cataract find that their close-up vision suddenly improves, but this is temporary. Vision is likely to get worse again as the cataract grows.

What Are the Different Types of Cataract?

- *Age-related cataract*: Most cataracts are related to aging.

- *Congenital cataract*: Some babies are born with cataracts or develop them in childhood, often in both eyes. These cataracts may not affect vision. If they do, they may need to be removed.

- *Secondary cataract*: Cataracts are more likely to develop in people who have certain other health problems, such as diabetes. Also, cataracts are sometimes linked to steroid use.

- *Traumatic cataract*: Cataracts can develop soon after an eye injury, or years later.

How Is a Cataract Detected?

To detect a cataract, an eye care professional examines the lens. A comprehensive eye examination usually includes:

- *Visual acuity test*: This eye chart test measures how well you see at various distances.

- *Pupil dilation*: The pupil is widened with eye drops to allow your eye care professional to see more of the lens and retina and look for other eye problems.

- *Tonometry*: This is a standard test to measure fluid pressure inside the eye. Increased pressure may be a sign of glaucoma.

Your eye care professional may also do other tests to learn more about the structure and health of your eye.

How Is It Treated?

For an early cataract, vision may improve by using different eyeglasses, magnifying lenses, or stronger lighting. If these measures don't help, surgery is the only effective treatment. This treatment involves removing the cloudy lens and replacing it with a substitute lens.

A cataract needs to be removed only when vision loss interferes with your everyday activities, such as driving, reading, or watching TV. You and your eye care professional can make that decision together. In most cases, waiting until you are ready to have cataract surgery will not harm your eye. If you decide on surgery, your eye care professional may refer you to a specialist to remove the cataract. If you have cataracts in both eyes, the doctor will not remove them both at the same time. You will need to have each done separately.

Sometimes, a cataract should be removed even if it doesn't cause problems with your vision. For example, a cataract should be removed if it prevents examination or treatment of another eye problem, such as age-related macular degeneration or diabetic retinopathy.

Is Cataract Surgery Effective?

Cataract removal is one of the most common operations performed in the United States today. It is also one of the safest and most effective. In about 90 percent of cases, people who have cataract surgery have better vision afterward.

How Is a Cataract Removed?

There are two primary ways to remove a cataract. Your doctor can explain the differences and help determine which is best for you:

- **Phacoemulsification, or phaco.** Your doctor makes a small incision on the side of the cornea, the clear, dome-shaped surface that covers the front of the eye. The doctor then inserts a tiny probe into the eye. This device emits ultrasound waves that soften and break up the cloudy center of the lens so it can be removed by suction. Most cataract surgery today is done by phaco, which is also called small incision cataract surgery.

- **Extracapsular surgery.** Your doctor makes a slightly longer incision on the side of the cornea and removes the hard center of the lens. The remainder of the lens is then removed by suction.

In most cataract surgeries, the removed lens is replaced by an intraocular lens (IOL). An IOL is a clear, artificial lens that requires no care and becomes a permanent part of your eye. With an IOL, you'll have improved vision because light will be able to pass through it to the retina. Also, you won't feel or see the new lens.

Some people cannot have an IOL. They may have problems during surgery, or maybe they have another eye disease. For these people, a soft contact lens may be suggested. For others, glasses that provide powerful magnification may be better.

What Happens before Surgery?

A week or two before surgery, your eye care professional will do some tests. These may include tests to measure the curve of the cornea and the size and shape of the eye. For patients who will receive an IOL, this information helps your doctor choose the right type of IOL. Also, doctors may ask you not to eat or drink anything after midnight the morning of your surgery.

What Happens during Surgery?

When you enter the hospital or clinic, you will be given eye drops to dilate the pupil. The area around your eye will be washed and cleansed.

The operation usually lasts less than 1 hour and is almost painless. Many people choose to stay awake during surgery, while others may need to be put to sleep for a short time. If you are awake, you will have an anesthetic to numb the nerves in and around your eye.

After the operation, a patch will be placed over your eye and you will rest for a while. You will be watched by your medical team to see if there are any problems, such as bleeding. Most people who have cataract surgery can go home the same day. Since you will not be able to drive, make sure you make arrangements for a ride.

What Happens after Surgery?

It's normal to feel itching and mild discomfort for a while after cataract surgery. Some fluid discharge is also common, and your eye may be sensitive to light and touch. If you have discomfort, your eye care professional may suggest a pain reliever every 4 to 6 hours. After 1 to 2 days, even moderate discomfort should disappear. In most cases, healing will take about 6 weeks.

After surgery, your doctor will schedule exams to check on your progress. For a few days after surgery, you may take eye drops or pills to help healing and control the pressure inside your eye. Ask your doctor how to use your medications, when to take them, and what effects they can have. You will also need to wear an eye shield or eyeglasses to help protect the eye. Avoid rubbing or pressing on your eye.

Problems after surgery are rare, but they can occur. These can include infection, bleeding, inflammation (pain, redness, swelling), loss of vision, or light flashes. With prompt medical attention, these problems usually can be treated successfully.

When you are home, try not to bend or lift heavy objects. Bending increases pressure in the eye. You can walk, climb stairs, and do light household chores.

When Will My Vision Be Normal Again?

You can quickly return to many everyday activities, but your vision may be blurry. The healing eye needs time to adjust so that it can focus properly with the other eye, especially if the other eye has a cataract. Ask your doctor when you can resume driving.

If you just received an IOL, you may notice that colors are very bright or have a blue tinge. Also, if you've been in bright sunlight, everything may be reddish for a few hours. If you see these color tinges, it is because your lens is clear and no longer cloudy. Within a few months after receiving an IOL, these colors should go away. And when you have healed, you will probably need new glasses.

What Is an After-Cataract?

Sometimes a part of the natural lens that is not removed during cataract surgery becomes cloudy and may blur your vision. This is called an after-cataract. An after-cataract can develop months or years later.

Unlike a cataract, an after-cataract is treated with a laser. In a technique called YAG laser capsulotomy, your doctor uses a laser beam to make a tiny hole in the lens to let light pass through. This is a painless outpatient procedure.

What Research Is Being Done?

Findings from the NEI-sponsored Age-Related Eye Disease Study (AREDS) showed that high levels of antioxidants and zinc has no significant effect on the development or progression of cataract.

Other research is focusing on new ways to prevent, diagnose, and treat cataracts. In addition, scientists are studying the role of genetics in the development of cataracts.

What Can You Do to Protect Your Vision?

Although we don't know how to protect against cataracts, people over the age of 60 are at risk for many vision problems. If you are age 60 or older, you should have an eye examination through dilated pupils at least every 2 years. This kind of exam allows your eye care professional to check for signs of age-related macular degeneration, glaucoma, cataracts, and other vision disorders.

For more information about cataracts, you may wish to contact:

Agency for Healthcare Research and Quality
2101 E. Jefferson St., Suite 501
Rockville, MD 20852
Phone: (301) 594-1364
Website: http://www.ahrq.gov

American Academy of Ophthalmology
P.O. Box 7424
San Francisco, CA 94120-7424
Phone: (415) 561-8500
Website: http://www.aao.org

American Optometric Association
243 North Lindbergh Blvd.
St. Louis, MO 63141
Phone: (314) 991-4100
Website: http://www.aoa.org

National Eye Institute
2020 Vision Place
Bethesda, MD 20892-3655
Phone: (301) 496-5248
Website: http://www.nei.nih.gov

Prevent Blindness America
500 E. Remington Rd.
Schaumburg, IL 60173
Toll-Free: (800) 331-2020
Phone: (847) 843-2020
Website: http://www.preventblindness.org

For more information about IOLs, contact:

U.S. Food and Drug Administration
5600 Fishers Lane
Rockville, MD 20857-0001
Toll-Free: (888) 463-6332
Website: http://www.fda.gov

Section 23.2

How Can a Cataract Be Treated?

The cataract may need no treatment at all if the vision is only a little blurry. A change in your eyeglass prescription may improve vision for a while. There are no medications, eye drops, exercises, or glasses that will cause cataracts to disappear once they have formed. When you are not able to see well enough to do the things you like to do, cataract surgery should be considered. Surgery is the only way to remove a cataract.

Cataracts cannot be removed with a laser, only through a surgical incision. In cataract surgery, the cloudy lens is removed from the eye. In most cases, the focusing power of the natural lens is restored by replacing it with a permanent intraocular lens implant.

What Can I Expect If I Decide to Have Surgery?

Before Surgery

Once you and your ophthalmologist (eye physician and surgeon) have decided that you will have your cataract removed, a physical examination is necessary so that he or she may be alerted to any special medical risks. Ask your ophthalmologist if you should continue your usual medications. Your eye will be measured to determine the proper power of the intraocular lens that will be placed in your eye during surgery.

The Day of Surgery

Surgery is usually done on an outpatient basis. You may be asked to skip breakfast, depending on the time of your surgery. Upon arrival for surgery, you will be given eye drops, and perhaps medications to help you relax. You will also be given an anesthetic (the type will depend on your particular situation) to numb the surgery site. Though you may see light and movement, you will not be able to see the surgery while it is happening, and will not have to worry about keeping your eye open or closed. The skin around your eye will be thoroughly cleansed, and sterile coverings will be placed around your head. When the operation is over, the surgeon will usually place a shield over your eye. After a short stay in the outpatient recovery area, you will be ready to go home. You should plan to have someone else drive you home.

Following Surgery

You will need to:

- Use the eye drops as prescribed.
- Be careful not to rub or press on your eye.
- Use over-the-counter pain medicine if necessary.
- Avoid very strenuous activities until the eye has healed.
- Continue normal daily activities and moderate exercise.
- Ask your doctor when you can begin driving.
- Wear eyeglasses or shield as advised by your doctor.

How Is the Surgery Done?

Under an operating microscope, a small incision is made into the eye. Microsurgical instruments are used to fragment and suction the cloudy lens from the eye. The back membrane of the lens (called the posterior capsule) is left in place. A plastic intraocular lens implant will be placed inside the eye to replace the natural lens that was removed. The incision is then closed. When stitches are used, they rarely need to be removed.

When Is the Laser Used?

The posterior capsule sometimes turns cloudy several months or years after the original cataract operation. If this blurs your vision, a clear opening can be made painlessly in the center of the membrane with a laser. Laser surgery is never part of the original cataract operation.

Will Cataract Surgery Improve My Vision?

Over 95 percent of cataract surgeries improve vision, but a small number of patients may have problems. Symptoms including infection, bleeding, and swelling or detachment of the retina are some of the more serious complications that may affect your vision. Call your ophthalmologist immediately if you have any of the following symptoms after surgery:

- Pain not relieved by non-prescription pain medication
- Loss of vision
- Nausea, vomiting or excessive coughing
- Injury to the eye

Pre-Existing Conditions

Even if the surgery itself is successful, the eye may still not see as well as you would like. Other problems with the eye, such as macular degeneration (aging of the retina), glaucoma, and diabetic damage may limit vision after surgery.

Even with such problems, cataract surgery may still be worthwhile. If the eye is healthy, the chances are excellent that you will have good vision following removal of your cataract.

Chapter 24

Glaucoma

Chapter Contents

Section 24.1

Facts about Glaucoma

"Facts about Glaucoma," National Eye Institute, available online at
http://www.nei.nih.gov, August 2001.

This chapter is designed to help people with glaucoma and their
families better understand the disease. It describes the causes, symptoms, diagnosis, and treatment of glaucoma. It is mainly about open-
angle glaucoma, the most common kind in the United States.

Glaucoma is a group of diseases that can lead to damage to the
eye's optic nerve and result in blindness.

Open-angle glaucoma, the most common form of glaucoma, affects
about 3 million Americans—half of whom don't know they have it. It
has no symptoms at first. But over the years it can steal your sight.
With early treatment, you can often protect your eyes against serious vision loss and blindness.

What Is the Optic Nerve?

The optic nerve is a bundle of more than 1 million nerve fibers. It
connects the retina, the light-sensitive layer of tissue at the back of
the eye, with the brain. A healthy optic nerve is necessary for good
vision.

How Does Glaucoma Damage the Optic Nerve?

In many people, increased pressure inside the eye causes glaucoma.
In the front of the eye is a space called the anterior chamber. A clear
fluid flows continuously in and out of this space and nourishes nearby
tissues.

The fluid leaves the anterior chamber at the angle where the cornea and iris meet. When the fluid reaches the angle, it flows through
a spongy meshwork, like a drain, and leaves the eye.

Open-angle glaucoma gets its name because the angle that allows
fluid to drain out of the anterior chamber is open. However, for unknown reasons, the fluid passes too slowly through the meshwork

drain. As the fluid builds up, the pressure inside the eye rises. Unless the pressure at the front of the eye is controlled, it can damage the optic nerve and cause vision loss.

Who Is at Risk?

Although anyone can get glaucoma, some people are at higher risk than others. They include:

• Blacks over age 40

• Everyone over age 60

• People with a family history of glaucoma

What Are the Symptoms of Glaucoma?

At first, open-angle glaucoma has no symptoms. Vision stays normal, and there is no pain. As glaucoma remains untreated, people may notice that although they see things clearly in front of them, they miss objects to the side and out of the corner of their eye.

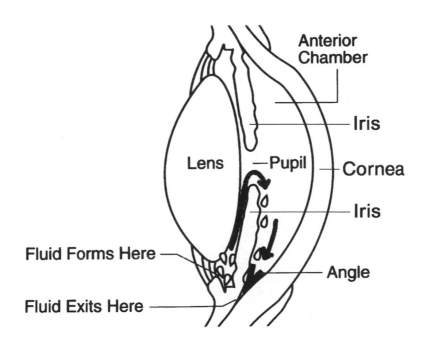

Figure 24.1. Flow of fluid through the anterior chamber.

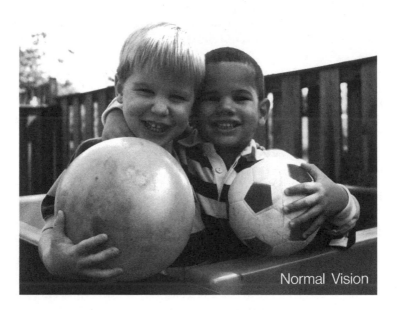

Figure 24.2. *Normal vision.*

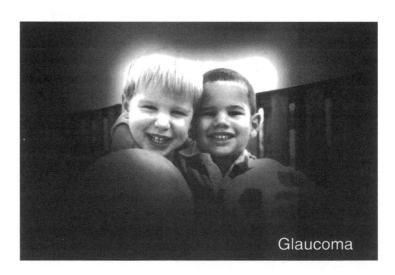

Figure 24.3. *The same scene as it might be viewed by a person with glaucoma.*

Without treatment, people with glaucoma may find that they suddenly have no side vision. It may seem as though they are looking through a tunnel. Over time, the remaining forward vision may decrease until there is no vision left.

How Is Glaucoma Detected?

Most people think that they have glaucoma if the pressure in their eye is increased. This is not always true. High pressure puts you at risk for glaucoma. It may not mean that you have the disease.

Whether or not you get glaucoma depends on the level of pressure that your optic nerve can tolerate without being damaged. This level is different for each person. Although normal pressure is usually between 12-21 mm Hg, a person might have glaucoma even if the pressure is in this range. That is why an eye examination is very important.

To detect glaucoma, your eye care professional will do the following tests:

- *Visual acuity*: This eye chart test measures how well you see at various distances.

- *Visual field*: This test measures your side (peripheral) vision. It helps your eye care professional find out if you have lost side vision, a sign of glaucoma.

- *Pupil dilation*: This examination provides your eye care professional with a better view of the optic nerve to check for signs of damage. To do this, your eye care professional places drops into the eye to dilate (widen) the pupil. After the examination, your close-up vision may remain blurred for several hours.

- *Tonometry*: This standard test determines the fluid pressure inside the eye. There are many types of tonometry. One type uses a purple light to measure pressure. Another type is the air puff test, which measures the resistance of the eye to a puff of air.

Can Glaucoma Be Treated?

Although you will never be cured of glaucoma, treatment often can control it. This makes early diagnosis and treatment important to protect your sight. Most doctors use medications for newly diagnosed glaucoma; however, new research findings show that laser surgery is a safe and effective alternative.

Glaucoma treatments include the following.

Medicine

Medicines are the most common early treatment for glaucoma. They come in the form of eye drops and pills. Some cause the eye to make less fluid. Others lower pressure by helping fluid drain from the eye.

Glaucoma drugs may be taken several times a day. Most people have no problems. However, some medicines can cause headaches or have side effects, which affect other parts of the body. Drops may cause stinging, burning, and redness in the eye. Ask your eye care professional to show you how to put the drops into your eye. In addition, tell your eye care professional about other medications you may be taking before you begin glaucoma treatment.

Many drugs are available to treat glaucoma. If you have problems with one medication, tell your eye care professional. Treatment using a different dosage or a new drug may be possible.

You will need to use the drops and/or pills as long as they help to control your eye pressure. This is very important. Because glaucoma often has no symptoms, people may be tempted to stop or may forget to take their medicine.

Laser Surgery

Laser surgery, also called laser trabeculoplasty, helps fluid drain out of the eye. Although your eye care professional may suggest laser surgery at any time, it is often done after trying treatment with medicines. In many cases, you will need to keep taking glaucoma drugs even after laser surgery.

Laser surgery is performed in an eye care professional's office or eye clinic. Before the surgery, your eye care professional will apply drops to numb the eye.

As you sit facing the laser machine, your eye care professional will hold a special lens to your eye. A high-energy beam of light is aimed at the lens and reflected onto the meshwork inside your eye.

You may see flashes of bright green or red light. The laser makes 50 to 100 evenly spaced burns. These burns stretch the drainage holes in the meshwork. This helps to open the holes and lets fluid drain better through them.

Your eye care professional will check your eye pressure shortly afterward. He or she may also give you some drops to take home for any soreness or swelling inside the eye. You will need to make several follow-up visits to have your pressure monitored.

Once you have had laser surgery over the entire meshwork, further laser treatment may not help. Studies show that laser surgery is very good at getting the pressure down. But its effects sometimes wear off over time. Two years after laser surgery, the pressure increases again in more than half of all patients.

Conventional Surgery

The purpose of surgery is to make a new opening for the fluid to leave the eye. Although your eye care professional may suggest it at any time, this surgery is often done after medicine and laser surgery have failed to control your pressure.

Surgery is performed in a clinic or hospital. Before the surgery, your eye care professional gives you medicine to help you relax and then small injections around the eye to make it numb.

The eye care professional removes a small piece of tissue from the white (sclera) of the eye. This creates a new channel for fluid to drain from the eye. But surgery does not leave an open hole in the eye. The white of the eye is covered by a thin, clear tissue called the conjunctiva. The fluid flows through the new opening, under the conjunctiva, and drains from the eye.

You must put drops in the eye for several weeks after the operation to fight infection and swelling. (The drops will be different than the eye drops you were using before surgery.) You will also need to make frequent visits to your eye care professional. This is very important, especially in the first few weeks after surgery.

In some patients, surgery is about 80 to 90 percent effective at lowering pressure. However, if the new drainage opening closes, a second operation may be needed. Conventional surgery works best if you have not had previous eye surgery, such as a cataract operation.

Keep in mind that while glaucoma surgery may save remaining vision, it does not improve sight. In fact, your vision may not be as good as it was before surgery.

Like any operation, glaucoma surgery can cause side effects. These include cataract, problems with the cornea, inflammation or infection inside the eye, and swelling of blood vessels behind the eye. However, if you do have any of these problems, effective treatments are available.

What Are Some Other Forms of Glaucoma?

Although open-angle glaucoma is the most common form, some people have other forms of the disease.

In low-tension or normal-tension glaucoma, optic nerve damage and narrowed side vision occur unexpectedly in people with normal eye pressure. People with this form of the disease have the same types of treatment as open-angle glaucoma.

In closed-angle glaucoma, the fluid at the front of the eye cannot reach the angle and leave the eye because the angle gets blocked by part of the iris. People with this type of glaucoma have a sudden increase in pressure. Symptoms include severe pain and nausea as well as redness of the eye and blurred vision. This is a medical emergency. The patient needs immediate treatment to improve the flow of fluid. Without treatment, the eye can become blind in as little as one or two days. Usually, prompt laser surgery can clear the blockage and protect sight.

In congenital glaucoma, children are born with defects in the angle of the eye that slow the normal drainage of fluid. Children with this problem usually have obvious symptoms such as cloudy eyes, sensitivity to light, and excessive tearing. Surgery is usually the suggested treatment, because medicines may have unknown effects in infants and be difficult to give to them. The surgery is safe and effective. If surgery is done promptly, these children usually have an excellent chance of having good vision.

Secondary glaucomas can develop as a complication of other medical conditions. They are sometimes associated with eye surgery or advanced cataracts, eye injuries, certain eye tumors, or uveitis (eye inflammation). One type, known as pigmentary glaucoma, occurs when pigment from the iris flakes off and blocks the meshwork, slowing fluid drainage. A severe form, called neovascular glaucoma, is linked to diabetes. Also, corticosteroid drugs—used to treat eye inflammations and other diseases—can trigger glaucoma in a few people. Treatment is with medicines, laser surgery, or conventional surgery.

What Research Is Being Done?

The National Eye Institute (NEI) is the Federal government's lead agency for vision research. The NEI is supporting many research studies both in the laboratory and with patients. This research should provide better ways in the future to detect, treat, and prevent vision loss in people with glaucoma.

For instance, researchers recently found a gene that causes a form of glaucoma that starts at a young age. This is the first glaucoma gene ever located. This finding could help us learn more about how glaucoma damages the eye.

The NEI is also supporting clinical studies that will tell us more about who is likely to get glaucoma, when to treat people with increased pressure, and which treatment to use first.

What Can You Do to Protect Your Vision?

If you are being treated for glaucoma, be sure to take your glaucoma medicine every day and see your eye care professional regularly.

You can also help protect the vision of family members and friends who may be at high risk for glaucoma—blacks over age 40 and everyone over age 60. Encourage them to have an eye examination through dilated pupils every two years.

For more information about glaucoma, you may wish to contact:

American Academy of Ophthalmology
P.O. Box 7424
San Francisco, CA 94120-7424
Phone: (415) 561-8500
Website: http://www.aao.org

American Optometric Association
243 North Lindbergh Blvd.
St. Louis, MO 63141
Phone: (314) 991-4100
Website: http://www.aoa.org

The Glaucoma Foundation
116 John Street
Suite 1605
New York, NY 10038
Phone: (212) 285-0080
E-mail: info@glaucoma-foundation.org
Website: http://www.glaucoma-foundation.org

Glaucoma Research Foundation
200 Pine Street
Suite 200
San Francisco, CA 94104
Toll-Free: (800) 826-6693
Phone: (415) 986-3162
Website: http://www.glaucoma.org

National Eye Institute
2020 Vision Place
Bethesda, MD 20892-3655
Phone: (301) 496-5248
E-mail: 2020@nei.nih.gov
Website: http://www.nei.nih.gov

Prevent Blindness America
500 East Remington Road
Schaumburg, IL 60173
Toll-Free: (800) 331-2020
Phone: (847) 843-2020
Website: http://preventblindness.org

Section 24.2

Who Is at Risk for Glaucoma?

From "Doctor, I Have a Question, Fourth Edition," © The Glaucoma
Foundation. Reprinted with permission. Available online at [http://
www.glaucomafoundation.org/education_content.php?i=12]; cited September 23, 2002.

Everyone should be concerned about glaucoma and its effects. It
is important for each of us, from infants to senior citizens, to have our
eyes checked regularly, because early detection and treatment of glaucoma are the only way to prevent vision impairment and blindness.
There are a few conditions related to this disease that tend to put some
people at greater risk:

- People over the age of 45: While glaucoma can develop in
  younger patients, it occurs more frequently as we get older.

- People who have a family history of glaucoma: Glaucoma appears to run in families. The tendency for developing glaucoma
  may be inherited. However, just because someone in your family

has glaucoma does not mean that you will necessarily develop the disease.

- People with abnormally high intraocular pressure (IOP): High IOP is the most important risk factor for glaucomatous damage.

- People of African descent: African-Americans have a greater tendency for developing primary open-angle glaucoma than do people of other races.

- People who have diabetes, myopia (nearsightedness), regular, long-term steroid/cortisone use, or a previous eye injury are at greater risk.

Section 24.3

Ocular Hypertension

Ocular hypertension is an increase in the pressure in your eyes that is above the range considered normal with no detectable changes in vision or damage to the structure of your eyes. The term is used to distinguish people with elevated pressure from those with glaucoma, a serious eye disease that causes damage to the optic nerve and vision loss.

Ocular hypertension can occur in people of all ages, but it occurs more frequently in African Americans, those over age 40, and those with family histories of ocular hypertension and/or glaucoma. It is also more common in those who are very nearsighted or who have diabetes.

Ocular hypertension has no noticeable signs or symptoms. Your doctor of optometry can check the pressure in your eyes with an instrument called a tonometer and can examine the inner structures of your eyes to assess your overall eye health.

Not all people with ocular hypertension will develop glaucoma. However, there is an increased risk of glaucoma among those with ocular hypertension, so regular comprehensive optometric examinations are essential to your overall eye health.

There is no cure for ocular hypertension, however, careful monitoring and treatment, when indicated, can decrease the risk of damage to your eyes.

Section 24.4

Elevated Risk of Glaucoma among African-Americans

Primary open-angle glaucoma is the leading cause of blindness among African-Americans. It occurs six to eight times more often among African-Americans than Caucasians, and often occurs earlier in life. Studies show that African-Americans between ages 45 and 65 are 14 to 17 times more likely to go blind from glaucoma than Caucasians with glaucoma in the same age group.

The reason for the higher rate of glaucoma and subsequent blindness among African-Americans is still uncertain. Reasons may include:

- a greater susceptibility to damage of the optic nerve (which is the cause of vision loss among those with glaucoma)

- a higher prevalence of earlier onset of intraocular pressure (thought to be a contributory cause of optic nerve damage)

- lower utilization of resources for detection and treatment of glaucoma

African-Americans can protect themselves against vision loss from glaucoma by being aware of their higher risk level for developing the disease, and by having regular eye examinations for glaucoma at appropriate intervals.

The American Academy of Ophthalmology recommends that African-Americans ages 20 to 39 without symptoms for glaucoma have a comprehensive eye examination every three to five years; and African-Americans over 40 have their eyes examined through dilated pupils at least every two years.

Section 24.5

Examination for Glaucoma

Because most people with glaucoma experience no noticeable symptoms, the eye examination for glaucoma is the single most important tool in preventing vision loss from the disease.

Glaucoma can be diagnosed only through a series of tests administered by trained personnel and interpreted by an ophthalmologist. An examination for glaucoma may include:

- History evaluation. The doctor or staff will ask questions about your medical and personal history, as well as your family's medical history.

- Measurement of intraocular pressure (IOP) using an instrument called a tonometer. The tonometer measures IOP using a pressure-sensitive tip placed gently near or against the eye (applanation or Schiotz tonometry), or by directing a brief puff of air gently onto the eye (air puff tonometry). Short-acting anesthetic drops may be used to numb the eye for this procedure.

- Inspection of the drainage angle. The ophthalmologist places a special lens on the eye in order to look at the area between the iris and the cornea to see if it is blocked. This procedure is called gonioscopy.

- Ophthalmoscopy. The ophthalmologist uses drops to dilate (or widen) the pupil so he or she look at the optic nerve using a special instrument called an ophthalmoscope. This allows the ophthalmologist to evaluate any optic nerve damage that may have occurred.

- Perimetry is used to test your visual field. The visual field is the outside area that can be seen by the eye when fixed straight ahead. This test can tell the ophthalmologist how much vision has been lost, even if you notice no impairment.

Some of these tests may not be necessary for every patient, but more tests may be added, or repeated more frequently if glaucoma is suspected or if glaucoma damage increases over time.

Because your eye may be dilated during your exam, you may want to bring sunglasses with you to your appointment. Dilation can make your eyes extra sensitive to light for a short time after your exam.

Everyone should have regular medical eye examinations, but those at risk for glaucoma need to have more frequent exams.

The American Academy of Ophthalmology recommends you have an examination:

- Every 3 to 5 years

  - if you are age 39 or over.

- Every 1 to 2 years

  - if you are age 50 or over
  - if a family member has glaucoma
  - if you are of African ancestry
  - if you have had a serious eye injury in the past
  - if you are taking steroid medication

Remember that early detection and treatment can prevent vision damage.

Section 24.6

Surgery for Glaucoma

For some people, surgery might be the best treatment for glaucoma.
Your ophthalmologist may suggest surgery as a first treatment, or
after trying medication to lower your IOP.

There are several different types of surgery for glaucoma. The kind
of surgery you and your ophthalmologist decide is right for you depends on many factors, including the type and severity of your glaucoma, and other eye problems or health conditions.

Glaucoma surgery may be performed using a laser (a concentrated
beam of light) or conventional surgical instruments.

Laser Surgery

Trabeculoplasty is used most often to treat open-angle glaucoma.
In trabeculoplasty, a laser is used to place spot welds in the drainage
area of the eye—also known as the trabecular meshwork—that allow
the aqueous to drain more freely.

Iridotomy is another kind of laser surgery used in treating glaucoma. It is frequently used to treat angle-closure glaucoma. In this
procedure, the surgeon uses the laser to make a small hole in the iris—
the colored part of the eye—which allows the aqueous to flow more freely
within the eye so the iris doesn't plug up the trabecular meshwork.

In cyclophotocoagulation, a laser beam is used to freeze selected
areas of the ciliary body—the part of the eye that produces aqueous
humor—to reduce the production of fluid. This procedure may be used
to treat more advanced or aggressive cases of glaucoma.

Most laser surgeries for glaucoma can be performed in the ophthalmologist's office or an outpatient surgical facility. Eye drops are used
to numb the eye for the duration of the procedure. Because there is
usually little discomfort during glaucoma surgery, this is often the only
anesthesia needed.

Little recuperation is needed after laser eye surgery. Patients may experience some local eye irritation, but can usually resume their normal activities a day or two after surgery.

In some cases, laser surgery is not the preferred surgical treatment for glaucoma. Sometimes, when vision loss is rapid, or medication and/ or laser surgery fails to lower IOP sufficiently, conventional incisional surgery is the best option.

Incisional Surgery

Filtering surgery is usually done in a hospital or outpatient surgery center, with local anesthesia, and sometimes, sedation. The surgeon uses very delicate instruments to remove a tiny piece of the wall of the eye (the sclera), leaving a tiny hole. The aqueous can then drain through the hole, reducing the intraocular pressure, and be reabsorbed into the bloodstream.

In some cases, the surgeon may place a small tube or valve in the eye through a tiny incision in the sclera. The valve acts a regulator for the buildup of aqueous within the eye. When the intraocular pressure reaches a certain level, the valve opens, allowing the fluid to flow out of the eye's interior, where it can be reabsorbed by the body. The procedure may take place in the ophthalmologist's office or outpatient surgical center, and can be done under local anesthesia.

The recuperative period following incisional glaucoma surgery is usually short. You may need to wear an eye patch for a few days after surgery, and to avoid activities which expose the eye to water, such as showering or swimming. The ophthalmologist may recommend you refrain from heavy exercise, straining or driving for a short time after surgery, to avoid complications.

Possible Complications

As with all surgery, there are risks associated with glaucoma surgery. Complications are unusual, but can include:

- infection
- bleeding
- undesirable changes in intraocular pressure
- loss of vision

Sometimes, a single surgical procedure is not effective in halting the progress of a person's glaucoma. In these cases, repeat surgery, and/or continued treatment with topical or oral medications may be necessary.

Your age, eye structure, type of glaucoma, and other medical conditions are all considerations when deciding how to treat your glaucoma.

The ophthalmologist, in partnership with the patient, is best able to make the appropriate treatment decisions.

If You Are Scheduled for Glaucoma Surgery

Before Your Surgery

Make sure you understand the risks and benefits of the surgery. Here are some questions you may want to ask your ophthalmologist:

- Why do you think surgery is the best treatment for my condition?

- What kind of surgery do you recommend for my condition, and why?

- Are there other treatment options I should consider?

- What do you think might happen if I don't have the surgery?

- Do you think I am likely to need further treatment after the surgery (i.e., medication or further surgery)?

- What change should I expect in my condition after surgery?

- What kind of anesthesia will you use for my surgery?

- Where will my surgery take place?

- Approximately how long will my surgery take?

- Should I discontinue any of my medications prior to surgery? If so, how long before my surgery should I stop taking them?

- Can I eat prior to my surgery?

You might find it helpful to write your questions down prior to your office visit, or to take notes during your appointment. This can help ensure you understand everything your ophthalmologist discusses with you.

If you have medical insurance, you should find out if your policy will cover your surgery, and how much—if anything—you should expect to pay out of pocket.

Most importantly, don't be afraid to ask your ophthalmologist questions. If you have any concerns, now is the time to discuss them with your doctor.

The Day of Your Surgery

If you've been told not to eat before surgery, it is very important that you follow that instruction. It can be dangerous to eat prior to undergoing some kinds of anesthesia.

Most hospitals and outpatient facilities recommend you leave valuables, such as money or jewelry at home. You may not be allowed to take those items into the procedure room.

If you are having your procedure in a hospital or outpatient surgery facility, make sure you get there in time to fill out any registration forms that may be required.

What Will Happen the Day of Surgery?

After you have registered or checked in, you may go to a waiting room or area prior to your surgery. You may be asked to change into a patient gown for your surgery. Depending on the kind of anesthesia you and your doctor selected for your procedure, an anesthesiologist may spend a few minutes talking with you to make sure it is the safest kind for you.

In the procedure room, you may be asked to sit in a special chair or lie on a table, depending on what kind of surgery you are having. In either case, special equipment will be used to make sure your head doesn't move during your procedure.

Your ophthalmologist or an assistant will probably put drops in your eyes to numb them. This is the only anesthesia necessary for many patients having glaucoma surgery. He or she may also give you one or more injections near your eye to help numb the whole area. This usually involves a minimum of discomfort.

If you and your ophthalmologist decide you need sedation—medication to make you less anxious—you may be given an injection or have an intravenous line (IV) placed in your arm. (This means a small needle will be placed in your arm and connected to some tubing and a bag of sterile solution and medication.) This usually doesn't hurt any more than getting a shot or giving blood.

If your surgery is a laser procedure, you will be seated in a special chair while the surgeon uses a beam of light to carry out the procedure. You will not be able to feel it, or to see it with the eye that is having the surgery.

If your surgery is an incisional procedure, the ophthalmologist or the assistant will place sterile cloth around your eye. You won't be able to feel the surgery, or see it with the eye having the surgery, but you may hear the tiny instruments while the ophthalmologist works.

Most glaucoma surgeries don't take very long—about an hour for most—but the time depends on many factors, such as your eye structure, the kind of surgery you're having and the difficulty of the procedure.

After Your Glaucoma Surgery

After your surgery, the ophthalmologist or assistant may put more drops in your eyes. You may be given medication for discomfort. You might need to wear an eye patch to protect the eye.

You will probably have to wait for a period after your surgery to make sure it's safe for you to return home. You may have to stay a little longer if you've had sedation.

Prior to leaving, you should be given instructions about:

- medications—when you should start taking them, and how often

- what to expect in the next few hours or days—i.e., how much discomfort or swelling you may have

- what signs to look out for that might indicate infection or another problem

- what activities you must refrain from, and for how long

- when you should return to the ophthalmologist for follow up

If you have any questions or concerns, ask your ophthalmologist or his/her assistant or nurse before you leave.

Make sure you have a friend or family member to drive you home after your procedure. You may have an eye patch or feel slightly groggy after your surgery.

Make sure you understand your ophthalmologist's instructions and follow them carefully. This will help ensure a speedy recovery and good outcome.

Keep your follow-up appointments, even if you have no sutures (stitches) to remove and are experiencing no complications.

Above all, take care of yourself and your eyes. Maintain a healthy diet—this is particularly important if you have a medical condition such as diabetes or hypertension (high blood pressure)—and get regular exercise. Wear sunglasses with adequate UV protection when you're in the sun, and make sure your eyes are protected when you play sports or use heavy machinery.

Section 24.7

Medications and Treatments for Glaucoma

There is no cure for glaucoma, but it can be controlled. Even when treatment is effective, people with glaucoma need to have their eyes checked regularly, and often need to continue treatment for the rest of their lives. This may seem like a burden, but it is preferable to losing your sight.

Treatment for glaucoma focuses on lowering intraocular pressure (IOP) to a level the ophthalmologist thinks is unlikely to cause further optic nerve damage. This level is sometimes known as the target pressure. (High IOP may damage your optic nerve, which can lead to vision loss.) That level differs from individual to individual, and one person's target pressure may change during the course of his or her lifetime.

Types of Medications

If you have open-angle glaucoma (the most common type) your ophthalmologist may prescribe medication to lower your intraocular pressure (IOP).

Medications may be topical, such as eye drops, inserts (wafer-like strips of medication you put in the corner of your eye) or eye ointments, or oral, such as pills or tablets. Topical medications reduce or control IOP in one of two ways.

Miotics increase the outflow of aqueous (liquid) from the eye. These include:

- Isopto Carpine®
- Pilocar®

- Ocusert®
- Pilopine®

Epinephrine compounds also increase the outflow of aqueous from the eye. These include:

- Epifrin®

- Propine®

Beta-blockers can reduce the amount of aqueous produced in the eye. These include:

- Betagan®
- Betoptic®
- OptiPranolol®

- Betimol®
- Ocupress®
- Timoptic®

Carbonic anhydrase inhibitors and alpha-adrenergic agonists also work to reduce the amount of aqueous the eye produces. These include:

- Alphagan®
- Trusopt®

- Iopidine®

In June 1996, the U.S. Food and Drug Administration (FDA) approved a new glaucoma medication, latanoprost (Xalatan®), for treatment of glaucoma. This medication is in a group of drugs called prostaglandin analogs. It works near the drainage area of the eye to increase the secondary route of outflow aqueous outflow to lower IOP.

Oral medication can also help control IOP. The most common oral medications are carbonic anhydrase inhibitors, which work to slow production of aqueous fluid in the eye. These pills include Daranide®, Diamox®, and Neptazane®.

The ophthalmologist may prescribe either topical or oral medication, or a combination of both. These may need to be taken several times a day in order to be effective.

Many of the same medications used to treat open-angle glaucoma are also used to treat angle-closure glaucoma.

This type of glaucoma can cause IOP to rise very quickly, and the ophthalmologist may need to lower the pressure rapidly to prevent vision loss. He or she may administer a sugar-based medication called a hyperosmotic agent either by mouth or by injection. This medication only lasts six to eight hours, so it is not used for long-term management of glaucoma.

Possible Side Effects

Any medication, including eye drops, may have side effects. Some people taking glaucoma medication may experience:

- Stinging or redness of eyes
- Blurred vision
- Headache
- Changes in pulse, heartbeat, or breathing
- Changes in sexual desire
- Mood changes
- Tingling of fingers and toes
- Drowsiness
- Loss of appetite
- Change of iris color (in people with light-colored eyes taking prostaglandin analogs)

Most side effects aren't serious and may disappear after a while. Not every patient will experience side effects with glaucoma medication. Since it is very important that people with glaucoma carefully follow their ophthalmologists' recommended treatments, any side effects of medication should be discussed with the doctor. If they become serious or intolerable, you and the ophthalmologist may decide to change medications or type of treatment.

Medication Tips

There are some things you should ask your ophthalmologist about your glaucoma medication:

- The name of the medication
- How to take it with food or on an empty stomach
- How often to take it (if several times per day, should you take it around the clock or only during waking hours)
- How to store it (i.e., in the refrigerator or a dark place)
- If you can take it with your other medications (make sure all your doctors are aware of all the medications you take, including non-prescription medication)

- What side effects you might experience
- What you should do if you experience side effects
- What you should do if you miss a dose

Section 24.8

Medical Developments in Glaucoma

From "Doctor, I Have a Question, Fourth Edition," © The Glaucoma Foundation. Reprinted with permission. Available online at [http://www.glaucoma-foundation.org/dihaq/app.htm]; cited August 29, 2002.

Latanoprost

Latanoprost received FDA approval in 1996. Marketed under the name Xalatan® by Pharmacia Corporation, it lowers intraocular pressure up to 20-40 percent both in people without glaucoma and in glaucoma patients, even when measured 24 hours after dosing. In three randomized, double-masked, multicenter trials, latanoprost 0.005 percent once a day was as effective or more effective than 0.5 percent timolol twice a day. Side effects such as burning, stinging, blurred vision, itching, foreign body sensation, tearing, or eye pain occurred infrequently in these trials. The mechanism of action of latanoprost is different from that of all other presently available glaucoma medications. It increases uveoscleral outflow, that is, outflow through the soft tissues of the front of the eye (iris and ciliary body).

Uveoscleral outflow is normally a minor route of aqueous outflow, accounting for about 10 percent of outflow in human beings, while 90 percent goes through the trabecular meshwork. Thus, latanoprost should prove to have an impact in addition to that of all other classes of antiglaucoma medications, which might be used in conjunction with it. There has been some publicity about the capacity of latanoprost to change eye color. In clinical trials, latanoprost produced an increase in iris pigmentation in 1-3 percent of patients and a possible increase in another few percent. Eyes prone to develop this complication typically are bicolored to begin with, the inner central portion of the iris (the sphincter) being brownish, and the remainder of the iris blue or green. In these cases, the peripheral iris darkens and the iris color becomes more uniform. The mechanism does not appear to be due to proliferation of melanocytes (mature pigment forming cells) but rather to stimulation of melanogenesis (melanin synthesis or melanin production) within iris melanocytes, so that the possibility of the origin, production or development of cancer appears most unlikely.

Please note: If you are interested in using latanoprost, you should consult your doctor.

Unoprostone Isopropyl Ophthalmic Solution, 0.15 percent

Unoprostone Isopropyl Ophthalmic Solution, 0.15 percent is a newly FDA-approved drug marketed under the name Rescula® by CIBA Vision, a Novartis company. According to clinical trial results, this drug increases aqueous fluid outflow in order to lower intraocular pressure (IOP).

Unoprostone differs from other treatments for open-angle glaucoma and ocular hypertension in that it contains a docosanoid (a new class of receptor) and uses a new mechanism of action not found in other glaucoma treatments. A docosanoid is similar to a naturally occurring substance in the eye that is considered an essential compound in the development and functioning of the retina. It is also believed that this drug has the potential to enhance blood flow to the optic nerve, a result that many doctors find promising because of the widespread belief that blood flow plays a role in glaucoma.

According to CIBA Vision, clinical trials involving more than 1,100 patients showed that unoprostone "consistently and safely" lowered IOP when used either by itself or as a part of a combination therapy (with other drugs). Additionally, using unoprostone in combination therapy was found to be as effective as many other combinations, while producing fewer side effects in patients than these combinations.

Unoprostone is generally dosed twice a day. The drug rapidly penetrates the cornea, achieving maximum effects in as soon as 24 hours. Importantly, clinical studies showed that unoprostone shows no loss in effectiveness over 12 months.

The studies also showed that Unoprostone has no impact on the cardiovascular system (common with beta blockers) and little effect on the pulmonary functions. The most commonly reported side effects (occurring in 10-25 percent of patients during clinical studies) include: burning and stinging upon instillation, dry eyes, itching, increased length of eyelashes, and redness. In a small number of cases, unoprostone has been reported to increase the amount of brown pigment in the iris, changing the color of the iris slowly and possibly permanently.

Please note: If you are interested in using unoprostone, you should consult your eye doctor.

Brinzolamide Ophthalmic Suspension, 1 percent

Brinzolamide is a newly FDA-approved drug marketed under the name Azopt® by Alcon Laboratories. Brinzolamide is a topical carbonic anhydrase inhibitor (CAI), meaning that it functions to reduce aqueous fluid flow into the eye, thereby lowering intraocular pressure (IOP). This drug is typically administered to patients with ocular hypertension or open-angle glaucoma.

Clinical trials have shown IOP reduction from brinzolamide to be equal to that of dorzolamide 2 percent (Trusopt®, manufactured by Merck & Co.), which is the only other topical CAI currently on the market; and the therapy was "demonstrated to be safe, and well tolerated." Patients in the study also found brinzolamide to be more comfortable than dorzolamide, as a result of the pH, and this could encourage patients to follow the course of treatment prescribed by doctors more stringently.

Oral carbonic anhydrase inhibitors have been used by glaucoma patients for over 3 decades. However, systemic side effects such as fatigue, gastrointestinal disturbances, and a feeling of general discomfort or uneasiness have often caused patients to request that their doctor change their drug treatment. In the topical form (eyedrops), CAIs are considered to be effective in lower doses, usually below the level which causes the above systemic side effects.

Brinzolamide is typically prescribed for use twice a day. Possible side effects of this topical drug include: allergy, altered taste sensation, stinging or burning of the eye, blurred vision, eye itching, and eye redness.

Please note: If you are interested in using brinzolamide, you should consult your eye doctor.

Dorzolamide Hydrochloride—Timolol® Maleate Ophthalmic Solution

Dorzolamide hydrochloride—timolol maleate ophthalmic solution is a new drug approved by the FDA within the last few months. Marketed under the name Cosopt® by Merck & Co., this drug represents the first combination drop treatment for patients with ocular hypertension or open-angle glaucoma who have had beneficial effects from the two drops given separately.

The drug consists of two components, dorzolamide and timolol, each of which works to decrease the aqueous (fluid) flow into the eye. The first component is a carbonic anhydrase inhibitor (CAI), marketed under the name Trusopt® and the second is a beta1 and beta2 (nonselective) adrenergic receptor, marketed under the name Timolol® by Merck & Co. Studies indicate that additional reduction of IOP with the use of this combination drug is possible, compared to using either of the drugs alone.

Using a combination drug treatment could reduce the need for multiple-bottle patient regimens, thereby assisting patients in following a simpler, less confusing treatment schedule. The combination drop is usually administered twice daily. Topical drugs can be absorbed systemically, meaning that they can affect the body generally. Accordingly, the same types of adverse reactions that are attributable to sulfonamides and/or systemic administration of beta-blockers may occur. During the manufacturer's trials, the most common side effects reported were: altered taste sensation, stinging or burning of the eye, blurred vision, eye itching and eye redness caused by congestion of blood vessels within the eye.

Please note: If you are interested in using dorzolamide hydrochloride—timolol maleate ophthalmic solution, you should consult your eye doctor.

Brimonidine Tartrate Ophthalmic Solution 0.2 percent

Brimonidine is a new drug marketed under the name Alphagan® by Allergan, Inc. Brimonidine is a highly selective alpha2-adrenoreceptor agonist, meaning it stimulates a class of cell surface receptors which reduce aqueous humor production. Instilled twice daily, the drug offers long term intraocular pressure (IOP) control for patients with glaucoma or ocular hypertension and it is currently the only alpha2-agonist to have received FDA approval for chronic treatment.

The IOP lowering capacity (mean 5.9 +/- 3.2 mmHg to 7.6 +/- 3.6 mmHg at peak) appears to be comparable to that of timolol 0.5 percent when used as the only therapy. These studies have shown a minimal drift in IOP within one year's time.

The drug appears to be generally well-tolerated by patients and has a favorable ocular and systemic safety profile, but, as with any new drug, this requires long-term follow-up. The potential for allergy, which is common in other common alpha agonists, has been clinically tested—and compared to apraclonidine, brimonidine .2 percent has a lower reported rate of ocular allergy.

Brimonidine is thought to have other characteristics that could benefit glaucoma research, but the clinical significance of these findings is unknown at present. It has been reported that alpha2-receptor agonists such as brimonidine have neuroprotective activity in models of cerebral ischemia (poor blood flow in the brain) and optic nerve injury, and therefore, could possibly offer a mechanism for delaying optic nerve degeneration, protecting retinal neurons from death, or stimulating regrowth of optic nerve fibers. The drug may also prove to be an appropriate choice as an additive agent for patients whose IOP is not adequately managed with other therapy. Further studies involving brimonidine in simultaneous use with other drugs are required to validate these approaches.

Please note: If you are interested in using brimonidine, you should consult your doctor.

Section 24.9

Glaucoma and Marijuana Use

"Workshop on the Medical Utility of Marijuana—Report to the Director, NIH," by the Ad Hoc Group of Experts, National Institutes of Health, National Eye Institute, http://www.nei.nih.gov, February 18, 1997.

Glaucoma is an eye disease usually associated with an increased fluid pressure inside the eyes, leading to vision loss or even blindness. The most common form of the disease—chronic, open-angle glaucoma—is a leading cause of blindness in the United States and the number one cause of blindness in African Americans.

Studies in the early 1970s showed that marijuana, when smoked, lowers intraocular pressure in people with normal pressure and those with glaucoma. In an effort to determine whether marijuana, or drugs derived from marijuana, might be effective as a glaucoma treatment, the National Eye Institute supported research studies from 1978 to

1984. These studies demonstrated that some derivatives of marijuana lowered intraocular pressure when administered orally, intravenously, or by smoking, but not when topically applied to the eye.

However, none of these studies demonstrated that marijuana—or any of its components—could safely and effectively lower intraocular pressure any more than a variety of drugs then on the market. As research with other potential glaucoma drugs has shown, simply lowering intraocular pressure does not necessarily control the disease. In addition, some potentially serious side effects were noted, including an increased heart rate and a decrease in blood pressure in studies using smoked marijuana.

A wide variety of therapies are currently used to treat glaucoma, including FDA-approved drugs and laser and conventional surgery. Several of these medications have just recently been approved by the FDA. Research to date has not investigated whether marijuana use offers any advantages over currently available glaucoma treatments or if it is useful when used in combination with standard therapies.

The identification of potentially serious side effects from smoked marijuana, coupled with the emergence of FDA-approved medications for glaucoma treatment, may have led to diminished interest in this research area. However, the National Eye Institute stands ready to evaluate any well-designed studies for treatment of eye diseases, including those involving marijuana for treatment of glaucoma.

Chapter 25

Age-Related Macular Degeneration (ARMD)

Chapter Contents

261

Section 25.1

Facts about Age-Related Macular Degeneration

"Facts about Age-Related Macular Degeneration," National Eye Institute, available online at http://www.nei.nih.gov, August 2002.

This chapter is designed to help people with age-related macular degeneration and their families better understand the disease. It describes the causes, symptoms, diagnosis, and treatment of age-related macular degeneration.

Age-related macular degeneration (AMD) is a disease that affects your central vision. It is a common cause of vision loss among people over age of 60. Because only the center of your vision is usually affected, people rarely go blind from the disease. However, AMD can sometimes make it difficult to read, drive, or perform other daily activities that require fine, central vision.

What Is the Macula?

The macula is in the center of the retina, the light-sensitive layer of tissue at the back of the eye. As you read, light is focused onto your macula. There, millions of cells change the light into nerve signals that tell the brain what you are seeing. This is called your central vision. With it, you are able to read, drive, and perform other activities that require fine, sharp, straight-ahead vision.

How Does AMD Damage Vision?

AMD occurs in two forms:

Dry AMD: Dry AMD affects about 90 percent of those with the disease. Its cause is unknown. Slowly, the light sensitive cells in the macula break down. With less of the macula working, you may start to lose central vision in the affected eye as the years go by. Dry AMD often occurs in just one eye at first. You may get the disease later in

262

the other eye. Doctors have no way of knowing if or when both eyes may be affected.

Wet AMD: Although only 10 percent of all people with AMD have this type, it accounts for 90 percent of all severe vision loss from the disease. It occurs when new blood vessels behind the retina start to grow toward the macula. Because these new blood vessels tend to be very fragile, they will often leak blood and fluid under the macula. This causes rapid damage to the macula that can lead to the loss of central vision in a short period of time.

Who Is at Risk for AMD?

Although AMD can occur during middle age, the risk increases as a person gets older. Results of a large study show that people in their 50s have about a two percent chance of getting AMD. This risk rises to nearly 30 percent in those over age 75. Besides age, other AMD risk factors include:

- Gender—Women may be at greater risk than men, according to some studies.

- Smoking—Smoking may increase the risk of AMD.

- Family History—People with a family history of AMD may be at higher risk of getting the disease.

- Cholesterol—People with elevated levels of blood cholesterol may be at higher risk for wet AMD.

What Are the Symptoms of AMD?

Neither dry nor wet AMD causes any pain. The most common symptom of dry AMD is slightly blurred vision. You may need more light for reading and other tasks. Also, you may find it hard to recognize faces until you are very close to them.

As dry AMD gets worse, you may see a blurred spot in the center of your vision. This spot occurs because a group of cells in the macula have stopped working properly. Over time, the blurred spot may get bigger and darker, taking more of your central vision.

People with dry AMD in one eye often do not notice any changes in their vision. With one eye seeing clearly, they can still drive, read, and see fine details. Some people may notice changes in their vision only if AMD affects both of their eyes.

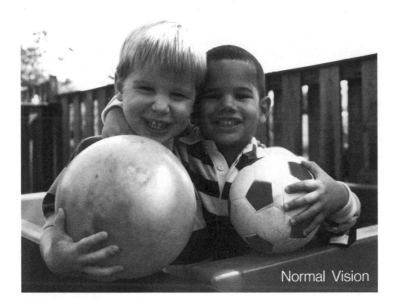

Figure 25.1. *Normal vision.*

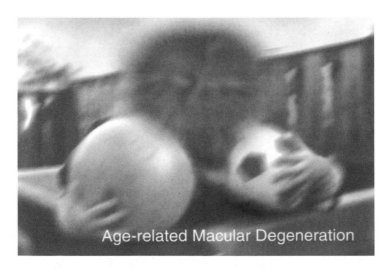

Figure 25.2. *The same scene as it might be viewed by a person with AMD.*

An early symptom of wet AMD is that straight lines appear wavy. This happens because the newly formed blood vessels leak fluid under the macula. The fluid raises the macula from its normal place at the back of the eye and distorts your vision. Another sign that you may have wet AMD is rapid loss of your central vision. This is different from dry AMD in which loss of central vision occurs slowly. As in dry AMD, you may also notice a blind spot.

If you notice any of these changes in your vision, contact your eye care professional at once for an eye exam.

How Is AMD Detected?

Eye care professionals detect AMD during an eye examination that includes:

- Visual acuity test: This eye chart test measures how well you see at various distances.

- Pupil dilation: This examination enables your eye care professional to see more of the retina and look for signs of AMD. To do this, drops are placed into the eye to dilate (widen) the pupil. After the examination, your vision may remain blurred for several hours.

One of the most common early signs of AMD is the presence of drusen. Drusen are tiny yellow deposits in the retina. Your eye care professional can see them during an eye examination. The presence of drusen alone does not indicate a disease, but it might mean that the eye is at risk for developing more severe AMD.

While conducting the examination, your eye care professional may ask you to look at an Amsler grid. This grid is a pattern that resembles a checkerboard. You will be asked to cover one eye and stare at a black dot in the center of the grid. While staring at the dot, you may notice that the straight lines in the pattern appear wavy to you. You may notice that some of the lines are missing. These may be signs of wet AMD.

If your eye care professional suspects you have wet AMD, you may need to have a test called fluorescein angiography. In this test, a special dye is injected into a vein in your arm. Pictures are then taken as the dye passes through the blood vessels in the retina. The photos help your eye care professional evaluate leaking blood vessels to determine whether they can be treated.

Figure 25.3 is what an Amsler grid normally looks like, and the illustration in Figure 25.4 is how it might look to someone with AMD.

These grids are reduced in size; ask your doctor for a full-size grid to use at home.

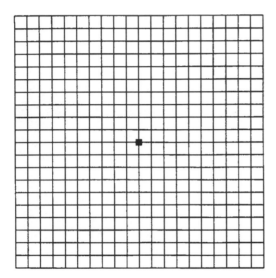

Figure 25.3. Amsler grid.

Figure 25.4. Amsler grid to someone with AMD.

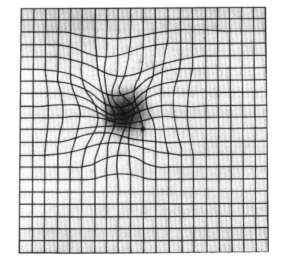

How Is AMD Treated?

Dry AMD currently cannot be treated. But this does not mean that you will lose your sight. Fortunately, dry AMD develops very slowly. You may lose some of your central vision over the years. However, most people are able to lead normal, active lives—especially if AMD affects only one eye.

Some cases of wet AMD can be treated with laser surgery. The treatment involves aiming a high energy beam of light directly onto the leaking blood vessels. Laser treatment is more effective if the leaky blood vessels have developed away from the fovea—the central part of the macula. But even if the blood vessels are growing right behind the fovea, the treatment can be of some value in stopping further vision loss.

How Is Laser Surgery Performed?

Laser surgery is performed in your eye care professional's office or eye clinic. Before the surgery, he or she will: (1) dilate your pupil and (2) apply drops to numb the eye. In some cases, he or she also may numb the area behind the eye to prevent any discomfort.

The lights in the office will be dim. As you sit facing the laser machine, your eye care professional will hold a special lens to your eye. You may see flashes of light.

You can leave the office once the treatment is done, but you will need someone to drive you home. Because your pupils will stay dilated for a few hours, you also should bring a pair of sunglasses.

For the rest of the day, your vision may be a little blurry. Your eye may also hurt a bit. This is easily controlled with drugs that your eye care professional can suggest.

You will need to make frequent follow-up visits. During each exam, you may have fluorescein angiography to make sure that the blood vessels are not still leaking, or that new blood vessels have not developed. If the vessels continue to leak, you might need some more laser surgery. It is important to realize that laser surgery is not a cure for AMD. It is only a treatment to help stop further vision loss. The risk of new blood vessels growing back after laser treatment is relatively high.

What Research Is Being Done?

The National Eye Institute (NEI) is the Federal government's lead agency for vision research. The NEI is supporting a number of research studies both in the laboratory and with patients to learn more about the cause of AMD. This research should provide better ways to detect, treat, and prevent vision loss in people with the disease.

Findings from the NEI-sponsored Age-Related Eye Disease Study (AREDS) showed that high levels of antioxidants and zinc significantly reduces the risk of advanced age- related macular degeneration (AMD) by about 25 percent.

Scientists have begun to study the possibility of transplanting healthy cells into a diseased retina. Although this work is at a very early stage and still experimental, someday it may help people keep their vision or restore some lost vision.

What Can You Do to Protect Your Vision?

If you have dry AMD, you should have your eyes examined through dilated pupils at least once a year. This will allow your eye care professional to monitor your condition and check for other eye diseases as well.

You should also obtain an Amsler grid from an eye care professional to use at home. This will provide you with a quick and inexpensive test to evaluate your vision each day for signs of wet AMD. It works best for people who still have good central vision. You should check each eye separately—cover one eye and look at the grid, then cover your other eye and look at the grid.

You also may want to check your vision by reading the newspaper, watching television, and just looking at people's faces. If you detect any changes, you should have an eye exam.

If you have wet AMD, it is important not to delay laser surgery if your eye care professional advises you to have it. After surgery, you will need to have frequent eye examinations to detect any recurrence of leaking blood vessels. Studies show that people who smoke have a greater risk of recurrence than those who don't.

In addition, you should continue to check your vision (at home with the Amsler grid or other methods) as described under dry AMD and schedule an eye exam immediately if you detect any changes.

What Can You Do if You Have Already Lost Vision to AMD?

Normal use of your eyes will not cause further damage to your vision. Even if you have lost sight to AMD, you should not be afraid to use your eyes for reading, watching TV, and other usual activities.

Low vision aids are available to help you make the most of your remaining vision. Low vision aids are special lenses or electronic systems that make images appear larger. If you need low vision aids, your eye care professional can often prescribe them or refer you to a low vision specialist. In addition, groups and agencies that offer information about counseling, training, and other special services are available. You may also want to contact a nearby school of medicine or optometry as well as a local agency devoted to helping the visually impaired.

For more information about low vision programs, contact:

American Foundation for the Blind
11 Penn Plaza, Suite 300
New York, NY 10001
Toll-Free: (800) 232-5463
Phone: (212) 502-7600
E-mail: afbinfo@afb.net
Website: http://www.afb.org

Lighthouse International
111 East 59th Street
New York, NY 10022
Toll-Free: (800) 829-0500
Phone: (212) 821-9200
Website: http://www.lighthouse.org

National Federation of the Blind
1800 Johnson Street
Baltimore, MD 21230
Phone: (410) 659-9314
Website: http://www.nfb.org

For more information about AMD, contact:

AMD Alliance International
1314 Bedford Avenue, Suite 113
Baltimore, Maryland 21208
Toll-Free: (877) 263-7171
Website: http://www.amdalliance.org

American Academy of Ophthalmology
P.O. Box 7424
San Francisco, CA 94120-7424
Phone: (415) 561-8500
Website: http://www.aao.org

American Optometric Association
243 North Lindbergh Blvd.
St. Louis, MO 63141
Phone: (314) 991-4100
Website: http://www.aoa.org

Association for Macular Diseases
210 East 64th Street, 8th Floor
New York, NY 10021
Phone: (212) 605-3719

Foundation Fighting Blindness
11435 Cronhill Drive
Owings Mills, MD 21117-2220
Toll-Free: (888) 394-3937
Phone: (410) 568-0150
Website: http://www.blindness.org

Macular Degeneration International
6700 North Oracle Road, Suite 505
Tucson, AZ 85704
Toll-Free: (800) 393-7634
Phone: (520) 797-2525

Macular Degeneration Partnership
8733 Beverly Boulevard, Suite 201
Los Angeles, CA 90048
Phone: (310) 423-6455
Website: http://www.macd.net

National Eye Institute
2020 Vision Place
Bethesda, MD 20892-3655
Phone: (301) 496-5248
Website: http://www.nei.nih.gov

Prevent Blindness America
500 E. Remington Rd.
Schaumburg, IL 60173
Toll-Free: (800) 331-2020
Phone: (847) 843-2020
Website: http://www.preventblindness.org

Section 25.2

Macular Degeneration: Medications to Use with Caution

From "Medications to Use with Caution." © 2001 American Macular Degeneration Foundation, P.O. Box 515, Northampton, MA 01061-0515, 1-888-MACULAR, www.macular.org. Reprinted with permission. The list of medications has been compiled by the National Registry of Drug-Induced Ocular Side Effects, Oregon Health Sciences University, 3181 S.W. Sam Jackson Park Road, Portland, OR 97219.

Few patients consider visual symptoms as being related to their medicine. However, when you realize that your eyes are really just an extension of your brain, an organ which is extremely sensitive to many drugs, it is not surprising that vision can be impaired by a host of medications.

Vision can be impaired by many medications. The National Registry of Drug-Induced Ocular Side Effects has published the following list of drugs which might be associated with macular degeneration. The drugs with more tenuous links to macular degeneration are followed by a question (?) mark. The generic name is followed by various proprietary names from around the world.

If you have any questions or want more information about any drug on this list and its possible links to macular degeneration, talk to your prescribing physician and/or ophthalmologist. You may also want to discuss whether the use of a drug on this list outweighs the increased risk of side effects compared with other treatments. Be sure to mention any prescribed or over-the-counter medications and other supplements you're taking. Describe any side effects you may have experienced. Remember, no summary can take the place of careful discussions with your health care professionals.

Macular Edema

Acetazolamide

Defiltran (Fr.), Diamox, Diazol (S. Afr.), Didoc (Jap.), Diuramid (Pol.), Glaucomide (Austral.), Glaupax (Swed.), Hydrazol

Allopurinol (?)

Bloxanth (Canad.), Epidropal (Germ.), Foligan (Germ.), Lopurin, Urosin (Germ.), Zyloprim, Zyloric (G.B.)

Aluminum Nicotinate

Nicalex

Betaxolol (?)

Betoptic

Broxyquinoline

Colipar (Fr.), Fenilor (Belg., Germ.)

Chymotrypsin (?)

Alpha Chymar, Alphacutanee (Fr.), Alphlozyme (Fr.), Catarase, Chymar (G.B.), Chymar-Zon (G.B.), Enzeon, Kimopsin (Austral., Jap.), Quimotrase (Canad.), Zolyse, Zonulyn (Canad.), Zonulysin (G.B.)

Diclorphenamide

Daranide, Oralcon (Swed.), Oratrol

Dipivefrin (?)

Propine

DPE (?)

Propine

Epinephrine

Adremad (Fr.), Adrenalin, Adrenaline (G.B.), Adrenatrate, Asmatane, Asmolin, Asthma Meter, Bronkaid, Dysne-Inhal (Canad.), Dyspne (Austral.), Glin-Epin (Austral.), Glycirenan (Germ.), Intranefrin (Canad.), Liadren (Ital.), Medihaler-Epi, Micronefrin, Primatene, Suprarenin, Sus-Phrine, Vaponefrin, Adrenaline (G.B.), El/2, E2, Epifrin, Epinal, Epitrate, Eppy, Glaucon, Glauconin (Swed.), Glaufrin (Swed.), Lyophrin (G.B.), Mistura E, Mytrate, Simplene (G.B.)

Ethoxzolamide

Ethamide

Griseofulvin

Fulcin (G.B.), Fulvicin-P/G, Fulvicin-U/F, Grifulvin V, Grisactin, Grisefuline (Fr.), Grisovin (G.B.), Grisowen, Gris-PEG, Lamoryl (Swed.), Likuden M (Germ.)

Hexamethonium

Hexamethonium

Indomethacin (Indometacin) (?)

Amuno (Germ.), Confortid (Swed.), Imbrilon (G.B.), Inacid (Span.), Indacin (Jap.), Indocid (G.B.), Indocin, Indomee (Swed.), Infrocin (Canad.), Metindol (Pol.), Mezolin (Jap.)

Iodide and Iodine Solutions and Compounds

Aqueous Iodine Solution (G.B.), Compound Iodine Solution, Iodex (G.B.), Jodex (Germ.), Lugol's Solution, Pima, Solute Iodo-Iodure Fort (Fr.), Strong Iodine Solution, Teinture d'Iode (Fr.), Trivajodan (Germ.), Weak Iodine Solution (G.B.), Iodine Solution

Iodochlorhydroxyquin

Budoform (Austral.), Chinoform (G.B.), Clioquinol (G.B.), Enteroquin (Austral.), Enteritan (Ital.), Entero-Valodon (G.B.), Entero-Vioform (G.B.), Iodochlorhydroxyquinoline (Ind.), Vioform

Iodoquinol (Diiodohydroxyquinoline)

Diiodohydroxyquin, Diodoquin, Direxiode (Austral., Fr.), Embequin (G.B.), Floraquin, Florequin (Swed.), Ioquin (Fr.), Moebiquin, Panaquin, Vaam-DHQ (Austral.), Yodoxin

Iothalamate Meglumine and/or Sodium

Angio-Conray, Cardio-Conray (Austral., G.B.), Conray, Contrix (Belg., Fr.), Cysto-Conray, Gastro-Conray (Austral., G.B.), Retro-Conray (Austral., G.B.), Sombril (Span.), Vascoray

Iothalamic Acid

Conray

Levobunolol (?)

Betagan

Methazolamide

Neptazane

Naproxen (?)

Anaprox, Naprosyn, Naxen (Mex.), Proxen (Aust., Germ., Switz.)

Niacin (Nicontic Acid)

Acidemel (S. Afr.), Diacin, Efacin, Niac, Nicangin (Swed.), Nico-400, Nicobid, Nicocap, Nicolar, Niconacid (Germ.), Ni Cord, Nico-Span, Nicotinex, Nicyl (Fr.), NiSpan, SK-Niacin, Span Niacin, Vasotherm, Wampocap

Niacinamide

Nicamid (Switz.), Nicobion (Fr., Germ.), Nicotamide (Fr.)

Nicotinyl Alcohol

Roniacol

Phenylephrine (?)

Neo-Synephrine, Ak-Dilate, Ak-Nefrin, Alcon-Efrin, Degest (Austral., Canad.), Dilatair, Efricel, I-Care (Austral.), Isopto Frin, Isopto Phenylephrine (Austral.), Mistura D, Mydfrin, Neo-Synephrine, Ocu-Phrin, Ocugestrin, Prefrin, Tear-Efrin

Quinine

Bi-quinate (Austral.), Coco-Quinine, Dentojel (Canad.), Quinamm, Quinate (Austral.), Quinbisan (Austral.), Quine, Quinsan (Austral.)

Radioactive iodides

Iodotope I-125, Iodotope I-131, Iodotope Therapeutic, Sodium Iodide (I-125), Sodium Iodide (I-131)

Tamoxifen

Nolvadex

Timolol (?)

Betim (G.B., Neth., Scand.), Blocadren, Blocanol (Fin.), Proflax (Arg.), Temserin (Germ., Gr.), Timacor (Denm., Fr.), Timoptic, Timoptol (Austral., Fr., G.B., Neth., N.Z., S. Afr.)

Macular or Paramacular Degeneration

Allopurinol (?)

Bloxanth (Canad.), Epidropal (Germ.), Foligan (Germ.), Lopurin, Urosin (Germ.), Zyloprim, Zyloric (G.B.)

Amodiaquinne

Basoquin (G.B.), Camoquin, Flavoquine (Fr.)

Broxyquinoline

Colipar (Fr.), Fenilor (Belg., Germ.)

Chloroquine

Aralen, Arechin (Pol.), Avoclor (G.B.), Chlorocon, Chlorquin (Austral.), Malaquin (Austral.), Malarex (Denm.), Malarivon (G.B.), Nivaquine (G.B.), Resochin (G.B.), Roquine, Siragan (Aust.), Tresochin (Swed.)

Clonidine (?)

Catapres, Catapresan (Germ., Swed.), Catapressan (Fr.), Dixarit (G.B.) Isoglaucon (Germ.)

Griseofulvin (?)

Fulcin (G.B.), Fulvicin-P/G, Fulvicin-U/F, Grifulvin V, Grisactin, Grisefuline (Fr.), Grisovin (G.B.), Grisowen, Gris-PEG, Lamoryl (Swed.), Likuden M (Germ.)

Hydroxychloroquine

Ercoquin (Norw., Swed.), Plaquenil, Plaquinol (Port.), Quensyl (Germ.)

Ibuprofen (?)

Advil, Algofen (Ital.), Amersol (Canad.), Andran (Jap.), Anflagen (Jap.), Apsifen (G.B.), Bluton (Jap.), Brufanic (Jap.), Brufen (Austral., Belg., Fr., G.B., Germ., Ital., Jap., Neth., S. Afr., Scand., Span., Swed., Switz.), Donjust B (Jap.), Ebufac (G.B.), Emodin (Arg.), Epobron (Jap.), Focus (Ital.), IB-100 (Jap.), Ibu-Slo (G.B.), Ibuprocin (Jap.), Inflam (Austral.), Inza (S. Afr.), Lamidon (Jap.), Liptan (Jap.), Medipren, Motrin, Mynosedin (Jap.), Nagifen-D (Jap.), Napacetin (Jap.), Nobfelon (Jap.), Nobgen (Jap.), Nuprin, Pantrop (Jap.), Rebugen (Ital.), Roidenin (Jap.), Rufen, Trendar

Indomethacin (Indometacin) (?)

Amuno (Germ.), Confortid (Swed.), Imbrilon (G.B.), Inacid (Span.), Indacin (Jap.), Indocid (G.B.), Indocin, Indomee (Swed.), Infrocin (Canad.), Metindol (Pol.), Mezolin (Jap.)

Iodochlorhydroxyquin

Budoform (Austral.), Chinoform (G.B.), Clioquinol (G.B.), Enteroquin (Austral.), Enteritan (Ital.), Entero-Valodon (G.B.), Entero-Vioform (G.B.), Iodochlorhydroxyquinoline (Ind.), Vioform

Iodoquinol

Diiodohydroxyquin, Diodoquin, Direxiode (Austral., Fr.), Embequin (G.B.), Floraquin, Florequin (Swed.), Ioquin (Fr.), Moebiquin, Panaquin, Vaam-DHQ (Austral.), Yodoxin

Quinine

Bi-quinate (Austral.), Coco-Quinine, Dentojel (Canad.), Quinamm, Quinate (Austral.), Quinbisan (Austral.), Quine, Quinsan (Austral.)

Section 25.3

Depression in People with Macular Degeneration

From "Depression in People with Macular Degeneration." © 2001
American Macular Degeneration Foundation, P.O. Box 515,
Northampton, MA 01061-0515, (888) MACULAR, www.macular.org.
Reprinted with permission.

The depressive response is accompanied by a set of typical physiological and emotional symptoms. Its adaptive function is to signal ourselves that there is an important problem that requires attention and resolution.

In preparation for this brief attempt to write something about depression that would be relevant and meaningful to individuals experiencing the visual acuity loss associated with macular degeneration, I tried to place myself directly in the shoes of one who has experienced such loss. Quickly, however, I sensed that losing a big part of such a crucial and taken-for-granted way of experiencing and relating to the world was virtually impossible for me to truly know from inside. Perhaps to experience such a loss, even within the safety of my imagination, was simply too threatening and might trigger my own painful and depressing crisis of the self.

What did get triggered at a gut level in this attempt at placing myself within the experience of you who know only too well what really having macular degeneration is like, was a wave of fear coursing through my body and soul—an old fear which we know now, from research, is a specific fear shared by more people than any other fear associated with losing one of our five senses—the fear of losing contact with the world through loss of sight. In re-exposing this usually suppressed fear within myself, I finally was able to come close to my original goal of empathy with macular degeneration's victims.

The first paragraph contains a phrase which I believe is key to any discussion about depression from whatever precipitating cause including macular degeneration, namely, crisis of the self. In fact, depression from both a layman's perspective and a psychiatric/clinical viewpoint can probably most usefully be defined as an unresolved crisis in the sense (image) of, security of, and esteem of one's self.

Let me digress a moment to acknowledge that as a psychiatrist, I am naturally aware of the currently prevailing professional and lay literature promoting a view of depression as a genetic disorder of chemical imbalance which a person gets or has, like one gets pneumonia or has diabetes or any number of other diseases and illnesses. This interesting, but unproved theory and literature seems partly based on the motivation to lift blame or concerns about personal weakness from depressed individuals or to bestow a medical/physical aura to what is basically emotional/psychological/spiritual suffering. It is based on recent research that has identified information transmitting chemicals in the brain that are involved in people's various emotional experiences and which antidepressant medication can often impact to improve the mood of some depressed individuals.

Cause and effect has often been poorly understood in this research. Increasingly, it is recognized that the changes (imbalances) in brain chemistry associated with depression, to the degree they exist at all, are primarily a result, not the cause, of the mood and thought changes inherent in the unresolved self in crisis (much as salty liquid discharges from the eyes (tears!) are the result, not the cause, of acute sadness or happiness).

How do you know if you are covered by the ADA [Americans with Disabilities Act]? You must be a qualified person with a disability. Because each person's disability and employment circumstance is different, you ultimately must consult a lawyer who specializes in disability law or other qualified professional for a definitive answer. However, the ADA sets forth the basic criteria against which all cases are measured.

As one who has worked in psychotherapy with many mildly and severely depressed individuals (frequently without utilizing antidepressant medication), I can attest to the significance of loss, in all its many manifestations, and the consequent emotional and thinking crises, fears, conflicts, and disruptions in sense of security, as the main cause of most, though perhaps not all, of the painful emotional and mental experience we call depression. Certainly, concepts such as blame, weakness, failure, badness, etc., have no place in any meaningful understanding of depression although they are almost inevitable factors in the experience of the self-in-crisis.

Another truth about depression that needs emphasis is that it is not pathological per se. This is related to the points made above. In fact, it is better viewed of as a normal, natural, built-in mental/emotional/physiological response of a person, which serves primarily a signaling and curative function (analogous, for instance, to fever in some physical illnesses).

To use macular degeneration as an example, when a person begins to experience the changes in central visual acuity, depth perception, contrast sensitivity, and glare sensitivity associated with the onset of macular degeneration, there follows an initial reaction of worry, concern, and perhaps anxiety which leads one to seek a medical evaluation, diagnosis, and (the usually expected) correction.

When the unexpected and devastating diagnosis of macular degeneration comes, one's world is suddenly topsy turvy (unless the psychological defense of total denial sets in to avoid emotional pain and protect the familiar self-image and sense of security). Even the sympathetic and encouraging words of a caring physician who understands both the limitations and continuities of sight that you may experience now and in the future, can often not be heard and emotionally processed at the moment of diagnosis. Your perception of yourself, and vision of your future is thrown into total disarray; you despairingly imagine a life of darkness, social isolation, dependency, risky treatments, loss of friends, hobbies, participation in activities of interest such as sports, theater, art and reading—in short, a kind of early death.

Before macular degeneration, you had already successfully made it through the crises of changes in self-image that occur in middle to later years of life and accepted the eventual, but still in some respects distant, inevitability of physical decline. But now this hits with all the same issues, only in spades, and with an immediacy that makes the present, and especially the future, seem very dim indeed. Loss (especially of control, mastery, and independence) seems the dominant factor in your life, your old self-image and assumptions are out the window, your secure world tumbles like a house of cards, and your self-esteem begins to crumble with it.

All permanent challenge or loss that we suffer in our view of ourselves and our world, especially as it relates to our future, includes the above experiences to greater or lesser degree. In general, the more sudden our awareness of the loss, and the more it threatens contact with that which is most meaningful, the more traumatic and disruptive the experience.

For no one is the experience painless—it always hurts—but for some the crisis will be more temporary than for others. This depends on many factors such as their interpersonal support network, previous experience in mastery of severe loss, general emotional resilience (possibly partially related to built-in temperament factors), the degree of acceptance and ability to express to others their grief, anger, and fear, and the directness to which the loss is related to the core of their self-identity and esteem.

For many, the process of readjustment and re-establishment of their self esteem, security, and positive picture of themselves, as well as the struggle to reinvolve themselves in previously meaningful activities, or to learn new ones, will take longer. During this phase they may be said to be depressed in the sense of having less interest in usual activities, lower energy, some social withdrawal, some loss of usual appetite and restful sleep, some irritability and easy frustration with others and themselves, some self-pity, periods of despair, and, of course, considerable sadness and tears. However, the good news is that this is not truly a state of illness, or malfunction. Such depression is the heart, mind, and body's sad and slowed down response to a traumatic crisis demanding new adaptation which requires much time and opportunity (some of which includes a need for aloneness, more wakefulness, and less food intake) for a great deal of thought about past, present, and future, and the processing of many feelings which must have their day. The fact, however, that this process is a natural and potentially curative one does not mean that family, friends, macular degeneration support groups, or professional therapists should not be a part of it.

One of the great fears and initial expectations during this regrouping process is that one is totally alone with this sight loss and that the loss will include separation from meaningful and loved people. Including such people in the expression of the loss and in the readjustment process is inherent in the optimal healing function of this level of depression. (It is most helpful, of course, if the significant others in this process do not discount, denigrate, or push for quick change in the periods of withdrawal, range of emotions expressed, and changes in physiological functions or habits through which the person-in-crisis is going.)

Depression, though a natural and potentially productive, even curative, response (or signal) to persons in need of realignment of their self-identity, image, security, and esteem, can, and sometimes does, like a fever, progress to the point of diminished returns and become unproductive and, itself, debilitating. Nevertheless, even then it should still be considered as a natural and potentially productive signal or message from oneself to oneself that further work and re-adaptation is necessary. However, if the individual is unable, for whatever reason, to hear or respond to that message, and slips into a malignant spiral of increasing self-incrimination, social avoidance, despair, hopelessness, loss of weight, loss of adequate rest, or suicidal preoccupation, then psychotherapy along with antidepressant medication, and even occasionally self-protective brief hospitalization is indicated and may become life saving.

The goal, however, even in the more extreme situation, is not just a return to a previous level of functioning, but a renewal process of personal growth that will enable the individual to achieve greater and richer experiences of meaning, self-esteem, relationships with others, and ability to cope with life's stresses than had been the case prior to the traumatic loss experience of macular degeneration.

On that latter point, I have to think of a friend of who actually is now able to express gratitude for the depression and subsequent life re-examination he was forced to undergo as a result of the onset of macular degeneration many years ago. Although he would not wish such an eye problem on anyone, he is keenly aware that, for him, it may have been the kind of loss and trauma that was needed for him to finally examine his then self-destructive life course and to gain the insight and personal healing necessary to find a life of meaning, self-esteem, family relatedness, and service to others which he subsequently accomplished. Although he could no longer see people and objects outside of himself with as much visual clarity, he gained an ability to see both them and himself with a clarity of reality, respect, and optimism heretofore absent from his sight.

No longer a helpless and bitter victim, he became a healing facilitator for others. He had heard his own healing potential calling from the depth of his loss, grief, anger, and depression.

In summary, I have attempted to share some thoughts on the near inevitability of greater or lesser degrees of depression as a result of being given a diagnosis of macular degeneration and a way of viewing and understanding depression that emphasizes its potentially productive meaning for us as a normal reaction to difficult life circumstances, and a useful first alert to get help toward a better life.

Further Thoughts on Depression in People with Macular Degeneration

Above, I discussed depression, including in people with macular degeneration, as a basic, normal, and potentially adaptive response whenever we perceive that a significant physical, psychological, or interpersonal effort of ours is failing in its purpose or coming to a halt.

This depressive response is accompanied by a set of typical physiological and emotional symptoms. Its adaptive function is to signal ourselves that there is an important problem that requires attention and resolution. Depression aids and protects concentration on the emotional and thinking readjustment that needs to be done to alter or cope with the situation or to recognize and accept a situation that cannot be changed. The potential result is renewal of one's self-esteem and a greater capacity to move forward in life on the basis of new, even if deeply unwanted, realities.

I will now respond to some questions that your editors have asked regarding depression in general, and as it relates to people with macular degeneration.

Is It Possible for Depression to Make Our Visual Problems Worse?

There is no evidence that depression can worsen the physiological and histological changes of macular degeneration. However, to the degree that depression temporarily narrows our attention, interest and involvement in the world around us, we might perceive a worsening in our visual acuity and sensitivity. An analogy would be the difference in brightness and color we experience in our surroundings when we are in a bright mood versus the dull or gray appearance that even a beautiful day may have to one who is blue. However, this will be transient and when the work of depression has been accomplished, there will be no permanent physical effects from this perceived worsening of vision.

How Long Will a Person Be Depressed and Is There Any Way of Predicting This?

For the most part, depressive responses arising from unexpected traumatic circumstances such as macular degeneration are relatively short in duration, perhaps a few weeks to a few months. The only way I know of predicting just how brief or long any particular individual is likely to experience depression is to look at his/her previous record in coping with the stresses of life.

Speaking generally, people who have enjoyed a previous high level of self-esteem, emotional resilience in the face of adversity, high levels of support from, and contact with, family and friends, etc., will show a quicker rebound from the initial devastating impact of their visual impairment. Those who, for whatever reason, have been more depression prone in the past and who are more dependent on everything in their life being ideal for their sense of their own self-worth and stability may take a longer time to hear and respond to the growth-demands inherent in their depression. Although we all feel good vision as very important to our lives, the degree to which visual acuity is central to one's career or hobbies can also affect the amount of personal threat one feels when faced with its complete or partial loss. It is important to remember that, for most people most of the time, depression is a time-limited experience with spontaneous recovery the rule.

Is There Anything You Can Advise a Person to Do, or Take, That May Alleviate Their Depression?

Most of us are not especially open to advice when we are in the depths of depression or despair. Usually we simply have to go through a healing process either alone, with the help of friends and family, or with the help of a therapist. However, there are some suggestions that can be made that might be helpful for some.

Acknowledge and accept the depressive feelings as real, true, natural, and as a signal of some personal adjustment and healing which needs to take place. Avoid the trap of thinking that your current emotional suffering, anger, and disinterest in life is a sign of personal weakness, badness, or failure. Accept it as a sign that the former path in life you were on may no longer go anywhere for you and a somewhat new path must be found. Find a trusted friend or family member with whom to share your feelings about your loss and ask them primarily just to listen and care, not to give you lots of advice or try to push you to feel better until you have gone through your own process of acceptance and adjustment. Don't be quick to pop every little pill or potion in your mouth that others say was a miracle cure for them! Keep up as many of your daily routines as possible and take good care of your body and spirit through daily exercise to the degree that you can feel motivated to do so.

Are There Any Over-the-counter Vitamins or Drugs That a Person with Depression Could Take That Might Help? Or Would They Need a Prescription?

In general, look not for help and healing through the oral and digestive system, but through the psychological/interpersonal system. Your soul has been wounded by loss in a personal sensory function that had tremendous value to your sense of your self and your contact with life. Such a soul wound heals with a combination of time, painful acceptance of what has happened, healing contact with people who care and try to understand, and gradual investment of time and energy in what can still be for you, rather than what can no longer be. This is an internal psychological process, not an oral or chemical process.

However, the process can be supported through continuing good nutrition (including vitamin supplements if one's loss of appetite diminishes good nutrition), regular physical exercise, and sometimes even prescription antidepressant medications. The latter, prescribed by a psychiatrist or your family physician, can for some people assist in re-establishing the balance and function of neurochemicals in the brain that have functioned less effectively as a result of prolonged emotional/psychological depression. They will not, however, be needed for most people dealing with depression in response to a life stress or trauma and should be seen as adjunctive (added to), rather than central, to the healing of the soul wound.

What Can Family and Friends Do to Help Alleviate the Depression?

Like the victim of macular degeneration themselves, family and friends can help most by not being alarmed at the initial depressive response but to recognize that this response creates, by its various reactions, a frame of mind and a physical state promoting the work of re-adaptation and regrouping. A caring and understanding ear should be offered rather than impatience at the individuals temporary withdrawal, loss of appetite and sleep, sadness, and anger. Working creatively together with the victim of macular degeneration to find treatment where indicated, and to find ways to support what vision the individual has as well as to compensate for what is lost will be helpful. The victim's need for maximum independence in the face of greater dependence in certain ways should be recognized and supported.

If the depression remains deep and unproductive for weeks on end or includes unrelenting suicidal thoughts, wishes, or behavior, a friend or family member should firmly press for professional help for the depressed person.

At What Point Should the Patient with Age-Related Macular Degeneration Seek Professional Help?

In most cases this won't be necessary as the potential for recovery is present in everyone, especially where solid interpersonal relationships exist prior to the onset of the macular degeneration. However, sometimes the traumatic situation and resulting depression or anxiety, including preoccupation with death and suicide, becomes so overwhelming and protracted that professional help is indicated. To seek such help when the frame of mind and physical reactions of depression have not spontaneously remitted is a sign of strength, not weakness.

Often, the very decision to get professional help or the first meeting with a professional expert who is experienced in helping people work through their loss and regain their interest and enthusiasm for life will already lead to relief from the worst feelings of hopelessness and despair. Generally speaking, it is better to be sooner rather than later in obtaining professional help as it becomes harder for most people to seek such help when their depression becomes severe and unproductive to the point of feelings of hopelessness and despair about future possibilities for meaning and happiness.

What Professional Options Are Available to the Patient? What Are Some Benefits and Drawbacks to Each Option?

If one has an ophthalmologist or family physician who is sensitive to the emotional experiences the patient is likely to go through who has just been diagnosed with macular degeneration, that physician can help a great deal by spending time listening about and discussing those typical emotional responses. Frequently, that is all the professional help that is needed. In addition, an ophthalmologist or family doctor who is experienced and judicious in the use of antidepressant medications may prescribe them when indicated.

If more intensive psychotherapy is indicated however, the patient should seek the assistance of a clinical social worker, psychologist, or psychiatrist who is trained and experienced in the special skills that good listening/interactive psychotherapy requires.

The current managed health care environment makes obtaining such psychotherapy over an extended time much less available to the average person, especially if done with a psychiatrist, but just pills or a session or two of advice will often be insufficient to help the person regain optimal psychological growth and health from their traumatic loss. A psychiatrist who is trained and experienced in psychotherapy offers the added benefit of being an expert on psycho-pharmacology, but many other mental health professionals are also highly skilled in offering individual, group, or family therapy. In some locations, the patient may also find excellent self-help groups led by either a professional or a skilled lay person who him/herself has experienced macular degeneration.

Are There Any Good Books or Articles on Depression That One Might Read?

Although depression is such a natural, common and universal response to unresolved loss or stress, it is also very unique in some respects for each individual because each person is unique. Therefore, I am not fond of recommending reading in the field for the person currently suffering the loss of traumas such as macular degeneration. The path of recovery will come, not from books and articles, but from one's own inner process, relationship with significant others, and, where indicated, a caring and skilled professional. For readers of this article who are interested in reading an excellent book written for professionals and educated laypersons, I would suggest *Productive and Unproductive Depression, Success or Failure of a Vital Process* by Emmy Gut, Basic Books, Inc., New York.

Brief Biographical Sketch

Dr. Arnold Wyse, a native of Michigan, is a board-certified psychiatrist and psychoanalyst who received his specialty training at The Institute of Living in Hartford, Connecticut, and at New York Medical College in New York City. After twenty years in private practice in Hartford and as associate clinical professor at both the University of Connecticut School of Medicine and New York Medical College, Arnie joined the Indian Health Service. From 1992 until 2000, Dr. Wyse served as Director of Mental Health Services and Medical Director at Northern Navajo Medical Center in Shiprock, New Mexico.

Part Four

Pediatric Eye Problems

Chapter 26

Amblyopia

The information provided in this chapter was developed by the National Eye Institute to help patients and their families search for general information about amblyopia. An eye care professional who has examined the patient's eyes and is familiar with his or her medical history is the best person to answer specific questions.

What Is Amblyopia?

The brain and the eye work together to produce vision. Light enters the eye and is changed into nerve signals that travel along the optic nerve to the brain. Amblyopia is the medical term used when the vision in one of the eyes is reduced because the eye and the brain are not working together properly. The eye itself looks normal, but it is not being used normally because the brain is favoring the other eye. This condition is also sometimes called lazy eye.

How Common Is Amblyopia?

Amblyopia is the most common cause of decreased vision in children. The condition affects approximately 2 or 3 out of every 100 children. It is estimated that as many as three percent of children in the U.S. have some degree of vision impairment due to amblyopia. Unless it is successfully treated in early childhood, amblyopia usually

"Amblyopia Resource Guide," National Eye Institute, available online at http://www.nei.nih.gov, April 2002.

persists into adulthood, and is the most common cause of monocular (one eye) visual impairment among children and young and middle-aged adults.

What Causes Amblyopia?

Amblyopia may be caused by any condition that affects normal visual development or use of the eyes. Amblyopia can be caused by strabismus, an imbalance in the positioning of the two eyes. Strabismus can cause the eyes to cross in (esotropia) or turn out (exotropia). Sometimes amblyopia is caused when one eye is more nearsighted, farsighted, or astigmatic than the other eye. Occasionally, amblyopia is caused by other eye conditions such as cataract.

How Is Amblyopia Treated in Children?

Amblyopia treatment is most effective when done early in the child's life, usually before age 7. Treating amblyopia involves making the child use the eye with the reduced vision (weaker eye). Currently, there are two ways used to do this:

Atropine

A drop of a drug called atropine is placed in the stronger eye once a day to temporarily blur the vision so that the child will prefer to use the eye with amblyopia. Treatment with atropine also stimulates vision in the weaker eye and helps the part of the brain that manages vision develop more completely.

Patching

An opaque, adhesive patch is worn over the stronger eye for weeks to months. This therapy forces the child to use the eye with amblyopia. Patching stimulates vision in the weaker eye and helps the part of the brain that manages vision develop more completely. To be effective, patching must usually be done for a minimum of six hours each day.

Can Amblyopia Be Treated in Adults?

During the first six to nine years of life, the visual system develops very rapidly. Complicated connections between the eye and the brain are created. We do not yet have the technology to create these eye-to-brain connections in older children and adults.

Scientists are exploring whether treatment for amblyopia in older children and adults can improve vision.

National Eye Institute–Supported Research

The National Eye Institute (NEI) is currently supporting the Amblyopia Treatment Study (ATS) to determine whether patching or eyedrops is a better treatment for amblyopia. Recent results for the ATS found that the atropine eyedrops, when placed in the unaffected eye once a day, work as well as eye patching and may encourage better compliance. The study was conducted at 47 clinical sites throughout North America.

The NEI is also supporting the Vision in Preschoolers (VIP) Study, a clinical study designed to develop an effective and efficient set of screening tests to identify those 3- and 4-year-old Head Start children in need of further vision care for amblyopia, strabismus, and/or significant refractive error.

Resources

The following organizations may be able to provide additional information on amblyopia:

National Eye Institute
2020 Vision Place
Bethesda, MD 20892-3655
Phone: (301) 496-5248
Website: http://www.nei.nih.gov

Conducts and supports vision research. Part of the National Institutes of Health.

American Academy of Ophthalmology
P.O. Box 7424
San Francisco, CA 94120-7424
Phone: (415) 561-8500
Website: http://www.aao.org

Represents board-certified ophthalmologists in the United States. Provides information for the public on amblyopia.

American Association for Pediatric Ophthalmology and Strabismus
P.O. Box 193832
San Francisco, CA 94119-3832

291

American Association for Pediatric Ophthalmology and Strabismus, continued

Phone: (415) 561-8505
Website: http://www.aapos.org

Represents ophthalmologists that specialize in providing eye care for children.

American Optometric Association

243 North Lindbergh Boulevard
St. Louis, MO 63141
Phone: (314) 991-4100
Website: http://www.aoa.org

Represents optometrists in the United States. Provides information for the public on amblyopia.

For additional information, you may wish to contact a local library.

Medical Literature

Below is a sample of the citations available through MEDLINE/ PubMed, a service of the National Library of Medicine. MEDLINE/ PubMed provides access to over 11 million medical literature citations from 1966 to the present and includes links to many sites providing full-text articles and other related resources. You can conduct your own free literature search by accessing MEDLINE through the Internet at http://medlineplus.nlm.nih.gov/hinfo.html. You can also get assistance with a literature search at a local library.

To obtain copies of any of the articles listed below, contact a local community, university, or medical library. If the library you visit does not have a copy of a desired article, you may usually obtain it through an inter-library loan.

Please keep in mind that articles in the medical literature are usually written in technical language. We encourage you to share any articles you order with a health care professional who can help you understand them.

A Randomized Trial of Atropine versus Patching for Treatment of Moderate Amblyopia in Children

The Pediatric Eye Disease Investigator Group. Jaeb Center for Health Research, Tampa FL. *Arch Ophthalmol* 120:268-278, 2002.

Amblyopia is the most common cause of monocular visual impairment in both children and young and middle-age adults. In a randomized clinical trial, 419 children younger than 7 years with amblyopia and visual acuity in the range of 20/40 to 20/100 were assisted to receive either patching or atropine eye drops at 47 clinical centers. Atropine and patching produce improvement of similar magnitude, and both are appropriate modalities for the initial treatment of moderate amblyopia in children aged 3 to less than 7 years.

The Amblyopia Treatment Study Visual Acuity Testing Protocol

Holmes JM, Beck RW, Repka MX, Leske DA, Kraker RT, Blair RC, Moke PS, Birch EE, Saunders RA, Hertle RW, Quinn GE, Simons KA, Miller JM and the Pediatric Eye Disease Investigator Group. Mayo Clinic, Rochester, MN. *Arch Ophthalmol* 119:1345-53, 2001.

This article evaluates the reliability of a new visual acuity testing protocol for children using isolated surrounded HOTV optotypes (letters used for testing). After initial pilot testing and modification, the protocol was evaluated using the Baylor-Video Acuity Tester (BVAT) to present isolated surrounded HOTV optotypes. At 6 sites, the protocol was evaluated for testability in 178 children aged 2 to 7 years and for reliability in a subset of 88 children. Twenty-eight percent of the 178 children were classified as having amblyopia. Using the modified protocol, testability ranged from 24 percent in 2-year-olds to 96 percent in 5- to 7-year-olds. Test-retest reliability was high (r = 0.82), with 93 percent of retest scores within 0.1 logMAR unit of the initial test score. The 95 percent confidence interval for an acuity score was calculated to be the score +/-0.125 logMAR unit. For a change between 2 acuity scores, the 95 percent confidence interval was the difference +/-0.18 logMAR unit. The visual acuity protocol had a high level of testability in 3- to 7-year-olds and excellent test-retest reliability. The protocol has been incorporated into the multicenter Amblyopia Treatment Study and has wide potential application for standardizing visual acuity testing in children.

Amblyopia: Detection, Prevention, and Rehabilitation

LaRoche GR. Division of Ophthalmology, IWK Health Center, Halifax, Nova Scotia, Canada. *Curr Opin Ophthalmol* 12(5):363-7, 2001.

This year's literature on the detection, prevention, and rehabilitation of amblyopia is again somewhat dominated by the topic of vision screening, specifically photoscreening and also by the therapeutic challenges of compliance and late treatment. Basic scientists also have added to our knowledge and understanding of certain interesting and clinically significant characteristics of the visual perception of people with amblyopia.

The Role of Drug Treatment in Children with Strabismus and Amblyopia

Chatzistefanou KI, Mills MD. Department of Ophthalmology and Visual Sciences, University of Wisconsin-Madison Medical School. *Paediatr Drugs* 2(2):91-100, 2000.

Strabismus, or misalignment of the eyes, is a common ophthalmic problem in childhood, affecting 2 to 5 percent of the preschool population. Amblyopia is an important cause of visual morbidity frequently associated with strabismus, and both conditions should be treated simultaneously. Pharmacological means for treating strabismus and amblyopia can be divided into 3 categories: paralytic agents (botulinum toxin) used directly on the extraocular muscles to affect eye movements; autonomic agents (atropine, miotics) used topically to manipulate the refractive status of the eye and thereby affect alignment, focus and amblyopia; and centrally acting agents, including levodopa and citicoline, which affect the central visual system abnormalities in amblyopia. In amblyopia therapy, atropine is used to blur vision in the non-amblyopic eye and offers a useful alternative to traditional occlusion therapy with patching, especially in older children who are not compliant with patching.

Successful Amblyopia Therapy Initiated after Age 7 Years: Compliance Cures

Mintz-Hittner HA, Fernandez KM. Department of Ophthalmology and Visual Science, University of Texas Houston Medical School. *Arch Ophthalmol* 118(11):1535-41, 2000.

This article reports successful therapy for anisometropic and strabismic amblyopia initiated after age 7 years. A consecutive series of 36 compliant children older than 7 years (range, 7.0 to 10.3 years; mean, 8.2 years) at initiation of amblyopia therapy for anisometropic (19 patients; mean age, 8.3 years), strabismic (9 patients; mean age, 8.0 years), or anisometropic and strabismic (8 patients; mean age, 8.0

years) amblyopia was studied. Initial (worst) visual acuities were between 20/50 and 20/400 (log geometric mean, -0.83 [antilog, 20/134] for all patients; -0.88 [antilog, 20/151] for anisometropic patients; -0.70 [antilog, 20/100] for strabismic patients; and -0.88 [antilog, 20/151] for anisometropic and strabismic patients). Initial (worst) binocularity was absent or reduced in all cases. Therapy consisted of (1) full-time standard occlusion (21 patients; mean age, 8.0 years), (2) total penalization (7 patients; mean age, 7.8 years), or (3) full-time occlusive contact lenses (8 patients; mean age, 8.8 years). Final (best) visual acuities were between 20/20 and 20/30 for all 36 patients. Final (best) binocularity was maintained or improved for 22 (61 percent) of 36 patients, including 16 anisometropic patients (84 percent), 2 strabismic patients (22 percent), and 4 anisometropic and strabismic patients (50 percent). Given compliance, therapy for anisometropic and strabismic amblyopia can be successful even if initiated after age 7 years.

The National Eye Institute (NEI), part of the National Institutes of Health (NIH), is the Federal Government's principal agency for conducting and supporting vision research. Inclusion of an item in this chapter does not imply the endorsement of the NEI or the NIH.

Chapter 27

Juvenile Macular Degeneration

Juvenile macular degeneration (JMD) is a broad term used to describe several eye disorders that primarily affect infants, children, and young adults. They all are associated with genetic mutations that affect the macula and cause malfunction and eventual death of cone cells, which are responsible for central vision.

Stargardt's disease is the most common type of JMD and affects one in 10,000 people. Symptoms usually develop between the ages of 7 and 12, although some people do not experience visual impairment until their 30s or 40s. Manifestation of Stargardt's includes yellow spots composed of the pigment lipofuscein, scarring of the macula, and central vision loss.

Most patients with Stargardt's experience central vision loss by the time they reach adulthood. The progression of visual loss varies, but one study found that by age 50, one half of participants had reached legal blindness. In late stages of the disease, color vision may also be impaired.

Stargardt's disease is an inherited autosomal recessive syndrome, which means that both parents carry the defective gene but have normal retinas. There is a 25 percent chance that their child will be born with Stargardt's disease. Children who are unaffected are unlikely to pass along the trait, unless they have a child with someone who has Stargardt's or carries the gene.

Reprinted with permission of Healthcommunities.com, from www.vision channel.net/maculardegeneration/juvenile.shtml. © 2002 Healthcommunities .com, Inc; updated September 2002. For further information, contact Nancy Gable Lucas, Editor, at nlucas@healthcommunities.com.

A variation of this disorder is fundus flavimaculatus. Symptoms are similar, but the eye shows yellow-white spots and flecks of various shapes and minimal changes in the macula. Fundus flavimaculatus has a more favorable prognosis and symptoms often do not develop until young adulthood.

Best's vitelliform retinal dystrophy is the second most common type of JMD. The age of onset and severity of symptoms vary greatly, even among family members and it is usually diagnosed during childhood or adolescence.

In its early stages, a large, yellow, cyst-like drusen resembling an egg yolk forms under the retinal pigment epithelial (RPE) cells. Despite the cyst, vision often remains normal, or nearly normal, for many years. Eventually the cyst ruptures and the fluid and yellow deposits spread beneath the macula.

Once the cyst ruptures, degeneration of the macula and RPE cells begins, causing vision loss. Central vision may deteriorate to about 20/100 later in life. Peripheral vision usually remains unaffected, and Best's does not always affect both eyes equally. Many patients retain good central vision in at least one eye and sometimes, Best's disease does not cause significant central vision loss.

It has an autosomal dominant pattern of inheritance, which means that an affected person has one Best gene, paired with one normal gene. Affected individuals have a 50 percent chance of passing the disease-causing gene to a child, even if their partner is unaffected.

Treatment and Prevention

There is no treatment for JMD disorders. The disorders that cause neovascularization and leakage may respond to laser treatment, but there are no standard therapies.

Genetic testing and counseling may assist with family planning.

Chapter 28

Learning Disabilities, Dyslexia, and Vision

Policy

Learning disabilities are common conditions in pediatric patients. The etiology of these difficulties is multifactorial, reflecting genetic influences and abnormalities of brain structure and function. Early recognition and referral to qualified educational professionals is critical for the best possible outcome. Visual problems are rarely responsible for learning difficulties. No scientific evidence exists for the efficacy of eye exercises, vision therapy, or the use of special tinted lenses in the remediation of these complex pediatric neurological conditions.

Background

Learning disabilities have become an increasing personal and public concern. Among the spectrum of issues of concern in learning disabilities is the inability to read and comprehend, which is a major obstacle to learning and may have long-term educational, social, and economic implications. Family concern for the welfare of children with dyslexia and learning disabilities has led to a proliferation of diagnostic and remedial treatment procedures, many of which are controversial or without clear scientific evidence of efficacy. Many educators, psychologists, and medical specialists concur that individuals who have learning disabilities should:

1. receive early comprehensive educational, psychological, and medical assessment

2. receive educational remediation combined with appropriate psychological and medical treatment

3. avoid remedies involving eye exercises, filters, tinted lenses, or other optical devices that have no know scientific proof of efficacy

This chapter addresses these issues.

Evaluation and Management

Reading involves the integration of multiple factors related to an individual's experience, ability, and neurological functioning. Research has shown that the majority of children and adults with reading difficulties experience a variety of problems with language[1-3] that stem from altered brain function and that such difficulties are not caused by altered visual function.[4-7] In addition, a variety of secondary emotional and environmental factors may have a detrimental effect on the learning process in such children.

Sometimes children may also have a treatable visual difficulty along with their primary reading or learning dysfunction. Routine vision screening examinations can identify most of those who have reduced visual acuity. Pediatricians and other primary care physicians, whose pediatric patients cannot pass vision screening according to national standards,[8,9] should refer these patients to an ophthalmologist who has experience in the care of children.

Role of the Eyes

Decoding of retinal images occurs in the brain after visual signals are transmitted from the eye via the visual pathways. Some vision care practitioners incorrectly attribute reading difficulties to one or more subtle ocular or visual abnormalities. Although the eyes are obviously necessary for vision, the brain performs the complex function of interpreting visual images. Currently no scientific evidence supports the view that correction of subtle visual defects can alter the brain's processing of visual stimuli. Statistically, children with dyslexia or related learning disabilities have the same ocular health as children without such conditions.[10-12]

Controversies

Eye defects, subtle or severe, do not cause the patient to experience reversal of letters, words, or numbers. No scientific evidence supports claims that the academic abilities of children with learning disabilities can be improved with treatments that are based on 1) visual training, including muscle exercises, ocular pursuit, tracking exercises, or training glasses (with or without bifocals or prisms);[13-15] 2) neurological organizational training (laterality training, crawling, balance board, perceptual training);[16-18] or 3) colored lenses.[18-20] These more controversial methods of treatment may give parents and teachers a false sense of security that a child's reading difficulties are being addressed, which may delay proper instruction or remediation. The expense of these methods is unwarranted, and they cannot be substituted for appropriate educational measures. Claims of improved reading and learning after visual training, neurological organization training, or use of colored lenses, are almost always based on poorly controlled studies that typically rely on anecdotal information. These methods are without scientific validation.[21] Their reported benefits can be explained by the traditional educational remedial techniques with which they are usually combined.

Early Detection

Pediatricians, primary care physicians, and educational specialists may use screening techniques to detect learning disabilities in preschool-age children but, in many cases, the learning disability is discovered after the child experiences academic difficulties. Learning disabilities can include dyslexia, problems with memory and language, and difficulty with mathematic computation. These difficulties are often complicated by attention deficit disorders. A family history of learning disabilities is common in such conditions. Children who are considered to be at risk for or suspected of having these conditions by their physician should be evaluated by more detailed study by educational and/or psychological specialists.

Role of the Physician

Ocular defects in young children should be identified as early as possible, and when they are correctable, they should be managed by an ophthalmologist, who is experienced in the care of children.[22] Treatable ocular conditions among others include refractive errors, focusing deficiencies, eye muscle imbalances, and motor fusion deficiencies. When children have learning problems, that are suspected to be associated with visual defects, the ophthalmologist may be consulted by the primary care pediatrician. If no ocular defect is found, the child needs no further vision care or treatment and should be referred for medical and appropriate special educational evaluation and services. Pediatricians have an important role in coordination of care between the family and other health care services provided by ophthalmologists, optometrists, and other health care professionals who may become involved in the treatment plan.

Multidisciplinary Approach

The management of a child who has learning disabilities requires a multidisciplinary approach for diagnosis and treatment that involves educators, psychologists, and physicians. Basic scientific and clinical research into the role of the brain's structure and function in learning disabilities has demonstrated a neural basis of dyslexia and other specific learning disabilities and not the result of an ocular disorder alone.[4-6]

The Role of Education

The teaching of children, adolescents, and adults with dyslexia and learning disabilities is a challenge for educators. Skilled educators use standardized educational diagnostic evaluations and professional judgment to design and monitor individualized remedial programs. Psychologists may help with educational diagnosis and classification. Physicians, including pediatricians, otolaryngologists, neurologists, ophthalmologists, mental health professionals and other appropriate medical specialists, may assist in treating the health problems of these patients. Since remediation may be more effective during the early years, prompt diagnosis is paramount.[20-21] Educators, with specialty training in learning disabilities, ultimately play a key role in providing help for the learning disabled or dyslexic child or adult.

Recommendations

1. For all children, clinicians should perform vision screening according to national standards.[8,9]

2. Any child who cannot pass the recommended vision screening test should be referred to an ophthalmologist, who has experience in the care of children.

3. Children with educational problems and normal vision screening should be referred for educational diagnostic evaluation and appropriate special educational evaluation and services.

4. Diagnostic and treatment approaches that lack objective, scientifically established efficacy should not be used.

Summary

Reading difficulties and learning disabilities are complex problems that have no simple solutions. The American Academy of Pediatrics, the American Academy of Ophthalmology, and the American Association for Pediatric Ophthalmology and Strabismus strongly support the need for early diagnosis and educational remediation. There is no known eye or visual cause for these learning disabilities and no known effective visual treatment.[23,24] Recommendations for multidisciplinary evaluation and management must be based on evidence of proven effectiveness demonstrated by objective scientific methodology.[23,24] It is important that any therapy for learning disabilities be scientifically established to be valid before it can be recommended for treatment.

The recommendations in this policy statement do not indicate an exclusive course of treatment or procedure to be followed. Variations, taking into account individual circumstances, may be appropriate.

References

1. Mattis T, French JH, Rapin I. Dyslexia in children and young adults: Three independent neuropsychological syndromes. *Dev Med Child Neurol* 1975;17:150-163.

2. Vellutino FR. Dyslexia. *Scientific American* 1987;256(3):34-41.

3. Council on Scientific Affairs. Dyslexia. *JAMA* 1989;261:2236-2239.

4. Petersen SE, Fox PT, Posner MI, Mintun M, Raichle ME. Positron emission tomographic studies of the cortical anatomy of single-word processing. *Nature* 1988;331:585-589.

5. Galaburda A. Ordinary and extraordinary brain development: Anatomical variation in developmental dyslexia. *Ann of Dyslexia* 1989;39:67-80.

6. Hynd GW, Semrud-Clikeman M, Lorys AR, Novey ES, Eliopulos D. Brain morphology in developmental dyslexia and attention deficit disorder/hyperactivity. *Arch Neurol* 1990;47:919-926.

7. Metzger RL, Werner DB. Use of visual training for reading disabilities: A review. *Pediatrics* 1984;73:824-829.

8. American Academy of Pediatrics, Committee on Practice and Ambulatory medicine and Section on Ophthalmology. Eye examination and vision screening in infants, children, and young adults. *Pediatrics* 1996;98:153-157.

9. American Academy of Ophthalmology and American Association for Pediatric Ophthalmology and Strabismus. Vision Screening for Infants and Children. 1996.

10. Golberg HK, Drash PW. The disabled reader. *J Pediatr Ophthalmol* 1968;5:11-24.

11. Helveston EM, Weber JC, Miller K, et al. Visual function and academic performance. *Am J. Ophthalmol* 1985;99:346-355.

12. Levine MD. Reading disability: Do the eyes have it? *Pediatrics* 1984;73:869-870.

13. Keogh B, Pelland M. Vision training revisited. *J Learn Disabil* 1985;18:228-236.

14. Beauchamp GR. Optometric vision training. *Pediatrics* 1986:77:121-124.

15. Cohen HJ, Birch HG, Taft LT. Some considerations for evaluating the Doman-Delacato "patterning method." *Pediatrics* 1970;45:302-314.

16. Kavale K, Mattson PD. One jumped off the balance beam: Meta-analysis of perceptual-motor training. *J Learn Disabil* 1983;16:165-173.

17. Black JL, Collins DWK, DeRoach JN, et al. A detailed study of sequential saccadic eye movements for normal and poor reading children. *Percept Mot Skills* 1984;59:423-434.

18. Solan HA. An appraisal of the Irlen technique of correcting reading disorders using tinted overlays and tinted lenses. *J Learn Disabil* 1990;23:621-623.

19. Hoyt CS. Irlen lenses and reading difficulties. *J Learn Disabil* 1990;23:624-626.

20. Sedun AA. Dyslexia at New York Times: (mis)understanding of parallel vision processing. *Arch of Ophth* 1992;110:933-934.

21. Bradley L. Rhyme recognition and reading and spelling in young children. In: Masland RL, Masland MW, eds. *Preschool Prevention of Reading Failure*. Parkton, MD: York Press; 1988;143-162.

22. Ogden S, Hindman S, Turner SD. Multisensory programs in the public schools: A brighter future for LD children. *Annals of Dyslexia* 1989;39:247-267.

23. Romanchuk KG. Skepticism about Irlen filters to treat learning disabilities. *CMAJ*. 1995;153:397.

24. Silver LB. Controversial therapies. *J Child Neurol*. 1995;10 Suppl 1:S96-100.

Chapter 29

Retinitis Pigmentosa

Retinitis pigmentosa (RP) is the name given to a group of inherited diseases that affect the retina. They are characterized by a gradual breakdown and degeneration of photoreceptor cells, which results in a progressive loss of vision. It is estimated that RP affects 100,000 individuals in the United States.

Clinical Description

RP causes degeneration of the retina, a delicate tissue composed of several cell layers that line the inside of the back of the eye and contain photoreceptor cells (rods and cones). The rods are concentrated outside the center of the retina, known as the macula, and are required for peripheral vision and for night vision. The cones are concentrated in the macula and are responsible for central and color vision. Together, rods and cones are the cells responsible for converting light into electrical impulses that transfer messages to the brain where seeing actually occurs.

The most common feature of all forms of RP is a gradual breakdown and degeneration of the rods and cones. Depending on which type of cell is predominantly affected, the symptoms vary, and include night blindness, lost peripheral vision (also referred to as tunnel vision), and loss of the ability to discriminate color before peripheral vision is diminished.

Reprinted with permission from "Retinitis Pigmentosa" by Tom Hoglund. © 1998 Foundation Fighting Blindness, 11435 Cronhill Drive, Owings Mills, MD 21117-2220, (888) 394-3937. Additional information is available at www.blindness.org.

Symptoms of RP are most often recognized in adolescents and young adults, with progression of the disease usually continuing throughout the individual's life. The rate of progression and degree of visual loss are variable.

Inheritance

RP can be passed to succeeding family generations by one of three genetic inheritance patterns: autosomal dominant, autosomal recessive, or X-linked inheritance.

Because RP is an inherited disorder, it can potentially affect other family members. There are also cases of isolated inherited RP as well. Individuals of an affected family may not experience the same intensity of symptoms and as a result may not recognize that they have RP and need medical consultation. If one member of a family is diagnosed with a hereditary retinal degeneration, it is strongly advised that all members of that family contact an ophthalmologist.

Treatment

As yet, there is no known cure for RP. However, intensive research is currently under way to discover the cause, prevention, and treatment of RP. At this time, RP researchers have identified a first step in managing RP. While not a cure, certain doses of vitamin A have been found to slightly slow the progression of RP in some individuals. An information packet on this research breakthrough is available from The Foundation.

Researchers have found some of the genes that cause RP. It is now possible, in some families with X-linked RP or autosomal dominant RP, to perform a test on genetic material from blood and other cells to determine if members of an affected family have one of several RP genes.

Related Diseases

There are other inherited retinal degenerative diseases that share some of the clinical symptoms of RP. Some of these conditions are complicated by other symptoms besides loss of vision. The most common of these is Usher syndrome, which causes both hearing and vision loss. Other rare syndromes that researchers are studying with funding from The Foundation Fighting Blindness include Bardet-Biedl (Laurence-Moon) syndrome, Best disease, choroideremia, gyrate-atrophy, Leber Congenital Amaurosis, and Stargardt's Disease.

Chapter 30

Retinopathy of Prematurity

Overview

Retinopathy of prematurity (ROP), also known as retrolental fibro-
plasia, is a potentially blinding condition affecting the retina of newborns. In the 1950's it was associated with the use of high amounts
of oxygen in neonatal units. Today, modern neonatal care has curbed
the incidence, yet because the survival rate of low birth weight infants is much higher, the exposure of surviving babies to required
oxygen levels is increasing. The factors that put infants at greatest
risk of developing ROP are low birth weight (less than 3.5 pounds)
and premature delivery (26 to 28 weeks).

In babies born prematurely, the growth and development of normal blood vessels in the retina are halted and abnormal vessels
may begin to develop. The problem with abnormal vessel growth,
known as neovascularization, is that it does not deliver adequate
oxygen supply to the retina. In addition, it may cause many secondary problems.

ROP is classified in five stages, depending on the extent of the disease. Progression of the disease to later stages can lead to the formation of scar tissue in the retina and complications such as retinal
detachment, vitreous hemorrhage, strabismus, and amblyopia. Many
children with ROP develop nearsightedness.

Reprinted with permission from www.stlukeseye.com, the website of The
St. Luke's Cataract & Laser Institute, Tarpon Springs, FL. © 2000.

Signs and Symptoms

Because newborns cannot communicate their symptoms, parents, neonatologists, pediatricians, and ophthalmologists are keenly aware of risk factors for ROP.

- Low birth weight (3.5 pounds or less)
- The need for any oxygen within the first week after birth
- Unstable health immediately after birth

Children with ROP as infants should be watched for the following symptoms that could signal underlying problems that may not surface until later:

- Holding objects very close
- Difficulty seeing distant objects
- Favoring or winking one eye
- Reluctance to use one eye
- Poor vision (previously undetected by the physician)
- Sudden decrease of vision
- Crossed or turned eye

Detection and Diagnosis

Infants at risk for ROP should have an ophthalmic examination at approximately 4 to 6 weeks of age. After instilling a series of dilating drops in each eye, the doctor examines the retina with an ophthalmoscope. The exam is often performed while a parent holds the child.

Regardless of whether treatment is required, children should be reexamined at recommended intervals to determine if the progression of the disease has halted or whether treatment is required.

Treatment

Some children who develop only stage 1 to 2 of the disease improve with no treatment. In other cases, treatment is required if it reaches threshold. This is a term that indicates the presence of stage 3 changes.

To prevent the proliferation of abnormal vascularization, areas of the retina may be frozen with a technique called cryotherapy. Alternatively, laser may be used for the same purpose. Both treatments leave permanent scars in the peripheral retina, but they are often successful in preserving central vision.

St. Luke's Cataract & Laser Institute provides this chapter for educational and communication purposes only and it should not be construed as personal medical advice. Information published in this chapter is not intended to replace, supplant, or augment a consultation with an eye care professional regarding the viewer/user's own medical care. St. Luke's disclaims any and all liability for injury or other damages that could result from use of the information obtained from this chapter.

Chapter 31

Strabismus

What is strabismus?

Strabismus is a deviation of the eyes. The term is used to describe eyes that are not straight or properly aligned.

What causes the misalignment?

The misalignment results from the failure of the eye muscles to work together. One eye, or sometimes both, may turn in (crossed eyes), turn out (wall eyes), turn up, or turn down. Sometimes more than one of the turns are present.

When strabismus is present, will the eyes always look misaligned?

The deviation may be constant or it may come and go. In young children strabismus may vary not only from day to day, but during the course of a day.

My infant's eyes roll all over. Should I be concerned?

At birth, an infant's eyes cannot always focus directly on objects. They may appear to move quite independently at first, sometimes

"Frequently Asked Questions about Strabismus," reprinted with permission from Prevent Blindness America. © 2000. For additional information, call the Prevent Blindness America toll-free information line at (800) 331-2020, or visit www.preventblindness.org.

crossing, and sometimes wandering outward. But by the age of three to four months, an infant's eyes should have the ability to focus on small objects and the eyes should be straight or parallel. A six-month-old infant should be able to focus on both distant and near objects.

What should I do if I notice wandering eyes in my four-month-old child?

If parents notice crossed or wall eyes persisting in a child four months of age, they should immediately take the child to an eye care professional for an examination. Early medical attention is recommended for another important reason—to rule out the presence of a serious disease, such as a tumor.

What if my baby appears completely healthy?

Prevent Blindness America recommends that all children have an eye exam by the age of six months.

Is strabismus present at birth?

Strabismus may be present at birth, it may become apparent at a later age, or it may appear at any time in life as a result of illness or accident.

How many children have strabismus?

Approximately two percent of the nation's children have strabismus. Half of them are born with the condition.

Is it important to detect strabismus early?

It is critical that this condition be diagnosed and corrected at an early age since children with uncorrected strabismus may go on to develop amblyopia.

What is false or pseudo-strabismus?

Certain children may appear to have strabismus when, in fact, they do not. An extra fold of skin near the inner eye, a broad, flat nose, or eyes that are unusually close together may also produce the effect of false (or pseudo) strabismus. False strabismus should disappear as the child's face grows.

After a professional examination, a parent's concern can be quickly dispelled if false strabismus is present.

What treatment is available for strabismus?

Strabismus cannot be outgrown, nor will it improve by itself. Treatment to straighten the eyes is required. The types of treatments may be used alone or in combination, depending on the type of strabismus and its cause.

- Glasses are commonly prescribed to improve focusing and redirect the line of sight, enabling the eyes to straighten.

- Medication in the form of eye drops or ointment may be used, with or without glasses. Injected medication may be used to selectively weaken an overactive eye muscle.

- Surgery may be performed on eye muscles to straighten the eyes if nonsurgical means are unsuccessful.

- Eye exercise, a limited form of treatment, may be recommended either before or after surgery to teach proper eye coordination.

To learn more about strabismus, please contact Prevent Blindness America or the Prevent Blindness affiliate near you.

Chapter 32

Tear-Duct Obstruction and Surgery

Many children are born with an underdeveloped tear-duct system, a problem that can lead to tear-duct blockage, excess tearing, and infection.

Blocked tear ducts are a fairly common problem in infants; as many as one third may be born with this condition. Fortunately, more than 90 percent of all cases resolve by the time children are 1 year old with little or no treatment. The earlier that blocked tear ducts are discovered, the less likely it is that infection will result or surgery will be necessary.

What Are Tear Ducts?

Our eyes are continually exposed to dust, bacteria, viruses, and other objects that could cause damage. The eyelids and eyelashes play a key role in preventing these objects from entering our eyes and hurting them. But besides serving as barriers, the lids and lashes also help our eyes stay moist. Without moisture, our corneas, which serve as protective domes for the front of the eyes, would dry out and could become cloudy or injured.

Working with our lids and lashes, the protective system of glands and ducts called the lacrimal system keeps our eyes from drying out.

This information was provided by KidsHealth, one of the largest resources online for medically reviewed health information written for parents, kids, and teens. For more articles like this one, visit www.KidsHealth.org or www.TeensHealth.org. © 2001 The Nemours Center for Children's Health Media, a division of The Nemours Foundation.

Small glands at the edge of the eyelid produce an oily film that mixes with the liquid part of our tears and keeps them from evaporating. Lacrimal (or tear-producing) glands secrete the watery part of tears. These glands are located under the brow bone behind the upper eyelid, at the edge of the eye socket, and in the lids.

Eyelids move tears across the eyes. Tears keep the eyes lubricated and clean and contain antibodies that protect the eyes from infection. They drain out of the eyes through two ducts called punctum or lacrimal ducts, one on each of the upper and lower lids. From these ducts, tears enter small tubes called canaliculi, which are located at the inner corner of the eyelids. They pass from the eyes into the lacrimal sac, a small sac that's located next to the inner corner of the eyes (between the eyes and the nose).

From the lacrimal sacs, tears move down through the nasolacrimal duct and drain into the back of the nose. (That's why you usually get a runny nose when you cry—your eyes are producing excess tears, and your nose can't handle the additional flow.) When you blink, the motion forces the lacrimal sacs to compress, squeezing tears out of them, away from the eyes, and into the nasolacrimal duct.

The nasolacrimal duct and the lacrimal ducts are also known as tear ducts. However, it's the nasolacrimal duct that's involved in tear-duct blockage.

What Causes a Blocked Tear Duct?

Many children are born without a fully developed nasolacrimal duct. This is called congenital nasolacrimal duct obstruction or dacryostenosis. Most commonly, an infant is born with a duct that is more narrow than usual and therefore does not drain properly or becomes blocked easily. The majority of children outgrow this condition by the time they are 1 year old. Less often, a child has a web of tissue over the end of the duct that didn't dissolve during fetal development. This condition is more likely to require surgical probing.

Other causes of blockage in children (especially older children) are rare. Some children have nasal polyps, which are cysts or growths of extra tissue in the nose at the end of the tear duct. A blockage can also be caused by a tumor in the nose, but again, this is unusual in children.

Trauma to the eye area or an eye injury that lacerates (cuts through) the tear ducts could also cause this condition, but reconstructive surgery at the time of the accident or injury may prevent blockage from happening.

318

Signs of Blocked Tear Ducts

Children with blocked tear ducts usually develop signs of the condition between birth and 12 weeks of age, although you may not realize your child has this problem until his eye becomes infected. The most common signs of blocked tear ducts are excessive tearing, even when a child is not crying (this is called epiphora). You may also notice pus in the corner of your child's eye, or he may wake up with a crust over the eyelid or in the eyelashes.

Children with blocked tear ducts may also develop an infection in their lacrimal sac called dacryocystitis. Signs of this infection include redness at the inner corner of the eye and a slight tenderness and swelling or bump at the side of the nose.

Another sign that the tear ducts may be blocked can be present at birth or soon after. Some infants are born with a swollen lacrimal sac, causing a blue bump called a dacryocystocele to appear next to the inside corner of the eye. Although this condition should be monitored closely by your child's doctor, it doesn't always lead to infection and can be treated at home with firm massage and topical antibiotics. However, if it becomes infected, the child is usually admitted to the hospital for intravenous antibiotics, followed by surgical probing of the duct.

When to Call Your Child's Doctor

If your child suffers from excessive tearing but shows no sign of infection, consult with your child's doctor or a pediatric ophthalmologist (eye specialist) to see if your child has a blocked tear duct. Early treatment can prevent the need for surgery. If signs of infection (such as redness, pus, or swelling) are present, call your child's doctor immediately because the infection can spread to other parts of the face or lead to an abscess if not treated.

Treating Blocked Tear Ducts

Children with blocked tear ducts often can be treated at home. Your child's doctor or pediatric ophthalmologist may recommend that you massage the eye several times daily for a couple of months. Before massaging the tear duct, wash your hands. Place your index finger on the side of your child's nose and firmly massage down toward the corner of the nose. You may also want to apply warm compresses to the eye to help promote drainage and ease any discomfort your child may have.

If your child develops an infection as a result of the tear-duct blockage, your child's doctor will prescribe antibiotic eye drops or ointment to treat the infection. It's important to remember that antibiotics will not get rid of the obstruction. Once the infection has cleared, you can continue massaging the tear duct as your child's doctor recommends.

If your child still has excess tearing after 6 to 8 months, develops a serious infection, or has repeated infections, the doctor may recommend that your child's tear duct be surgically probed. This procedure has an 85 percent to 95 percent success rate for children who are one year old or younger; the success rate drops as children age.

Surgical probing may be repeated if it's not initially successful. If your child continues to experience blockage, your child's doctor may also recommend surgery to widen the tear ducts using tubes that are implanted in your child's tear ducts for 6 months, or a balloon that stretches the tear duct. Both of these surgical procedures have high success rates.

What Happens before and during Surgery?

Surgery should be performed by a pediatric ophthalmologist who is familiar with the procedure—your child's doctor should be able to refer you to such a specialist. All three surgical procedures are done on an outpatient basis (unless your child is suffering from a severe infection and has already been admitted to the hospital) under general anesthesia.

When a child is referred for a blocked tear duct because of an infection or excessive tearing, a pediatric ophthalmologist will do a complete eye exam to make sure that a blocked tear duct is actually the cause of the problem. That's because lashes rubbing on the eye, inflammation of the eye, or congenital glaucoma could cause some of the same symptoms.

A dye disappearance test may also help determine the cause of the problem. This involves placing fluorescein dye in the eye and then examining the tear film (the amount of tear in the eye) to see if it's greater than it should be. Or the doctor will wait to see if dye has drained properly by having the child blow his nose and then checking to see if any of the dye exited through the nose.

A surgical probe takes about 10 minutes. A thin, blunt metal wire is gently passed through the tear duct to open any obstruction. Sterile saline is then irrigated through the duct into the nose to make sure that there is now an open path. Infants experience no pain after the probing.

If surgical probing is unsuccessful, your child's doctor may recommend further surgical treatment. The more traditional form of treatment is called silicone tube intubation. In this procedure, silicone tubes are placed in your child's tear ducts to stretch them. The tubes are left in place for 6 months and then removed in another short surgical procedure.

A newer form of treatment is balloon catheter dilation (DCP) or LacriCATH. In this procedure, a balloon is inserted through an opening in the corner of the eye and into the tear duct. The balloon is inflated with a sterile solution to expand the tear duct for 90 seconds. It is then deflated and reinflated for 60 seconds before being repositioned slightly higher in the duct and inflated twice again. It's then deflated and removed.

Both of these procedures are fairly short—your child will be in surgery for less than an hour. Success rates are not as well documented with these two procedures, although they are both considered to be generally successful.

Taking Care of Your Child after Surgery

It may take up to a week after surgery before your child's symptoms improve. Your child's doctor will give you antibiotic ointment or drops along with specific instructions on how to care for your child.

Note: All information on KidsHealth is for educational purposes only. For specific medical advice, diagnoses, and treatment, consult your doctor.

Part Five

Disorders with Eye-Related Complications

Chapter 33

Behçet's Disease of the Eye

The information provided in this chapter was developed by the National Eye Institute to help patients and their families in searching for general information about Behçet's disease. An eye care professional who has examined the patient's eyes and is familiar with his or her medical history is the best person to answer specific questions.

What Is Behçet's Disease?

Behçet's disease is an autoimmune disease that results from damage to blood vessels throughout the body, particularly veins. In an autoimmune disease, the immune system attacks and harms the body's own tissues.

What Causes Behçet's Disease?

The exact cause is unknown. It is believed that an autoimmune reaction may cause blood vessels to become inflamed, but it is not clear what triggers this reaction.

What Are the Symptoms of Behçet's Disease?

Behçet's disease affects each person differently. The four most common symptoms are mouth sores, genital sores, inflammation inside

"Behçet's Disease of the Eye Resource Guide," National Eye Institute, available online at http://www.nei.nih.gov, September 2002.

of the eye, and skin problems. Inflammation inside of the eye (uveitis, retinitis, and iritis) occurs in more that half of those with Behçet's disease and can cause blurred vision, pain, and redness.

Other symptoms may include arthritis, blood clots, and inflammation in the central nervous system and digestive organs.

How Is Behçet's Disease Treated?

There is no cure for Behçet's disease. Treatment typically focuses on reducing discomfort and preventing serious complications.

Corticosteroids and other medications that suppress the immune system may be prescribed to treat inflammation.

What Is the Prognosis for Someone with Behçet's Disease?

Behçet's is a chronic disease that recurs. However, patients may have periods of time when symptoms go away temporarily (remission).

How severe the disease is varies from patient to patient. Some patients may live normal lives, but others may become blind or severely disabled.

NEI-Supported Research

A Study to Investigate the Safety and Efficacy of HAT to Treat the Ocular Complications Related to Behçet's Disease

The National Eye Institute is evaluating the safety and effectiveness of Zenapax in controlling recurrent eye inflammations associated with Behçet's disease. Zenapax was previously studied in 10 patients with uveitis with positive results. The patients were able to reduce the other medicines they were taking with minimal side effects. This study is currently recruiting patients. For additional information, please contact NIH Patient Recruitment and Public Liaison Office at (800) 411-1222.

Other Resources

The following organizations may be able to provide additional information on Behçet's disease:

National Institute of Arthritis and Musculoskeletal and Skin Diseases (NIAMS)

1 AMS Circle
Bethesda, MD 20892-3675
Phone: (301) 496-8188
Website: http://www.nih.gov/niams

Conducts and supports research on the many forms of arthritis and diseases of the musculoskeletal system (bones) and the skin. Provides information on Behçet's disease.

American Behçet's Disease Association

P.O. Box 15247
Chattanooga, TN 37415-0240
Toll-Free: (800) 723-4238
Website: http://www.behcets.com

Provides support and information to people with Behçet's disease, publishes a quarterly newsletter, distributes patient pamphlets, and coordinates a pen pal/phone pal network. Provides physician referrals, coordinates a network of local support groups, and holds an annual international conference.

National Organization for Rare Disorders, Inc. (NORD)

P.O. Box 8923
New Fairfield, CT 06812-8923
Toll-Free: (800) 999-6673
Phone: (203) 746-6481
Website: http://www.rarediseases.org

Provides information about rare disorders and connects families with similar disorders with each other for mutual support. Serves people with orphan diseases who are not otherwise represented. Maintains information on Behçet's disease in the Rare Disease Database.

For additional information, you may also wish to contact a local library.

Medical Literature

Below is a sample of the citations available through MEDLINE/ PubMed, a service of the National Library of Medicine. MEDLINE/ PubMed provides access to over 11 million medical literature citations from 1966 to the present and includes links to many sites providing full text articles and other related resources. You can conduct your own free literature search by accessing MEDLINE through the Internet at http://medlineplus.nlm.nih.gov/hinfo.html. You can also get assistance with a literature search at a local library.

To obtain copies of any of the articles listed below, contact a local community, university, or medical library. If the library you visit does not have a copy of a desired article, you may usually obtain it through an inter-library loan.

Please keep in mind that articles in the medical literature are usually written in technical language. We encourage you to share any articles you order with a health care professional who can help you understand them.

Behçet's Disease: Immunopathologic and Therapeutic Aspects

Meador R, Ehrlich G, Von Feldt JM: *Current Rheumatology Reports* 4(1):47-54, February 2002.

Behçet's disease (BD) is a systemic inflammatory disease of unknown etiology. The disease is strongly associated with the human leukocyte antigen (HLA) B51. BD has a chronic course with periodic exacerbations and progressive deterioration. There are no specific diagnostic laboratory tests, although recurrent oral ulceration is an obligatory manifestation for diagnosis. The treatment, which includes local, systemic, or surgical therapies, is based on the severity of the illness; the most appropriate management requires a multidisciplinary approach. This paper summarizes all aspects of BD with particular emphasis on the latest immunologic and treatment aspects.

Behçet's Disease: An Update

Ehrlich GE University of Pennsylvania School of Medicine. *Comprehensive Therapy* 25(4):216-20, April 1999.

This article reviews current therapies for Behçet's disease, although no diagnostic laboratory test or cure has been found. Genetic studies have identified those most at risk, and newer molecular biologic investigations further clarify its etiology and shed light on potential triggers.

Ocular Immunopathology of Behçet's Disease

George RK, Chan CC, Whitcup SM, Nussenblatt RB. Madigan Army Medical Center, Tacoma, Washington. *Survey of Ophthalmology* 42(2):157-62, 1997.

This article describes a patient who developed progressive, severe, recurrent iridocyclitis in both eyes, retinal vasculitis, and hemorrhagic infarction of the retina that led to blindness despite immunosuppressive therapy. Histopathology revealed marked nongranulomatous uveitis with a predominantly CD4+ T-lymphocytic infiltration, as well as B-cell and plasma cell aggregation.

Extensive expression of adhesion molecules was found on vascular endothelial cells. This finding suggests that adhesion molecules play an important role in the vasculitic process that is the hallmark of Behçet's disease. The ocular pathology and the therapeutic approach to Behçet's disease are briefly reviewed as well.

The National Eye Institute, part of the National Institutes of Health, is the Federal government's principal agency for conducting and supporting vision research. Inclusion of an item in this chapter does not imply the endorsement of the National Eye Institute or the National Institutes of Health.

Chapter 34

Diabetic Retinopathy

Chapter Contents

Section 34.1

Facts about Diabetic Retinopathy

"Facts about Diabetic Retinopathy," National Eye Institute, available
online at http://www.nei.nih.gov, March 2000.

This chapter has been written to help people with diabetic retinopathy and their families and friends better understand the disease. It describes the cause, symptoms, diagnosis, and treatment of diabetic retinopathy.

Diabetic retinopathy is a potentially blinding complication of diabetes that damages the eye's retina. It affects half of all Americans diagnosed with diabetes.

At first, you may notice no changes in your vision. But don't let diabetic retinopathy fool you. It could get worse over the years and threaten your good vision. With timely treatment, 90 percent of those with advanced diabetic retinopathy can be saved from going blind.

The National Eye Institute (NEI) is the Federal government's lead agency for vision research. The NEI urges all people with diabetes to have an eye examination through dilated pupils at least once a year.

What Is the Retina?

The retina is a light-sensitive tissue at the back of the eye. When light enters the eye, the retina changes the light into nerve signals. The retina then sends these signals along the optic nerve to the brain. Without a retina, the eye cannot communicate with the brain, making vision impossible.

How Does Diabetic Retinopathy Damage the Retina?

Diabetic retinopathy occurs when diabetes damages the tiny blood vessels in the retina. At this point, most people do not notice any changes in their vision.

Some people develop a condition called macular edema. It occurs when the damaged blood vessels leak fluid and lipids onto the macula, the part of the retina that lets us see detail. The fluid makes the macula swell, blurring vision.

As the disease progresses, it enters its advanced, or proliferative, stage. Fragile, new blood vessels grow along the retina and in the clear, gel-like vitreous that fills the inside of the eye. Without timely treatment, these new blood vessels can bleed, cloud vision, and destroy the retina.

Who Is at Risk for This Disease?

All people with diabetes are at risk—those with Type I diabetes (juvenile onset) and those with Type II diabetes (adult onset).

During pregnancy, diabetic retinopathy may also be a problem for women with diabetes. It is recommended that all pregnant women with diabetes have dilated eye examinations each trimester to protect their vision.

What Are Its Symptoms?

Diabetic retinopathy often has no early warning signs. At some point, though, you may have macular edema. It blurs vision, making it hard to do things like read and drive. In some cases, your vision will get better or worse during the day.

As new blood vessels form at the back of the eye, they can bleed (hemorrhage) and blur vision. The first time this happens it may not be very severe. In most cases, it will leave just a few specks of blood, or spots, floating in your vision. They often go away after a few hours.

These spots are often followed within a few days or weeks by a much greater leakage of blood. The blood will blur your vision. In extreme cases, a person will only be able to tell light from dark in that eye. It may take the blood anywhere from a few days to months or even years to clear from the inside of your eye. In some cases, the blood will not clear. You should be aware that large hemorrhages tend to happen more than once, often during sleep.

How Is It Detected?

Diabetic retinopathy is detected during an eye examination that includes:

- Visual acuity test: This eye chart test measures how well you see at various distances.

333

- Pupil dilation: The eye care professional places drops into the eye to widen the pupil. This allows him or her to see more of the retina and look for signs of diabetic retinopathy. After the examination, close-up vision may remain blurred for several hours.

- Ophthalmoscopy: This is an examination of the retina in which the eye care professional: (1) looks through a device with a special magnifying lens that provides a narrow view of the retina, or (2) wearing a headset with a bright light, looks through a special magnifying glass and gains a wide view of the retina.

- Tonometry: A standard test that determines the fluid pressure inside the eye. Elevated pressure is a possible sign of glaucoma, another common eye problem in people with diabetes.

Your eye care professional will look at your retina for early signs of the disease, such as: (1) leaking blood vessels, (2) retinal swelling, such as macular edema, (3) pale, fatty deposits on the retina—signs of leaking blood vessels, (4) damaged nerve tissue, and (5) any changes in the blood vessels.

Should your doctor suspect that you need treatment for macular edema, he or she may ask you to have a test called fluorescein angiography.

In this test, a special dye is injected into your arm. Pictures are then taken as the dye passes through the blood vessels in the retina. This test allows your doctor to find the leaking blood vessels.

How Is It Treated?

There are two treatments for diabetic retinopathy. They are very effective in reducing vision loss from this disease. In fact, even people with advanced retinopathy have a 90 percent chance of keeping their vision when they get treatment before the retina is severely damaged.

These two treatments are laser surgery and vitrectomy. It is important to note that although these treatments are very successful, they do not cure diabetic retinopathy.

Laser Surgery

Laser surgery is performed in a doctor's office or eye clinic. Before the surgery, your ophthalmologist will: (1) dilate your pupil and (2) apply drops to numb the eye. In some cases, the doctor also may numb the area behind the eye to prevent any discomfort.

The lights in the office will be dim. As you sit facing the laser machine, your doctor will hold a special lens to your eye. During the procedure, you may see flashes of light. These flashes may eventually create a stinging sensation that makes you feel a little uncomfortable.

You may leave the office once the treatment is done, but you will need someone to drive you home. Because your pupils will remain dilated for a few hours, you also should bring a pair of sunglasses.

For the rest of the day, your vision will probably be a little blurry. If your eye hurts a bit, your eye care professional can suggest a way to control this.

Doctors will perform laser surgery to treat severe macular edema and proliferative retinopathy.

Macular Edema

Timely laser surgery can reduce vision loss from macular edema by half. But you may need to have laser surgery more than once to control the leaking fluid.

During the surgery, your doctor will aim a high-energy beam of light directly onto the damaged blood vessels. This is called focal laser treatment. This seals the vessels and stops them from leaking.

Generally, laser surgery is used to stabilize vision, not necessarily to improve it.

Proliferative Retinopathy

In treating advanced diabetic retinopathy, doctors use the laser to destroy the abnormal blood vessels that form at the back of the eye.

Rather than focus the light on a single spot, your eye care professional will make hundreds of small laser burns away from the center of the retina. This is called scatter laser treatment. The treatment shrinks the abnormal blood vessels. You will lose some of your side vision after this surgery to save the rest of your sight.

Laser surgery may also slightly reduce your color and night vision. Once you have proliferative retinopathy, you will always be at risk for new bleeding. This means you may need treatment more than once to protect your sight.

Vitrectomy

Instead of laser surgery, you may need an eye operation called a vitrectomy to restore your sight. A vitrectomy is performed if you have a lot of blood in the vitreous. It involves removing the cloudy vitreous and replacing it with a salt solution. Because the vitreous is mostly water, you will notice no change between the salt solution and the normal vitreous.

Studies show that people who have a vitrectomy soon after a large hemorrhage are more likely to protect their vision than someone who waits to have the operation.

Early vitrectomy is especially effective in people with insulin-dependent diabetes, who may be at greater risk of blindness from a hemorrhage into the eye.

Vitrectomy is often done under local anesthesia. This means that you will be awake during the operation. The doctor makes a tiny incision in the sclera, or white of the eye. Next, a small instrument is placed into the eye. It removes the vitreous and inserts the salt solution into the eye.

You may be able to return home soon after the vitrectomy. Or, you may be asked to stay in the hospital overnight. Your eye will be red and sensitive. After the operation, you will need to wear an eye patch for a few days or weeks to protect the eye. You will also need to use medicated eye drops to protect against infection.

What Research Is Being Done?

The NEI is currently supporting a number of research studies in both the laboratory and with patients to learn more about the cause of diabetic retinopathy. This research should provide better ways to detect, treat, and prevent vision loss in people with diabetes.

For example, it is likely that in the coming years researchers will develop drugs that turn off enzyme activity that has been shown to cause diabetic retinopathy. Some day, these drugs will help people to control the disease and reduce the need for laser surgery.

What Can You Do to Protect Your Vision?

The NEI urges all people with diabetes to have an eye examination through dilated pupils at least once a year. If you have more serious retinopathy, you may need to have a dilated eye examination more often.

A recent study, the Diabetes Control and Complications Trial (DCCT), showed that better control of blood sugar levels slows the onset and progression of retinopathy and lessens the need for laser surgery for severe retinopathy.

The study found that the group that tried to keep their blood sugar levels as close to normal as possible, had much less eye, kidney, and nerve disease. This level of blood sugar control may not be best for everyone, including some elderly patients, children under 13, or people with heart disease. So ask your doctor if this program is right for you.

For more information about diabetic retinopathy or diabetes, you may wish to contact:

American Academy of Ophthalmology
P.O. Box 7424
San Francisco, CA 94120-7424
Phone: (415) 561-8500
Website: http://www.aao.org

American Optometric Association
243 North Lindbergh Blvd.
St. Louis, MO 63141
Phone: (314) 991-4100
Website: http://www.aoa.org

American Diabetes Association
1701 North Beauregard Street
Alexandria, VA 22314
Toll-free: (800) 342-2383
Phone: (703) 549-1500
Website: http://www.diabetes.org

Juvenile Diabetes Foundation International
432 Park Avenue South
New York, NY 10016
Phone: (212) 889-7575
Website: http://www.jdfcare.com

National Diabetes Information Clearinghouse
National Institute of Diabetes and Digestive and Kidney Diseases
1 Information Way
Bethesda, MD 20892-3560
Phone: (301) 654-3327
Website: http://www.niddk.nih.gov

National Eye Institute
2020 Vision Place
Bethesda, MD 20892-3655
Phone: (301) 496-5248
Website: http://www.nei.nih.gov

Prevent Blindness America
500 E. Remington Rd.
Schaumburg, IL 60173
Toll-Free: (800) 331-2020
Phone: (847) 843-2020
Website: http://www.preventblindness.org

Section 34.2

Prevent Diabetes Problems: Keep Your Eyes Healthy

"Prevent Diabetes Problems—Keep Your Eyes Healthy," National Institutes of Health Publication No. 00-4279, National Institute of Digestive and Diabetes and Kidney Disorders, available online at http://www.niddk.nih.gov, May 2000.

What Are Diabetes Problems?

Too much sugar in the blood for a long time causes diabetes problems. This high blood sugar can damage many parts of the body, such as the eyes, heart, and blood vessels. Diabetes problems can be scary, but there is a lot you can do to prevent them or slow them down.

This chapter is about eye problems caused by diabetes. You will learn the things you can do each day and during each year to stay healthy and prevent diabetes problems.

What Should I Do Each Day to Stay Healthy with Diabetes?

- Follow the healthy eating plan that you and your doctor or dietitian have worked out. Eat your meals and snacks at around the same times each day.

- Be active a total of 30 minutes most days. Ask your doctor what activities are best for you.

- Take your diabetes medicine at the same times each day.

- Check your blood sugar every day. Each time you check your blood sugar, write the number in your record book. Call your doctor if your numbers are too high or too low for two to three days.

- Check your feet every day for cuts, blisters, sores, swelling, redness, or sore toenails.

- Brush and floss your teeth and gums every day.

- Don't smoke.

What Can I Do to Prevent Diabetes Eye Problems?

- Keep your blood sugar and blood pressure as close to normal as you can.

- Have an eye doctor examine your eyes once a year. Have this exam even if your vision is OK. The eye doctor will use drops to make the black part of your eyes (pupils) bigger. This is called dilating your pupil, which allows the doctor to see your retina. Finding eye problems early and getting treatment right away will help prevent more serious problems later on.

- Ask your eye doctor to check for signs of cataracts and glaucoma.

- If you are pregnant and have diabetes, see an eye doctor during your first three months.

- If you are planning to get pregnant, ask your doctor if you should have an eye exam.

- Don't smoke.

How Can Diabetes Hurt My Eyes?

High blood sugar and high blood pressure from diabetes can hurt four parts of your eye:

- Retina: The retina is the lining at the back of the eye. The retina's job is to sense light coming into the eye.

- Vitreous: The vitreous is a jelly-like fluid that fills the back of the eye.

- Lens: The lens is at the front of the eye and it focuses light on the retina.

- Optic nerve: The optic nerve is the eye's main nerve to the brain.

How Can Diabetes Hurt the Retinas of My Eyes?

Retina damage happens slowly. Your retinas have tiny blood vessels that are easy to damage. Having high blood sugar and high blood pressure for a long time can damage these tiny blood vessels.

First, these tiny blood vessels swell and weaken. Some blood vessels then become clogged and do not let enough blood through. At first, you might not have any loss of sight from these changes. This is why you need to have a dilated eye exam once a year even if your sight seems fine.

One of your eyes may be damaged more than the other. Or both eyes may have the same amount of damage. Diabetic retinopathy is the medical term for the most common diabetes eye problem.

What happens as diabetes retina problems get worse? As diabetes retina problems get worse, new blood vessels grow. These new blood vessels are weak. They break easily and leak blood into the vitreous of your eye. The leaking blood keeps light from reaching the retina.

You may see floating spots or almost total darkness. Sometimes the blood will clear out by itself. But you might need surgery to remove it. Over the years, the swollen and weak blood vessels can form scar tissue and pull the retina away from the back of the eye. If the retina becomes detached, you may see floating spots or flashing lights.

You may feel as if a curtain has been pulled over part of what you are looking at. A detached retina can cause loss of sight or blindness if you don't take care of it right away.

Call your doctor right away if you think you have a detached retina.

What Can I Do about Diabetes Retina Problems?

First, keep your blood sugar and blood pressure as close to normal as you can. Your eye doctor may suggest laser treatment, which is when a light beam is aimed into the retina of the damaged eye. The beam closes off leaking blood vessels. It may stop blood and fluid from leaking into the vitreous. Laser treatment may slow the loss of sight.

If a lot of blood has leaked into your vitreous and your sight is poor, your eye doctor might suggest you have surgery called a vitrectomy.

340

A vitrectomy removes blood and fluids from the vitreous of your eye. Then clean fluid is put back into the eye. The surgery often makes your eyesight better.

How Do I Know if I Have Retina Damage from Diabetes?

You may not get any signs of diabetes retina damage or you may get one or more signs:

- Blurry or double vision
- Rings, flashing lights, or blank spots
- Dark or floating spots
- Pain or pressure in one or both of your eyes
- Trouble seeing things out of the corners of your eyes

Does Diabetes Cause Other Eye Problems?

Yes. You can get two other eye problems—cataracts and glaucoma. People without diabetes can get these eye problems, too. But people with diabetes get them more often and at a younger age.

A cataract is a cloud over the lens of your eye, which is usually clear. The lens focuses light onto the retina. A cataract makes everything you look at seem cloudy. You need surgery to remove the cataract. During surgery your lens is taken out and a plastic lens, like a contact lens, is put in. The plastic lens stays in your eye all the time. Cataract surgery helps you see clearly again.

Glaucoma starts from pressure building up in the eye. Over time, this pressure damages your eye's main nerve—the optic nerve. The damage first causes you to lose sight from the sides of your eyes. Without treatment, you can go blind. Treating glaucoma is usually simple. Your eye doctor will give you special drops to use every day to lower the pressure in your eye. Or your eye doctor may want you to have laser surgery.

For More Information

National Diabetes Information Clearinghouse
1 Information Way
Bethesda, MD 20892-3560
Phone: (301) 654-3327
Fax: (301) 907-8906
E-mail: ndic@info.niddk.nih.gov

The National Diabetes Information Clearinghouse (NDIC) is a service of the National Institute of Diabetes and Digestive and Kidney Diseases (NIDDK). NIDDK is part of the National Institutes of Health under the U.S. Department of Health and Human Services. Established in 1978, the clearinghouse provides information about diabetes to people with diabetes and to their families, health care professionals, and the public. NDIC answers inquiries; develops, reviews, and distributes publications; and works closely with professional and patient organizations and Government agencies to coordinate resources about diabetes.

Publications produced by the clearinghouse are carefully reviewed for scientific accuracy, content, and readability.

Chapter 35

Histoplasmosis

What Is Histoplasmosis?

Histoplasmosis is a disease caused when airborne spores of the fungus *Histoplasma capsulatum* are inhaled into the lungs, the primary infection site. This microscopic fungus, which is found throughout the world in river valleys and soil where bird or bat droppings accumulate, is released into the air when soil is disturbed by plowing fields, sweeping chicken coops, or digging holes.

Histoplasmosis is often so mild that it produces no apparent symptoms. Any symptoms that might occur are often similar to those from a common cold. In fact, if you had histoplasmosis symptoms, you might dismiss them as those from a cold or flu, since the body's immune system normally overcomes the infection in a few days without treatment.

However, histoplasmosis, even mild cases, can later cause a serious eye disease called ocular histoplasmosis syndrome (OHS), a leading cause of vision loss in Americans ages 20 to 40.

How Does Histoplasmosis Cause Ocular Histoplasmosis Syndrome?

Scientists believe that *Histoplasma capsulatum* (histo) spores spread from the lungs to the eye, lodging in the choroid, a layer of blood

"Histoplasmosis Resource Guide," National Eye Institute, available online at http://www.nei.nih.gov, June 2002.

343

vessels that provides blood and nutrients to the retina. The retina is the light-sensitive layer of tissue that lines the back of the eye. Scientists have not yet been able to detect any trace of the histo fungus in the eyes of patients with ocular histoplasmosis syndrome. Nevertheless, there is good reason to suspect the histo organism as the cause of OHS.

How Does OHS Develop?

OHS develops when fragile, abnormal blood vessels grow underneath the retina. These abnormal blood vessels form a lesion known as choroidal neovascularization (CNV). If left untreated, the CNV lesion can turn into scar tissue and replace the normal retinal tissue in the macula. The macula is the central part of the retina that provides the sharp, central vision that allows us to read a newspaper or drive a car. When this scar tissue forms, visual messages from the retina to the brain are affected, and vision loss results.

Vision is also impaired when these abnormal blood vessels leak fluid and blood into the macula. If these abnormal blood vessels grow toward the center of the macula, they may affect a tiny depression called the fovea. The fovea is the region of the retina with the highest concentration of special retinal nerve cells, called cones, that produce sharp, daytime vision. Damage to the fovea and the cones can severely impair, and even destroy, this straight-ahead vision. Early treatment of OHS is essential; if the abnormal blood vessels have affected the fovea, controlling the disease will be more difficult. Since OHS rarely affects side, or peripheral vision, the disease does not cause total blindness.

What Are the Symptoms of OHS?

OHS usually has no symptoms in its early stages; the initial OHS infection usually subsides without the need for treatment. This is true for other histo infections; in fact, often the only evidence that the inflammation ever occurred are tiny scars called histo spots, which remain at the infection sites. Histo spots do not generally affect vision, but for reasons that are still not well understood, they can result in complications years—sometimes even decades—after the original eye infection. Histo spots have been associated with the growth of the abnormal blood vessels underneath the retina.

In later stages, OHS symptoms may appear if the abnormal blood vessels cause changes in vision. For example, straight lines may appear crooked or wavy, or a blind spot may appear in the field of vision. Because these symptoms indicate that OHS has already progressed enough to affect vision, anyone who has been exposed to histoplasmosis and perceives even slight changes in vision should consult an eye care professional.

Who Is at Risk for OHS?

Although only a tiny fraction of the people infected with the histo fungus ever develops OHS, any person who has had histoplasmosis should be alert for any changes in vision similar to those described above. Studies have shown the OHS patients usually test positive for previous exposure to histoplasmosis.

In the United States, the highest incidence of histoplasmosis occurs in a region often referred to as the Histo Belt, where up to 90 percent of the adult population has been infected by histoplasmosis.

This region includes all of Arkansas, Kentucky, Missouri, Tennessee, and West Virginia as well as large portions of Alabama, Illinois, Indiana, Iowa, Kansas, Louisiana, Maryland, Mississippi, Nebraska, Ohio, Oklahoma, Texas, and Virginia. Since most cases of histoplasmosis are undiagnosed, anyone who has ever lived in an area known to have a high rate of histoplasmosis should consider having their eyes examined for histo spots.

How Is OHS Diagnosed?

An eye care professional will usually diagnose OHS if a careful eye examination reveals two conditions: (1) the presence of histo spots, which indicate previous exposure to the histo fungus spores; and (2) swelling of the retina, which signals the growth of new, abnormal blood vessels. To confirm the diagnosis, a dilated eye examination must be performed. This means that the pupils are enlarged temporarily with special drops, allowing the eye care professional to better examine the retina.

If fluid, blood, or abnormal blood vessels are present, an eye care professional may want to perform a diagnostic procedure called fluorescein angiography. In this procedure, a dye, injected into the patient's arm, travels to the blood vessels of the retina. The dye allows a better view of the CNV lesion, and photographs can document the location and extent to which it has spread. Particular attention is paid to how close the abnormal blood vessels are to the fovea.

How Is OHS Treated?

The only proven treatment for OHS is a form of laser surgery called photocoagulation. A small, powerful beam of light destroys the fragile, abnormal blood vessels, as well as a small amount of the overlying retinal tissue. Although the destruction of retinal tissue during the procedure can itself cause some loss of vision, this is done in the hope of protecting the fovea and preserving the finely tuned vision it provides.

How Effective Is Laser Surgery?

Controlled clinical trials, sponsored by the National Eye Institute, have shown that photocoagulation can reduce future vision loss from OHS by more than half. The treatment is most effective when:

- The CNV has not grown into the center of the fovea, where it can affect vision.

- The eye care professional is able to identify and destroy the entire area of CNV.

Does Laser Surgery Restore Lost Vision?

Laser photocoagulation usually does not restore lost vision. However, it does reduce the chance of further CNV growth and any resulting vision loss.

Does Laser Surgery Cure OHS?

No. OHS cannot be cured. Once contracted, OHS remains a threat to a person's sight for their lifetime. People with OHS who experience one bout of abnormal blood vessel growth may have recurrent CNV. Each recurrence can damage vision and may require additional laser therapy. It is crucial to detect and treat OHS as early as possible before it causes significant visual impairment.

Is There a Simple Way to Check for Signs of OHS Damage to the Macula?

Yes. A person can check for signs of damage to the macula by looking at a printed pattern called an Amsler grid. If the macula has been damaged, the vertical and horizontal lines of the grid may appear curved, or a blank spot may seem to appear.

Many eye care professionals advise patients who have received treatment for OHS, as well as those with histo spots, to check their vision daily with the Amsler grid one eye at a time. Patients with OHS in one eye are likely to develop it in the other.

What Help Is Available for People Who Have Already Lost Significant Vision from OHS?

Scientists and engineers have developed many useful devices to help people with severe visual impairment in both eyes. These devices, called low vision aids, use special lenses or electronics to create enlarged visual images. An eye care professional can suggest sources that provide information on counseling, training, and special services for people with low vision. Many organizations for people who are blind also serve those with low vision.

What Research Is Being Conducted on the Ocular Histoplasmosis Syndrome?

The National Eye Institute (NEI) supports research aimed at learning more about the relationship between histoplasmosis and OHS and how to treat OHS effectively. One such multicenter clinical study is called the Submacular Surgery Trials (SST). This clinical study is examining whether CNV in the fovea, which cannot be treated by laser photocoagulation, can be successfully removed through traditional surgery. Patients with OHS who would like to receive more information about the Submacular Surgery Trials should call the SST Chairman's Office toll-free at (888) 554-0412. Information on the Submacular Surgery Trials is also available on the NEI Website at http://www.nei.nih.gov/neitrials/index.htm.

Where Can I Obtain More Information?

Information on systemic histoplasmosis can be obtained from:

The National Institute of Allergy and Infectious Diseases (NIAID)
The National Institutes of Health
Building 31, Room 7A50
31 Center Drive, MSC 2520
Bethesda, MD 20892-2520
Phone: (301) 496-5717
Website: http://www.niaid.nih.gov

347

Chapter 36

Sjögren's Syndrome

What Is Sjögren's Syndrome?

Sjögren's syndrome is an autoimmune disease in which the body's immune system mistakenly attacks its own moisture-producing glands. Sjögren's is one of the most prevalent autoimmune disorders, striking as many as 4,000,000 Americans. Nine out of ten patients are women. The average age of onset is late 40s although Sjögren's occurs in all age groups in both women and men.

About 50% of the time Sjögren's syndrome occurs alone, and 50% of the time it occurs in the presence of another connective tissue disease, such as rheumatoid arthritis, lupus, or scleroderma. Sometimes researchers refer to the first type as primary Sjögren's and the second as secondary Sjögren's. All instances of Sjögren's syndrome are systemic, affecting the entire body.

The hallmark symptoms are dry eyes and dry mouth. Sjögren's may also cause dryness of other organs, affecting the kidneys, GI tract, blood vessels, lung, liver, pancreas, and the central nervous system. Many patients experience debilitating fatigue and joint pain. Symptoms can plateau, worsen, or go into remission. While some people experience mild symptoms, others suffer debilitating symptoms that greatly impair their quality of life.

This chapter includes "What Is Sjögren's Syndrome?" "Diagnosis," "Treatment," and "Treatment Centers," reprinted with permission from www.sjogrens.org, the website of the Sjögren's Syndrome Foundation. © 2002.

Diagnosis

Early diagnosis and treatment are important for preventing complications. The symptoms of Sjögren's syndrome may overlap with or mimic those of other diseases including lupus, rheumatoid arthritis, fibromyalgia, chronic fatigue syndrome, and multiple sclerosis. Furthermore, dryness can occur for other reasons, such as a side effect of medication like anti-depressants or high blood pressure medication.

Additionally, because all symptoms are not always present at the same time and because Sjögren's can involve several body systems, physicians and dentists sometimes treat each symptom individually and do not recognize that a systemic disease is present. The average time from onset of symptoms to diagnosis is over six years. Rheumatologists have primary responsibility for diagnosing and managing Sjögren's syndrome.

Once Sjögren's syndrome is suspected, a physician will request a series of blood tests, including:

- **ANA** (Anti-Nuclear Antibody): ANAs are a group of antibodies that react against normal components of a cell nucleus. About 70% of Sjögren's patients have a positive ANA test result.

- **SSA and SSB**: The antibodies SSA (or RO) and SSB (or LA) are often found in Sjögren's syndrome; 70% of patients are positive for SSA and 40% are positive for SSB.

- **RF** (Rheumatoid Factor): This antibody test is indicative of a rheumatic disease. In Sjögren's patients, 60-70% have a positive RF.

- **ESR** (Erythrocyte Sedimentation Rate): This test measures inflammation. An elevated ESR can indicate an inflammatory disorder, including Sjögren's syndrome.

- **IGs** (Immunoglobulins): These are normal blood proteins. They are usually elevated in Sjögren's.

The physician is likely to refer the patient to an ophthalmologist for further tests and to an oral pathologist or dentist for additional procedures.

The ophthalmologic tests include:

- **Schirmer Test**: Measures tear production.

- **Rose Bengal and Lissamine Green**: Uses dyes to observe abnormal cells on the surface of the eye.

- **Slit-Lamp Exam**: Indicates the volume of tears by magnifying the eye and viewing it in its resting state.

The dental tests include:

- **Parotid Gland Flow**: Measures the amount of saliva produced over a certain period of time.

- **Salivary Scintigraphy**: Measures salivary gland function.

- **Sialography**: An x-ray of the salivary-duct system.

- **Lip Biopsy**: Used to confirm lymphocytic infiltration of the minor salivary glands.

Treatment

Early diagnosis and high quality professional dental and eye care are extremely important.

Many symptoms and problems of Sjögren's syndrome can be treated with over-the-counter medications. And there are non-medication strategies for dealing with the various symptoms of Sjögren's syndrome including use of a humidifier and protective gear such as goggles. Often, patients learn the most from one another in support groups. The feeling of isolation, of not knowing another person with Sjögren's, can be overcome easily.

The over-the-counter (OTC) products include preservative-free artificial tears, artificial salivas, unscented skin lotions, saline nasal sprays, and vaginal lubricants. The Sjögren's Syndrome Foundation maintains an updated list of these products. The Foundation also offers tips for daily living in *The New Sjögren's Syndrome Handbook* and in its *Moisture Seekers®* newsletter.

One prescription product, Lacriserts®, is used by some to alleviate dry eyes. Two prescription medications, Salagen® (pilocarpine hydrochloride) and Evoxac® (cevimeline), are available to treat dry mouth. Depending on the nature and severity of symptoms, other medications are available, including non-steroidal anti-inflammatory drugs (NSAIDs), steroids, and immunosuppressive drugs.

Treatment Centers

The following facilities have diagnostic and treatment programs for Sjögren's syndrome. The list is NOT comprehensive. Please contact the Sjögren's Syndrome Foundation for information about treatment providers in your area.

California

Sjögren's Syndrome Clinic
University of California—San Francisco
San Francisco, CA
Phone: (415) 476-2045

The Scripps Research Institute
La Jolla, CA
Phone: (858) 784-1000

Connecticut

University of Connecticut Health Center
Farmington, CT
Phone: (860) 679-3605

Florida

Center for Orphaned Autoimmune Disorders
University of Florida—Gainesville
Gainesville, FL
Phone: (800) 749-7424

Maryland

Sjögren's Syndrome Clinic
National Institute of Dental and Craniofacial Research
Bethesda, MD

Massachusetts

New England Dry Mouth Clinic
Boston, MA
Phone: (617) 636-6790

Schepens Eye Research Institute
Harvard Medical School
Boston, MA
Phone: (617) 912-0100

Minnesota

Xerostomia Clinic
Department of Oral Medicine, University of Minnesota
Minneapolis, MN
Phone: (612) 625-0693

New York

Lowenstein Foundation Sjögren's Center
Mount Sinai Medical Center
New York, NY
Phone: (212) 241-3173

Sjögren's Syndrome Center
Hospital for Joint Diseases
New York, NY
Phone: (212) 598-6518

Salivary Dysfunction Center
University of Rochester
Rochester, NY
Phone: (716) 275-7978

North Carolina

Duke University Eye Center
Duke University Health System
Durham, NC
Phone: (919) 684-6611

Oregon

Casey Eye Institute
Oregon Health & Sciences University
Phone: (503) 494-5023

Pennsylvania

Sjögren's Syndrome and Dry Mouth Treatment Center
Thomas Jefferson University Hospital
Philadelphia, PA
Phone: (215) 955-8430

Texas

Sjögren's Multi-Specialty Referral Center
Baylor College of Dentistry, Baylor University Medical Center and the
University of Texas Southwestern Medical Center at Dallas
Dallas, TX
Phone: (214) 828-8145

Salivary Dysfunction Clinic
Baylor College of Dentistry
Dallas, TX
Phone: (214) 828-8100

Sjögren's Syndrome Clinic
University of Texas Health Science Center at San Antonio
Department of Clinical Medicine and Immunology
San Antonio, TX
Phone: (210) 567-4073

Chapter 37

Thyroid Eye Disease

Graves' disease and the associated eye changes (Graves' orbit-opathy) are perplexing to the affected patient. The eye symptoms usually occur at the same time as thyroid disease, however they may precede or follow the obvious symptoms of the thyroid abnormality. Most patients with thyroid abnormalities will never be affected by eye disease and some patients only mildly so. Although the incidence of eye disease associated with thyroid dysfunction is higher and more severe in smokers, there is no way to predict which thyroid patients will be affected. In addition, while eye disease may be brought on by thyroid dysfunction, successful treatment of the thyroid gland does not guarantee that the eye disease will improve as well, and no particular thyroid treatment can minimize the chances that the eyes will deteriorate. Once inflamed, the eye disease may remain active from several months to as long as three years.

Subsequently, there may be a gradual or, in some cases, a complete improvement. While rare, recurrence of the eye disease is not unknown and may coincide with inadequate control of thyroid hormone levels.

Medical Treatment

Early eye symptoms, which may include dryness, redness, itching, swelling of the lids, and inability to wear contact lenses, are usually mild. Some patients find these symptoms to be particularly irritating at night, and environments with air conditioning, hot air heating, and windy days tend to be particularly troublesome. A few patients will develop double vision (diplopia), which is the result of asymmetric scarring and inflammation of the eye movement muscles.

Since most patients develop mild symptoms, they are often misdiagnosed with an ocular allergy. Therefore, Graves' disease patients should be followed by an ophthalmologist familiar with the conditions and available treatments. Patients with mild symptoms can often be successfully treated with frequent application of lubricating eye drops and eye covers at night. Humidification of room air can prevent drying of the eyes, and wrap-around polarizing sunglasses can also help relieve glare. Diplopia can be alleviated with prism lenses while awaiting either spontaneous improvement or surgical correction. Temporary plastic prisms are available which are applied to glasses and changed as needed. Prednisone, a steroid medication, may be taken orally to provide temporary relief from pain, swelling and redness, although side effects of the medication may limit the use of prednisone and related drugs.

Vision loss due to pressure on the optic nerve is the most severe form of the disease. Fortunately, this condition is rare, affecting less than 5% of patients with Graves' orbitopathy. Treatment with prednisone, radiotherapy, and/or surgery may be required to restore vision. Overall, it is important to keep in mind that eye disease associated with Graves' disease will only improve gradually.

Surgical Management

If the eye condition does not improve or deteriorates despite treatment, surgery may be required. Retracted and puffy eyelids can alter a person's appearance and increase the risk of cornea drying. Corrective eyelid surgery can alleviate the problem through adjustable loosening of the eyelid muscles, as well as removal of scar tissue, excessive fatty tissue, and skin to place the eyelids into a more normal position. Surgery may also be necessary to correct diplopia when this problem has not resolved either spontaneously or with prism lenses. This surgery entails detaching and repositioning the eye movement muscles on the eyeball to improve ocular alignment and minimize double vision.

The enlargement of tissue behind the eye may sometimes cause significant forward protrusion of the eye (exophthalmos), which produces the disfigurement, worsens the symptoms, and causes ocular exposure. Swelling in the orbit may actually contribute to vision loss as pressure increases on the optic nerve. Surgical procedures to relieve pressure on the optic nerve improve vision and allow the eye to settle back to a more normal position. Orbital decompression is indicated in patients with significant exophthalmos, visual loss, or severe exposure of the corneas. Sometimes careful resection of fat behind the eyeball is performed in conjunction with, or in place of bone decompression. For most patients, surgery is performed under general anesthesia and usually requires an overnight hospital stay.

Chapter 38

Usher Syndrome

The information provided in this chapter was developed by the National Eye Institute (NEI) to help patients and their families in searching for general information about Usher syndrome. An eye care professional who has examined the patient's eyes and is familiar with his or her medical history is the best person to answer specific questions.

What Is Usher Syndrome?

Usher syndrome is an inherited condition that causes 1) a serious hearing loss that is usually present at birth or shortly thereafter and 2) progressive vision loss caused by retinitis pigmentosa (RP). RP is a group of inherited diseases that cause night-blindness and peripheral (side) vision loss through the progressive degeneration of the retina, the light-sensitive tissue at the back of the eye that is crucial for vision.

Researchers have described three types of Usher syndrome—type I, type II, and type III.

- Individuals with Usher syndrome type I are nearly or completely deaf and experience problems with balance from a young age. They usually begin to exhibit signs of RP in early adolescence.

"Usher Syndrome Resource Guide," National Eye Institute, available online at http://www.nei.nih.gov, April 2002.

- Individuals with Usher syndrome type II experience moderate to severe hearing impairment, have normal balance, and experience symptoms of RP later in adolescence.

- Individuals with Usher syndrome type III are born with normal hearing but develop RP and then progressive hearing loss.

How Is Usher Syndrome Inherited?

The Usher syndrome types are inherited as an autosomal recessive trait. This means that an affected person receives one abnormal gene from each of his or her parents. A person who inherits a gene from only one parent will be a carrier, but will not develop the disease.

A person with Usher syndrome must pass on one disease gene to each of his or her children. However, unless the person has children with another carrier of Usher genes, the individual's children are not at risk for developing the disease. Currently we cannot reasonably test everyone for carrier status, but this may change in the years ahead.

How Is Usher Syndrome Diagnosed?

Since individuals with Usher syndrome have both hearing and visual symptoms, we perform testing of both systems. This testing includes:

- visual function tests: visual fields and electroretinogram (ERG)
- a retinal examination
- hearing tests
- balance tests for all patients age ten years and older

Although some of the genes that cause Usher syndrome have been identified, the diagnosis is still based on ocular and clinical testing.

Is Genetic Testing for Usher Syndrome Available?

At this time, genetic testing for Usher syndrome is done only as part of research projects. This is due to many factors. Usher syndrome is not caused by only one gene. So far, 10 Usher genes have been mapped: 7 for type I, 3 for type II, and 1 for type 3. There are still more genes to find. A few of these genes have been sequenced and

described. These are MYO7A, harmonin, CDH23, PCDH15, all causing type I. The usherin gene causes type II disease.

Finding the genes is a very important advance in the fight against
Usher syndrome. Further study is required to characterize these
genes, and determine how the mutated genes cause Usher syndrome.
Additional genes that cause Usher syndrome also need to be identified. Several researchers throughout the world are working on Usher
syndrome. Findings from this research may one day allow treatments
for Usher syndrome to be developed.

National Eye Institute Research

Researchers at of the National Eye Institute have been following
individuals with Usher syndrome (Research Protocol # 93-EI-0161).
They are available for patient examination and consultation. The vision and hearing of each patient is evaluated. In addition, samples of
blood from each patient are studied to better understand the genes
involved in Usher syndrome.

Other Resources

Individuals with Usher syndrome may find the following organizations useful for more information on the disease and rehabilitation:

National Eye Institute
2020 Vision Place
Bethesda, MD 20892-3655
Phone: (301) 496-5248
E-mail: 2020@nei.nih.gov
Website: http://www.nei.nih.gov

Foundation Fighting Blindness
1143 Cronhill Drive
Owings Mills, MD 21117-2220
Toll-Free: (800) 683-5551
TDD: (410) 363-7139
Phone: (410) 568-0150
Website: http://www.blindness.org

Funds research to discover the causes, treatments, preventions, and
cures for retinitis pigmentosa, macular degeneration, Usher syndrome, and other related retinal degenerations.

American Association of the Deaf-Blind
814 Thayer Avenue, Room 302
Silver Spring, MD 20910
Toll-Free: (800) 735-2258
TTY: (301) 588-6545
Website: http://www.tr.wou.edu/dblink/aadb.htm

Encourages independent living for individuals who are deaf-blind. Provides technical assistance to persons who are deaf-blind, families, educators, and service providers.

DB-LINK: National Information Clearinghouse on Children Who are Deaf-Blind
345 N Monmouth Avenue
Monmouth, Oregon 97361
Toll-Free: (800) 438-9376
TTY: (800) 854-7013
Website: http://www.tr.wosc.osshe.edu/dblink/index.htm

Offers information that assists education, medical, and service personnel in providing comprehensive services infants, toddlers, children, and youth who are deaf-blind in the United States.

Helen Keller National Center for Deaf-Blind Youths and Adults
111 Middle Neck Road
Sands Point, NY 11050
Phone: (516) 944-8900
TTY: (516) 944-8637
Website: http://www.helenkeller.org

Seeks to enable each person who is deaf-blind to live and work in his or her community of choice. Provides a comprehensive vocational rehabilitation training program.

National Family Association for Deaf-Blind
111 Middle Neck Road
Sands Point, New York 11050
Toll-Free: (800) 255-0411, ext. 275
TTY: (516) 944-8637
Website: http://www.nfadb.org

Serves as the largest national network of families focusing on issues surrounding deaf blindness.

National Institute on Deafness and Other Communication Disorders (NIDCD)
31 Center Drive, MSC 2320
Bethesda, MD 20892-2320
Phone: (301) 496-7243
TTY: (301) 402-0252
Website: http://www.nidcd.nih.gov

Conducts and supports research on diseases and disorders affecting hearing, balance, smell, taste, voice, speech, and language. Publishes an online fact sheet on Usher syndrome.

For additional information, you may also wish to contact a local library.

Medical Literature

Below is a sample of the citations available through MEDLINE/ PubMed, a service of the National Library of Medicine. MEDLINE/ PubMed provides access to over 11 million medical literature citations from 1966 to the present and includes links to many sites providing full text articles and other related resources. You can conduct your own free literature search by accessing MEDLINE through the Internet at http://medlineplus.nlm.nih.gov/hinfo.html. You can also get assistance with a literature search at a local library.

To obtain copies of any of the articles listed below, contact a local community, university, or medical library. If the library you visit does not have a copy of a particular article, you may usually obtain it through an inter-library loan.

Please keep in mind that articles in the medical literature are usually written in technical language. We encourage you to share any articles you order with a health care professional who can help you understand them.

The Usher Syndromes

Keats BJ, Corey, DP. LSU Medical Center, New Orleans, LA. *American Journal of Medical Genetics* 89(3):158-166, 1999.

This article reviews the information known by 1999 about the different types of Usher syndromes and the different genes found that cause them. It concentrates mainly on the MYO7A gene.

Genetic Heterogeneity of Usher Syndrome: Analysis of 151 Families with Usher Type I.

Astuto, LM, et al. *American Journal of Human Genetics* 67:1569-1574, 2000.

This article gives genetic information about 151 Usher I families studied. It provides a better idea of the percentage of Usher I caused by each of the 6 genes that have been mapped so far. MYO7A accounted for the largest percentage of families in their study.

Early Diagnosis of Usher Syndrome in Children.

Mets, MB, et al. Northwestern University Medical School, Chicago, IL. *Trans Am Ophthalmol Soc* 98:237-242, 2000.

This article reports the results of a screening study on children with severe to profound, preverbal hearing-impaired children for Usher syndrome by examination and ERG testing. They found that 10% of such children were diagnosed with Usher syndrome and conclude that all children with severe to profound, preverbal hearing impairment should be screened for Usher syndrome.

The National Eye Institute, part of the National Institutes of Health, is the Federal government's principal agency for conducting and supporting vision research. Inclusion of an item in this chapter does not imply the endorsement by the National Eye Institute or the National Institutes of Health.

Part Six

Other Eye Disorders and Problems

Chapter 39

Anophthalmia and Microphthalmia

The information provided in this chapter was developed by the National Eye Institute to help patients and their families in searching for general information about anophthalmia and microphthalmia. An eye care professional who has examined the patient's eyes and is familiar with his or her medical history is the best person to answer specific questions.

What Are Anophthalmia and Microphthalmia?

Anophthalmia and microphthalmia are often used interchangeably. Microphthalmia is a disorder in which one or both eyes are abnormally small, while anophthalmia is the absence of one or both eyes. These rare disorders develop during pregnancy and can be associated with other birth defects.

What Causes Anophthalmia and Microphthalmia?

Causes of these conditions may include genetic mutations and abnormal chromosomes. Researchers also believe that environmental factors, such as exposure to X-rays, chemicals, drugs, pesticides, toxins, radiation, or viruses, increase the risk of anophthalmia and microphthalmia, but research is not conclusive. Sometimes the cause in an individual patient cannot be determined.

"Anophthalmia and Microphthalmia Resource Guide," National Eye Institute, available online at http://www.nei.nih.gov, April 2002.

Can Anophthalmia and Microphthalmia Be Treated?

There is no treatment for severe anophthalmia or microphthalmia that will create a new eye or restore vision. However, some less severe forms of microphthalmia may benefit from medical or surgical treatments. In almost all cases improvements to a child's appearance are possible. Children can be fitted for a prosthetic (artificial) eye for cosmetic purposes and to promote socket growth. A newborn with anophthalmia or microphthalmia will need to visit several eye care professionals, including those who specialize in pediatrics, vitreoretinal disease, orbital and oculoplastic surgery, ophthalmic genetics, and prosthetic devices for the eye. Each specialist can provide information and possible treatments resulting in the best care for the child and family. The specialist in prosthetic diseases for the eye will make conformers, plastic structures that help support the face and encourage the eye socket to grow. As the face develops, new conformers will need to be made. A child with anophthalmia may also need to use expanders in addition to conformers to further enlarge the eye socket. Once the face is fully developed, prosthetic eyes can be made and placed. Prosthetic eyes will not restore vision.

How Do Conformers and Prosthetic Eyes Look?

A painted prosthesis that looks like a normal eye is usually fitted between ages one and two. Until then, clear conformers are used. When the conformers are in place the eye socket will look black. These conformers are not painted to look like a normal eye because they are changed too frequently. Every few weeks a child will progress to a larger size conformer until about two years of age. If a child needs to wear conformers after age two, the conformers will be painted like a regular prosthesis, giving the appearance of a normal but smaller eye. The average child will need three to four new painted prostheses before the age of 10.

How Is Microphthalmia Managed If There Is Residual Vision in the Eye?

Children with microphthalmia may have some residual vision (limited sight). In these cases, the good eye can be patched to strengthen vision in the microphthalmic eye. A prosthesis can be made to cap the microphthalmic eye to help with cosmetic appearance, while preserving the remaining sight.

Resources

The following organizations may be able to provide additional information on anophthalmia and microphthalmia:

National Eye Institute
2020 Vision Place
Bethesda, MD 20892-3655
Phone: (301) 496-5248
E-mail: 2020@nei.nih.gov
Website: http://www.nei.nih.gov

American Society of Ocularists
E-mail: aso@ocularist.org
Website: http://www.ocularist.org

Represents technicians specializing in making and fitting of custom artificial eyes.

American Society of Ophthalmic Plastic and Reconstructive Surgery
1133 West Morse Blvd. #201
Winter Park, FL 32789
Phone: (407) 647-8839
Website: http://www.asoprs.org

Represents ophthalmologists who specialize in reconstructive surgery involving the eye and surrounding structures. Publishes a fact sheet on anophthalmos and orbital implants.

International Children's Anophthalmia Network (ican)
Genetics, Levy 2
Albert Einstein Medical Center
5501 Old York Road
Philadelphia, PA 19141
Toll-Free: (800) 580-4226
Phone: (215) 456-8722
Website: http://www.ioi.com/ican

Provides information on anophthalmia and microphthalmia. Coordinates a patient registry. Offers referrals to local resources. Coordinates gatherings for people with anophthalmia and microphthalmia and their families. Publishes a newsletter, *The Conformer*.

Additional resources for parents and teachers of children with visual impairments can be found on the National Eye Institute's website at http://www.nei.nih.gov/health/organizations.htm#resources. For additional information, you may also wish to contact a local library.

Medical Literature

Below is a sample of the citations available through MEDLINE/ PubMed, a service of the National Library of Medicine. MEDLINE/ PubMed provides access to over 11 million medical literature citations from 1966 to the present and includes links to many sites providing full text articles and other related resources. You can conduct your own free literature search by accessing MEDLINE through the Internet at http://medlineplus.nlm.nih.gov/hinfo.html. You can also get assistance with a literature search at a local library.

To obtain copies of the article listed below, contact a local community, university, or medical library. If the library you visit does not have a copy of a desired article, you may usually obtain it through an interlibrary loan.

Please keep in mind that articles in the medical literature are usually written in technical language. We encourage you to share any articles you order with a health care professional who can help you understand them.

The Ocularists' Management of Congenital Microphthalmos and Anophthalmos

Dootz GL. *Advanced Ophthalmic Plastic Reconstructive Surgery* 1992; 9:41-56. 1992.

Early socket stimulation is crucial for management of congenital anophthalmos and microphthalmos among infants. Progressive sized hard conformers and lid expansion devices can expand the small socket in these patients. The ocularists' management of these two conditions is discussed and techniques are introduced.

The National Eye Institute (NEI), part of the National Institutes of Health (NIH), is the Federal government's principal agency for conducting and supporting vision research. Inclusion of an item in this chapter does not imply the endorsement of the NEI or the NIH.

Chapter 40

Anterior Uveitis

Anterior uveitis is an inflammation of the middle layer of the eye, which includes the iris (colored part of the eye) and adjacent tissue, known as the ciliary body. If untreated, it can cause permanent damage and loss of vision from the development of glaucoma, cataract, or retinal edema [swelling]. It usually responds well to treatment; however, there may be a tendency for the condition to recur. Treatment usually includes prescription eye drops, which dilate the pupils, in combination with anti-inflammatory drugs. Treatment usually takes several days, or up to several weeks, in some cases.

Anterior uveitis can occur as a result of trauma to the eye, such as a blow or foreign body penetrating the eye. It can also be a complication of other eye disease, or it may be associated with general health problems such as rheumatoid arthritis, rubella, and mumps. In most cases, there is no obvious underlying cause.

Signs/symptoms may include a red, sore, and inflamed eye, blurring of vision, sensitivity to light, and a small pupil. Since the symptoms of anterior uveitis are similar to those of other eye diseases, your optometrist will carefully examine the inside of your eye, under bright light and high magnification, to determine the presence and severity of the condition. Your optometrist may also perform or arrange for other diagnostic tests to help pinpoint the cause.

Chapter 41

Blepharitis

The information provided in this chapter was developed by the National Eye Institute (NEI) to help patients and their families in searching for general information about blepharitis. An eye care professional who has examined the patient's eyes and is familiar with his or her medical history is the best person to answer specific questions.

What Is Blepharitis?

Blepharitis is a common condition that causes inflammation of the eyelids. The condition can be difficult to manage because it tends to recur.

What Causes Blepharitis?

Blepharitis occurs in two forms.

Anterior blepharitis affects the outside front of the eyelid, where the eyelashes are attached. The two most common causes of anterior blepharitis are bacteria (Staphylococcus) and scalp dandruff.

Posterior blepharitis affects the inner eyelid (the moist part that makes contact with the eye) and is caused by problems with the oil (meibomian) glands in this part of the eyelid. Two skin disorders can cause this form of blepharitis: acne rosacea, which leads to red and inflamed skin, and scalp dandruff (seborrheic dermatitis).

"Blepharitis Resource Guide," National Eye Institute, available online at http://www.nei.nih.gov, April 2002.

What Are the Symptoms of Blepharitis?

Symptoms of either form of blepharitis include a foreign body or burning sensation, excessive tearing, itching, sensitivity to light (photophobia), red and swollen eyelids, redness of the eye, blurred vision, frothy tears, dry eye, or crusting of the eyelashes on awakening.

What Other Conditions Are Associated with Blepharitis?

Complications from blepharitis include:

Stye: A red tender bump on the eyelid that is caused by an acute infection of the oil glands of the eyelid.

Chalazion: This condition can follow the development of a stye. It is a usually painless firm lump caused by inflammation of the oil glands of the eyelid. Chalazion can be painful and red if there is also an infection.

Problems with the tear film: Abnormal or decreased oil secretions that are part of the tear film can result in excess tearing or dry eye. Because tears are necessary to keep the cornea healthy, tear film problems can make people more at risk for corneal infections.

How Is Blepharitis Treated?

Treatment for both forms of blepharitis involves keeping the lids clean and free of crusts. Warm compresses should be applied to the lid to loosen the crusts, followed by a light scrubbing of the eyelid with a cotton swab and a mixture of water and baby shampoo.

Because blepharitis rarely goes away completely, most patients must maintain an eyelid hygiene routine for life. If the blepharitis is severe, an eye care professional may also prescribe antibiotics or steroid eyedrops.

When scalp dandruff is present, a dandruff shampoo for the hair is recommended as well. In addition to the warm compresses, patients with posterior blepharitis will need to massage their eyelids to clean the oil accumulated in the glands. Patients who also have acne rosacea should have that condition treated at the same time.

Medical Literature

Below is a sample of the citations available in MEDLINE, a comprehensive medical literature database coordinated by the National

Library of Medicine (NLM). MEDLINE contains information on medical journal articles published from 1966 to the present. You can conduct your own free literature search by accessing MEDLINE through the Internet at http://medlineplus.nlm.nih.gov. You can also get assistance with a literature search at a local library.

To obtain copies of any of the articles listed below, contact a local community, university, or medical library. If the library you visit does not have a copy of a particular article, you may usually obtain it through an inter-library loan.

Please keep in mind that articles in the medical literature are usually written in technical language. We encourage you to share any articles you order with a health care professional who can help you understand them.

Meibomian Gland Dysfunction

Driver PJ; Lemp MA. Eye Institute at Cooper Hospital/University Medical Center, Camden, NJ. *Survey of Ophthalmology* 40(5):343-67, March-April 1996.

This article concentrates on posterior blepharitis that usually involves disorders of the meibomian glands. The article provides information on the history of meibomian gland dysfunction and also describes the population most commonly affected, symptoms of gland dysfunction and associated conditions. Problems that can affect the meibomian glands including the role bacteria and other organisms play in meibomian gland dysfunction are described. Treatments such as lid hygiene and antibiotics are also discussed.

Chronic Blepharitis: A Review

Smith RE; Flowers CW Jr. Department of Ophthalmology, University of Southern California, School of Medicine, Los Angeles, CA. *Contact Lens Association of Ophthalmologists, Inc. Journal* 21(3): 200-7, July 1995.

This article discusses various classification systems for blepharitis, explains the possible causes of blepharitis and details the methods of treatment for both anterior and posterior forms of this difficult-to-treat disorder.

Blepharitis

Raskin EM; Speaker MG; Laibson PR. Cornea Services, New York Eye and Ear Infirmary, New York, NY. *Infectious Disease Clinics of North America* 6(4):777-87, December 1992.

This article starts by describing blepharitis and its symptoms. The article explains different types of classifications for blepharitis, associated disorders (such as chalazion), other diseases that can be confused with blepharitis, possible causes of blepharitis, and the various treatments available.

The National Eye Institute (NEI), part of the National Institutes of Health (NIH), is the Federal government's principal agency for conducting and supporting vision research. Inclusion of an item in this chapter does not imply the endorsement by the NEI or the NIH.

Chapter 42

Blepharospasm

The information provided in this chapter was developed by the National Eye Institute (NEI) to help patients and their families search for general information about blepharospasm. An eye care professional who has examined the patient's eyes and is familiar with his or her medical history is the best person to answer specific questions.

What Is Blepharospasm?

Blepharospasm is an abnormal, involuntary blinking or spasm of the eyelids.

What Causes Blepharospasm?

Blepharospasm is associated with an abnormal function of the basal ganglion from an unknown cause. The basal ganglion is the part of the brain responsible for controlling the muscles. In rare cases, heredity may play a role in the development of blepharospasm.

What Are the Symptoms of Blepharospasm?

Most people develop blepharospasm without any warning symptoms. It may begin with a gradual increase in blinking or eye irritation. Some people may also experience fatigue, emotional tension, or

"Blepharospasm," National Eye Institute, available online at http://www.nei.nih.gov, August 2002.

sensitivity to bright light. As the condition progresses, the symptoms become more frequent, and facial spasms may develop. Blepharospasm may decrease or cease while a person is sleeping or concentrating on a specific task.

How Is Blepharospasm Treated?

To date, there is no successful cure for blepharospasm, although several treatment options can reduce its severity.

In the United States and Canada, the injection of Oculinum (botulinum toxin, or Botox®) into the muscles of the eyelids is an approved treatment for blepharospasm. Botulinum toxin, produced by the bacterium *Clostridium botulinum*, paralyzes the muscles of the eyelids.

Medications taken by mouth for blepharospasm are available but usually produce unpredictable results. Any symptom relief is usually short term and tends to be helpful in only 15 percent of the cases.

Myectomy, a surgical procedure to remove some of the muscles and nerves of the eyelids, is also a possible treatment option. This surgery has improved symptoms in 75 to 85 percent of people with blepharospasm.

Alternative treatments may include biofeedback, acupuncture, hypnosis, chiropractic, and nutritional therapy. The benefits of these alternative therapies have not been proven.

Research

The Doxil® Blepharospasm Treatment Trial

Doxorubicin injections in the eyelids are being studied as a way of relieving muscle spasms. Patients who participated in this study have experienced symptom relief since their last injection. No definite conclusions have been reached at this time. For additional information about this clinical trial, please visit the University of Minnesota Department of Ophthalmology website at http://www.med.umn.edu/ophthalmology/dbnews.html or contact:

Jonathan D. Wirtschafter, M.D.
Department of Ophthalmology
University of Minnesota—FUMC Box 493
420 Delaware Street SE
Minneapolis, MN 55455-0501
Phone: (612) 625-4400
E-mail: wirtsch@tc.umn.edu

Other Resources

The following resources may provide additional information on blepharospasm:

National Institute of Neurological Disorders and Stroke (NINDS)
National Institutes of Health
P.O. Box 5801
Bethesda, MD 20824
Toll-Free: (800) 352-9424
Distributes an information page on benign essential blepharospasm.

Benign Essential Blepharospasm Research Foundation, Inc.
P.O. Box 12468
Beaumont, TX 77726-2468
Phone: (409) 832-0788
Promotes research into the cause, treatment, and potential cure of benign essential blepharospasm and other disorders of the facial musculature. Acts as a clearinghouse for information on these disorders and distributes materials, including printed brochures, bimonthly newsletters, and fact sheets.

Office of Medical Applications of Research
National Institutes of Health
Building 31, Room 1B03
31 Center Drive, MSC 2082
Bethesda, MD 20892-2082
Phone: (301)-496-5641

For additional information, you may also wish to contact a local library.

Medical Literature

Below is a sample of the citations available in MEDLINE, a comprehensive medical literature database coordinated by the National Library of Medicine (NLM). MEDLINE contains information on medical journal articles published from 1966 to the present. You can conduct your own free literature search by accessing MEDLINE through the Internet at http://medlineplus.nlm.nih.gov/. You can also get assistance with a literature search at a local library.

To obtain copies of any of the articles listed below, contact a local community, university, or medical library. If the library you visit does not have a copy of a particular article, you may usually obtain it through an inter-library loan.

Please keep in mind that articles in the medical literature are usually written in technical language. We encourage you to share any articles you order with a health care professional who can help you understand them.

Blepharospasm: Report of a Workshop

Hallett M, Darof, R. Bethesda, Maryland. *Neurology*; 46(5):1213-1218, May 1996.

This article discusses the anatomy and physiology of the eyelid, clinical aspects of blepharospasm, and treatment options.

Pharmacotherapy with Botulinum Toxin: Harnessing Nature's Most Potent Neurotoxin

Bell MS, Vermeulen LC, Sperling KB. *Pharmacotherapy* 20(9):1079-91, September 2000.

This article begins with a brief overview of the use of botulinum toxin. Following is a discussion of the past uses of the botulinum toxin and the advances that have been made in its use as a pharmacological treatment for neurological disorders. The article also provides information on the safety and the efficacy of botulinum toxin.

The National Eye Institute (NEI), part of the National Institutes of Health (NIH), is the Federal government's principal agency for conducting and supporting vision research. Inclusion of an item in this chapter does not imply the endorsement by the NEI or the NIH.

Chapter 43

Color Blindness

What Is Color Blindness?

More correctly called color vision deficiency, color blindness describes a number of problems in identifying various colors and shades. Abnormal color vision may vary from only a slight difficulty distinguishing among different shades of the same color to the rare inability to distinguish any colors.

Who Is Affected by Color Vision Deficiency?

It's estimated that eight percent of males, and fewer than one percent of females, have some difficulty with color vision. Most types of color vision problems are present at birth.

But some people have color vision problems that aren't due to heredity. One common problem occurs with the normal aging of the eye's lens. Although our lenses are clear at birth, the aging process causes them to darken. Older adults may have trouble distinguishing one dark color from another. Also, certain medications and retinal or optic nerve disease may disrupt normal color vision.

"Frequently Asked Questions about Color Blindness," reprinted with permission from Prevent Blindness America. © 2000. For additional information, call the Prevent Blindness America toll-free information line at (800) 331-2020, or visit www.preventblindness.org.

Who Should Be Tested for Color Vision Deficiency?

Any child who is having difficulty in school should be checked for potential vision problems, including color vision. Others include those who have a family history of color vision deficiency, are considering occupations that require fine color discrimination, or are having problems identifying colors.

What Can Be Done about Faulty Color Vision?

Unfortunately, there is no cure for hereditary color vision deficiency, although some measures can be taken to compensate for the problem. For example, people can develop their own system or be taught to recognize colors by other means, such as by brightness or location. Specially tinted eyeglasses may help some people with color vision deficiency distinguish between confusing colors.

If you suspect that you may not be seeing as well as you should, the best advice is to explore it together with your eye doctor.

To learn more about color vision deficiency, please contact Prevent Blindness America or the Prevent Blindness affiliate near you.

Chapter 44

Corneal Disease

What Is the Cornea?

The cornea is the eye's outermost layer. It is the clear, dome-shaped surface that covers the front of the eye.

Structure of the Cornea

Although the cornea is clear and seems to lack substance, it is actually a highly organized group of cells and proteins. Unlike most tissues in the body, the cornea contains no blood vessels to nourish or protect it against infection. Instead, the cornea receives its nourishment from the tears and aqueous humor that fills the chamber behind it. The cornea must remain transparent to refract light properly, and the presence of even the tiniest blood vessels can interfere with this process. To see well, all layers of the cornea must be free of any cloudy or opaque areas.

The corneal tissue is arranged in five basic layers, each having an important function. These five layers are:

Epithelium

The epithelium is the cornea's outermost region, comprising about 10 percent of the tissue's thickness. The epithelium functions prima-

"Facts about the Cornea and Corneal Disease," National Eye Institute, available online at http://www.nei.nih.gov, June 2001.

rily to: (1) Block the passage of foreign material, such as dust, water, and bacteria, into the eye and other layers of the cornea; and (2) Provide a smooth surface that absorbs oxygen and cell nutrients from tears, then distributes these nutrients to the rest of the cornea. The epithelium is filled with thousands of tiny nerve endings that make the cornea extremely sensitive to pain when rubbed or scratched. The part of the epithelium that serves as the foundation on which the epithelial cells anchor and organize themselves is called the basement membrane.

Bowman's Layer

Lying directly below the basement membrane of the epithelium is a transparent sheet of tissue known as Bowman's layer. It is composed of strong layered protein fibers called collagen. Once injured, Bowman's layer can form a scar as it heals. If these scars are large and centrally located, some vision loss can occur.

Stroma

Beneath Bowman's layer is the stroma, which comprises about 90 percent of the cornea's thickness. It consists primarily of water (78 percent) and collagen (16 percent), and does not contain any blood vessels. Collagen gives the cornea its strength, elasticity, and form. The collagen's unique shape, arrangement, and spacing are essential in producing the cornea's light-conducting transparency.

Descemet's Membrane

Under the stroma is Descemet's membrane, a thin but strong sheet of tissue that serves as a protective barrier against infection and injuries. Descemet's membrane is composed of collagen fibers (different from those of the stroma) and is made by the endothelial cells that lie below it. Descemet's membrane is regenerated readily after injury.

Endothelium

The endothelium is the extremely thin, innermost layer of the cornea. Endothelial cells are essential in keeping the cornea clear. Normally, fluid leaks slowly from inside the eye into the middle corneal layer (stroma). The endothelium's primary task is to pump this excess fluid out of the stroma. Without this pumping action, the stroma would swell with water, become hazy, and ultimately opaque. In a healthy eye, a perfect balance is maintained between the fluid moving into the cornea and fluid being pumped out of the cornea. Once endothelium cells are destroyed by disease or trauma, they are lost forever. If too many endothelial cells are destroyed, corneal edema and blindness ensue, with corneal transplantation the only available therapy.

Refractive Errors

About 120 million people in the United States wear eyeglasses or contact lenses to correct nearsightedness, farsightedness, or astigmatism. These vision disorders—called refractive errors—affect the cornea and are the most common of all vision problems in this country.

Refractive errors occur when the curve of the cornea is irregularly shaped (too steep or too flat). When the cornea is of normal shape and curvature, it bends, or refracts, light on the retina with precision. However, when the curve of the cornea is irregularly shaped, the cornea bends light imperfectly on the retina. This affects good vision. The refractive process is similar to the way a camera takes a picture. The cornea and lens in your eye act as the camera lens. The retina is similar to the film. If the image is not focused properly, the film (or retina) receives a blurry image. The image that your retina sees then goes to your brain, which tells you what the image is.

When the cornea is curved too much, or if the eye is too long, faraway objects will appear blurry because they are focused in front of the retina. This is called myopia, or nearsightedness. Myopia affects over 25 percent of all adult Americans.

Hyperopia, or farsightedness, is the opposite of myopia. Distant objects are clear, and close-up objects appear blurry. With hyperopia, images focus on a point beyond the retina. Hyperopia results from an eye that is too short.

Astigmatism is a condition in which the uneven curvature of the cornea blurs and distorts both distant and near objects. A normal cornea is round, with even curves from side to side and top to bottom. With astigmatism, the cornea is shaped more like the back of a spoon, curved more in one direction than in another. This causes light rays to have more than one focal point and focus on two separate areas of the retina, distorting the visual image. Two thirds of Americans with myopia also have astigmatism.

Refractive errors are usually corrected by eyeglasses or contact lenses. Although these are safe and effective methods for treating refractive errors, refractive surgeries are becoming an increasingly popular option.

What Is the Function of the Cornea?

Because the cornea is as smooth and clear as glass but is strong and durable, it helps the eye in two ways:

1. It helps to shield the rest of the eye from germs, dust, and other harmful matter. The cornea shares this protective task with the eyelids, the eye socket, tears, and the sclera, or white part of the eye.

2. The cornea acts as the eye's outermost lens. It functions like a window that controls and focuses the entry of light into the eye. The cornea contributes between 65 to 75 percent of the eye's total focusing power.

When light strikes the cornea, it bends—or refracts—the incoming light onto the lens. The lens further refocuses that light onto the retina, a layer of light-sensing cells lining the back of the eye that starts the translation of light into vision. For you to see clearly, light rays must be focused by the cornea and lens to fall precisely on the retina. The retina converts the light rays into impulses that are sent through the optic nerve to the brain, which interprets them as images.

The refractive process is similar to the way a camera takes a picture. The cornea and lens in the eye act as the camera lens. The retina is similar to the film. If the image is not focused properly, the film (or retina) receives a blurry image.

The cornea also serves as a filter, screening out some of the most damaging ultraviolet (UV) wavelengths in sunlight. Without this protection, the lens and the retina would be highly susceptible to injury from UV radiation.

How Does the Cornea Respond to Injury?

The cornea copes very well with minor injuries or abrasions. If the highly sensitive cornea is scratched, healthy cells slide over quickly and patch the injury before infection occurs and vision is affected. If the scratch penetrates the cornea more deeply, however, the healing process will take longer, at times resulting in greater pain, blurred vision, tearing, redness, and extreme sensitivity to light. These symptoms require professional treatment. Deeper scratches can also cause corneal scarring, resulting in a haze on the cornea that can greatly impair vision. In this case, a corneal transplant may be needed.

What Are Some Diseases and Disorders Affecting the Cornea?

Some diseases and disorders of the cornea are:

Allergies

Allergies affecting the eye are fairly common. The most common allergies are those related to pollen, particularly when the weather is warm and dry. Symptoms can include redness, itching, tearing, burning, stinging, and watery discharge, although they are not usually severe enough to require medical attention. Antihistamine decongestant eye drops can effectively reduce these symptoms, as does rain and cooler weather, which decreases the amount of pollen in the air.

An increasing number of eye allergy cases are related to medications and contact lens wear. Also, animal hair and certain cosmetics, such as mascara, face creams, and eyebrow pencil, can cause allergies that affect the eye. Touching or rubbing eyes after handling nail polish, soaps, or chemicals may cause an allergic reaction. Some people have sensitivity to lip gloss and eye makeup. Allergy symptoms are temporary and can eliminated by not having contact with the offending cosmetic or detergent.

Conjunctivitis (Pink Eye)

This term describes a group of diseases that cause swelling, itching, burning, and redness of the conjunctiva, the protective membrane that lines the eyelids and covers exposed areas of the sclera, or white of the eye. Conjunctivitis can spread from one person to another and affects millions of Americans at any given time. Conjunctivitis can be caused by a bacterial or viral infection, allergy, environmental irritants, a contact lens product, eye drops, or eye ointments.

At its onset, conjunctivitis is usually painless and does not adversely affect vision. The infection will clear in most cases without requiring medical care. But for some forms of conjunctivitis, treatment will be needed. If treatment is delayed, the infection may worsen and cause corneal inflammation and a loss of vision.

Corneal Infections

Sometimes the cornea is damaged after a foreign object has penetrated the tissue, such as from a poke in the eye. At other times, bacteria or fungi from a contaminated contact lens can pass into the

387

cornea. Situations like these can cause painful inflammation and corneal infections called keratitis. These infections can reduce visual clarity, produce corneal discharges, and perhaps erode the cornea. Corneal infections can also lead to corneal scarring, which can impair vision and may require a corneal transplant.

As a general rule, the deeper the corneal infection, the more severe the symptoms and complications. It should be noted that corneal infections, although relatively infrequent, are the most serious complication of contact lens wear.

Minor corneal infections are commonly treated with antibacterial eye drops. If the problem is severe, it may require more intensive antibiotic or antifungal treatment to eliminate the infection, as well as steroid eye drops to reduce inflammation. Frequent visits to an eye care professional may be necessary for several months to eliminate the problem.

Dry Eye

The continuous production and drainage of tears is important to the eye's health. Tears keep the eye moist, help wounds heal, and protect against eye infection. In people with dry eye, the eye produces fewer or less quality tears and is unable to keep its surface lubricated and comfortable.

The tear film consists of three layers—an outer, oily (lipid) layer that keeps tears from evaporating too quickly and helps tears remain on the eye; a middle (aqueous) layer that nourishes the cornea and conjunctiva; and a bottom (mucin) layer that helps to spread the aqueous layer across the eye to ensure that the eye remains wet. As we age, the eyes usually produce fewer tears. Also, in some cases, the lipid and mucin layers produced by the eye are of such poor quality that tears cannot remain in the eye long enough to keep the eye sufficiently lubricated.

The main symptom of dry eye is usually a scratchy or sandy feeling as if something is in the eye. Other symptoms may include stinging or burning of the eye; episodes of excess tearing that follow periods of very dry sensation; a stringy discharge from the eye; and pain and redness of the eye. Sometimes people with dry eye experience heaviness of the eyelids or blurred, changing, or decreased vision, although loss of vision is uncommon.

Dry eye is more common in women, especially after menopause. Surprisingly, some people with dry eye may have tears that run down their cheeks. This is because the eye may be producing less of the lipid and mucin layers of the tear film, which help keep tears in the eye. When this happens, tears do not stay in the eye long enough to thoroughly moisten it.

Dry eye can occur in climates with dry air, as well as with the use of some drugs, including antihistamines, nasal decongestants, tranquilizers, and antidepressant drugs. People with dry eye should let their health care providers know all the medications they are taking, since some of them may intensify dry eye symptoms.

People with connective tissue diseases, such as rheumatoid arthritis, can also develop dry eye. It is important to note that dry eye is sometimes a symptom of Sjögren's syndrome, a disease that attacks the body's lubricating glands, such as the tear and salivary glands. A complete physical examination may diagnose any underlying diseases.

Artificial tears, which lubricate the eye, are the principal treatment for dry eye. They are available over-the-counter as eye drops. Sterile ointments are sometimes used at night to help prevent the eye from drying. Using humidifiers, wearing wrap-around glasses when outside, and avoiding outside windy and dry conditions may bring relief. For people with severe cases of dry eye, temporary or permanent closure of the tear drain (small openings at the inner corner of the eyelids where tears drain from the eye) may be helpful.

Fuchs' Dystrophy

Fuchs' dystrophy is a slowly progressing disease that usually affects both eyes and is slightly more common in women than in men. Although doctors can often see early signs of Fuchs' dystrophy in people in their 30s and 40s, the disease rarely affects vision until people reach their 50s and 60s.

Fuchs' dystrophy occurs when endothelial cells gradually deteriorate without any apparent reason. As more endothelial cells are lost over the years, the endothelium becomes less efficient at pumping water out of the stroma. This causes the cornea to swell and distort vision. Eventually, the epithelium also takes on water, resulting in pain and severe visual impairment.

Epithelial swelling damages vision by changing the cornea's normal curvature, and causing a sight-impairing haze to appear in the tissue. Epithelial swelling will also produce tiny blisters on the corneal surface. When these blisters burst, they are extremely painful.

At first, a person with Fuchs' dystrophy will awaken with blurred vision that will gradually clear during the day. This occurs because the cornea is normally thicker in the morning; it retains fluids during sleep that evaporate in the tear film while we are awake. As the disease worsens, this swelling will remain constant and reduce vision throughout the day.

When treating the disease, doctors will try first to reduce the swelling with drops, ointments, or soft contact lenses. They also may instruct a person to use a hair dryer, held at arm's length or directed across the face, to dry out the epithelial blisters. This can be done two or three times a day.

When the disease interferes with daily activities, a person may need to consider having a corneal transplant to restore sight. The short-term success rate of corneal transplantation is quite good for people with Fuchs' dystrophy. However, some studies suggest that the long-term survival of the new cornea can be a problem.

Corneal Dystrophies

A corneal dystrophy is a condition in which one or more parts of the cornea lose their normal clarity due to a buildup of cloudy material. There are over 20 corneal dystrophies that affect all parts of the cornea. These diseases share many traits:

- They are usually inherited.

- They affect the right and left eyes equally.

- They are not caused by outside factors, such as injury or diet.

- Most progress gradually.

- Most usually begin in one of the five corneal layers and may later spread to nearby layers.

- Most do not affect other parts of the body, nor are they related to diseases affecting other parts of the eye or body.

- Most can occur in otherwise totally healthy people, male or female.

Corneal dystrophies affect vision in widely differing ways. Some cause severe visual impairment, while a few cause no vision problems and are discovered during a routine eye examination. Other dystrophies may cause repeated episodes of pain without leading to permanent loss of vision.

Some of the most common corneal dystrophies include Fuchs' dystrophy, keratoconus, lattice dystrophy, and map-dot-fingerprint dystrophy.

Herpes Zoster (Shingles)

This infection is produced by the varicella zoster virus, the same virus that causes chicken pox. After an initial outbreak of chicken pox (often during childhood), the virus remains inactive within the nerve cells of the central nervous system. But in some people, the varicella zoster virus will reactivate at another time in their lives. When this occurs, the virus travels down long nerve fibers and infects some part of the body, producing a blistering rash (shingles), fever, painful inflammations of the affected nerve fibers, and a general feeling of sluggishness.

Varicella zoster virus may travel to the head and neck, perhaps involving an eye, part of the nose, cheek, and forehead. In about 40 percent of those with shingles in these areas, the virus infects the cornea. Doctors will often prescribe oral antiviral treatment to reduce the risk of the virus infecting cells deep within the tissue, which could inflame and scar the cornea. The disease may also cause decreased corneal sensitivity, meaning that foreign matter, such as eyelashes, in the eye are not felt as keenly. For many, this decreased sensitivity will be permanent.

Although shingles can occur in anyone exposed to the varicella zoster virus, research has established two general risk factors for the disease: (1) Advanced age; and (2) A weakened immune system. Studies show that people over age 80 have a five times greater chance of having shingles than adults between the ages of 20 and 40. Unlike herpes simplex I, the varicella zoster virus does not usually flare up more than once in adults with normally functioning immune systems.

Be aware that corneal problems may arise months after the shingles are gone. For this reason, it is important that people who have had facial shingles schedule follow-up eye examinations.

Iridocorneal Endothelial Syndrome

More common in women and usually diagnosed between ages 30 to 50, iridocorneal endothelial (ICE) syndrome has three main features: (1) Visible changes in the iris, the colored part of the eye that regulates the amount of light entering the eye; (2) Swelling of the cornea; and (3) The development of glaucoma, a disease that can cause severe vision loss when normal fluid inside the eye cannot drain properly. ICE is usually present in only one eye.

ICE syndrome is actually a grouping of three closely linked conditions: iris nevus (or Cogan-Reese) syndrome; Chandler's syndrome;

and essential (progressive) iris atrophy (hence the acronym ICE). The most common feature of this group of diseases is the movement of endothelial cells off the cornea onto the iris. This loss of cells from the cornea often leads to corneal swelling, distortion of the iris, and variable degrees of distortion of the pupil, the adjustable opening at the center of the iris that allows varying amounts of light to enter the eye. This cell movement also plugs the fluid outflow channels of the eye, causing glaucoma.

The cause of this disease is unknown. While we do not yet know how to keep ICE syndrome from progressing, the glaucoma associated with the disease can be treated with medication, and a corneal transplant can treat the corneal swelling.

Keratoconus

This disorder—a progressive thinning of the cornea—is the most common corneal dystrophy in the United States, affecting one in every 2,000 Americans. It is more prevalent in teenagers and adults in their 20s. Keratoconus arises when the middle of the cornea thins and gradually bulges outward, forming a rounded cone shape. This abnormal curvature changes the cornea's refractive power, producing moderate to severe distortion (astigmatism) and blurriness (nearsightedness) of vision. Keratoconus may also cause swelling and a sight-impairing scarring of the tissue.

Studies indicate that keratoconus stems from one of several possible causes:

- An inherited corneal abnormality. About seven percent of those with the condition have a family history of keratoconus.

- An eye injury, i.e., excessive eye rubbing or wearing hard contact lenses for many years.

- Certain eye diseases, such as retinitis pigmentosa, retinopathy of prematurity, and vernal keratoconjunctivitis.

- Systemic diseases, such as Leber's congenital amaurosis, Ehlers-Danlos syndrome, Down syndrome, and osteogenesis imperfecta.

Keratoconus usually affects both eyes. At first, people can correct their vision with eyeglasses. But as the astigmatism worsens, they must rely on specially fitted contact lenses to reduce the distortion and provide better vision. Although finding a comfortable contact lens can be an extremely frustrating and difficult process, it is crucial because a poorly fitting lens could further damage the cornea and make wearing a contact lens intolerable.

In most cases, the cornea will stabilize after a few years without ever causing severe vision problems. But in about 10 to 20 percent of people with keratoconus, the cornea will eventually become too scarred or will not tolerate a contact lens. If either of these problems occur, a corneal transplant may be needed. This operation is successful in more than 90 percent of those with advanced keratoconus. Several studies have also reported that 80 percent or more of these patients have 20/40 vision or better after the operation.

The National Eye Institute is conducting a natural history study— called the Collaborative Longitudinal Evaluation of Keratoconus Study—to identify factors that influence the severity and progression of keratoconus.

Lattice Dystrophy

Lattice dystrophy gets its name from an accumulation of amyloid deposits, or abnormal protein fibers, throughout the middle and anterior stroma. During an eye examination, the doctor sees these deposits in the stroma as clear, comma-shaped overlapping dots and branching filaments, creating a lattice effect. Over time, the lattice lines will grow opaque and involve more of the stroma. They will also gradually converge, giving the cornea a cloudiness that may also reduce vision.

In some people, these abnormal protein fibers can accumulate under the cornea's outer layer—the epithelium. This can cause erosion of the epithelium. This condition is known as recurrent epithelial erosion. These erosions: (1) Alter the cornea's normal curvature, resulting in temporary vision problems; and (2) Expose the nerves that line the cornea, causing severe pain. Even the involuntary act of blinking can be painful.

To ease this pain, a doctor may prescribe eye drops and ointments to reduce the friction on the eroded cornea. In some cases, an eye patch may be used to immobilize the eyelids. With effective care, these erosions usually heal within three days, although occasional sensations of pain may occur for the next six-to-eight weeks.

By about age 40, some people with lattice dystrophy will have scarring under the epithelium, resulting in a haze on the cornea that can greatly obscure vision. In this case, a corneal transplant may be needed. Although people with lattice dystrophy have an excellent chance for a successful transplant, the disease may also arise in the donor cornea in as little as three years. In one study, about half of the transplant patients with lattice dystrophy had a recurrence of the disease from between two to 26 years after the operation. Of these, 15 percent required a second corneal transplant. Early lattice and recurrent lattice arising in the donor cornea responds well to treatment with the excimer laser.

Although lattice dystrophy can occur at any time in life, the condition usually arises in children between the ages of two and seven.

Map-Dot-Fingerprint Dystrophy

This dystrophy occurs when the epithelium's basement membrane develops abnormally (the basement membrane serves as the foundation on which the epithelial cells, which absorb nutrients from tears, anchor and organize themselves). When the basement membrane develops abnormally, the epithelial cells cannot properly adhere to it. This, in turn, causes recurrent epithelial erosions, in which the epithelium's outermost layer rises slightly, exposing a small gap between the outermost layer and the rest of the cornea.

Epithelial erosions can be a chronic problem. They may alter the cornea's normal curvature, causing periodic blurred vision. They may also expose the nerve endings that line the tissue, resulting in moderate to severe pain lasting as long as several days. Generally, the pain will be worse on awakening in the morning. Other symptoms include sensitivity to light, excessive tearing, and foreign body sensation in the eye.

Map-dot-fingerprint dystrophy, which tends to occur in both eyes, usually affects adults between the ages of 40 and 70, although it can develop earlier in life. Also known as epithelial basement membrane dystrophy, map-dot-fingerprint dystrophy gets its name from the unusual appearance of the cornea during an eye examination. Most often, the affected epithelium will have a map-like appearance, i.e., large, slightly gray outlines that look like a continent on a map. There may also be clusters of opaque dots underneath or close to the map-like patches. Less frequently, the irregular basement membrane will form concentric lines in the central cornea that resemble small fingerprints.

Typically, map-dot-fingerprint dystrophy will flare up occasionally for a few years and then go away on its own, with no lasting loss of vision. Most people never know that they have map-dot-fingerprint dystrophy, since they do not have any pain or vision loss. However, if treatment is needed, doctors will try to control the pain associated with the epithelial erosions. They may patch the eye to immobilize it, or prescribe lubricating eye drops and ointments. With treatment, these erosions usually heal within three days, although periodic flashes of pain may occur for several weeks thereafter. Other treatments include anterior corneal punctures to allow better adherence of cells; corneal scraping to remove eroded areas of the cornea and allow regeneration of healthy epithelial tissue; and use of the excimer laser to remove surface irregularities.

Ocular Herpes

Herpes of the eye, or ocular herpes, is a recurrent viral infection that is caused by the herpes simplex virus and is the most common infectious cause of corneal blindness in the U.S. Previous studies show that once people develop ocular herpes, they have up to a 50 percent chance of having a recurrence. This second flare-up could come weeks or even years after the initial occurrence.

Ocular herpes can produce a painful sore on the eyelid or surface of the eye and cause inflammation of the cornea. Prompt treatment with anti-viral drugs helps to stop the herpes virus from multiplying and destroying epithelial cells. However, the infection may spread deeper into the cornea and develop into a more severe infection called stromal keratitis, which causes the body's immune system to attack and destroy stromal cells. Stromal keratitis is more difficult to treat than less severe ocular herpes infections. Recurrent episodes of stromal keratitis can cause scarring of the cornea, which can lead to loss of vision and possibly blindness.

Like other herpetic infections, herpes of the eye can be controlled. An estimated 400,000 Americans have had some form of ocular herpes. Each year, nearly 50,000 new and recurring cases are diagnosed in the United States, with the more serious stromal keratitis accounting for about 25 percent. In one large study, researchers found that recurrence rate of ocular herpes was 10 percent within one year, 23 percent within two years, and 63 percent within 20 years. Some factors believed to be associated with recurrence include fever, stress, sunlight, and eye injury.

The National Eye Institute supported the Herpetic Eye Disease Study, a group of clinical trials that studied various treatments for severe ocular herpes.

Pterygium

A pterygium is a pinkish, triangular-shaped tissue growth on the cornea. Some pterygia grow slowly throughout a person's life, while others stop growing after a certain point. A pterygium rarely grows so large that it begins to cover the pupil of the eye.

Pterygia are more common in sunny climates and in the 20 to 40 age group. Scientists do not know what causes pterygia to develop. However, since people who have pterygia usually have spent a significant time outdoors, many doctors believe ultraviolet (UV) light from the sun may be a factor. In areas where sunlight is strong, wearing protective eyeglasses, sunglasses, and/or hats with brims are suggested. While some studies report a higher prevalence of pterygia in men than in women, this may reflect different rates of exposure to UV light.

Because a pterygium is visible, many people want to have it removed for cosmetic reasons. It is usually not too noticeable unless it becomes red and swollen from dust or air pollutants. Surgery to remove a pterygium is not recommended unless it affects vision. If a pterygium is surgically removed, it may grow back, particularly if the patient is less than 40 years of age. Lubricants can reduce the redness and provide relief from the chronic irritation.

Stevens-Johnson Syndrome

Stevens-Johnson Syndrome (SJS), also called erythema multiforme major, is a disorder of the skin that can also affect the eyes. SJS is characterized by painful, blistery lesions on the skin and the mucous membranes (the thin, moist tissues that line body cavities) of the mouth, throat, genital region, and eyelids. SJS can cause serious eye problems, such as severe conjunctivitis; iritis, an inflammation inside the eye; corneal blisters and erosions; and corneal holes. In some cases, the ocular complications from SJS can be disabling and lead to severe vision loss.

Scientists are not certain why SJS develops. The most commonly cited cause of SJS is an adverse allergic drug reaction. Almost any drug—but most particularly sulfa drugs—can cause SJS. The allergic reaction to the drug may not occur until 7 to 14 days after first using it. SJS can also be preceded by a viral infection, such as herpes or the mumps, and its accompanying fever, sore throat, and sluggishness. Treatment for the eye may include artificial tears, antibiotics, or corticosteroids. About one-third of all patients diagnosed with SJS have recurrences of the disease.

SJS occurs twice as often in men as women, and most cases appear in children and young adults under 30, although it can develop in people at any age.

What Is a Corneal Transplant? Is It Safe?

A corneal transplant involves replacing a diseased or scarred cornea with a new one. When the cornea becomes cloudy, light cannot penetrate the eye to reach the light-sensitive retina. Poor vision or blindness may result.

In corneal transplant surgery, the surgeon removes the central portion of the cloudy cornea and replaces it with a clear cornea, usually donated through an eye bank. A trephine, an instrument like a cookie cutter, is used to remove the cloudy cornea. The surgeon places the new cornea in the opening and sews it with a very fine thread. The thread stays in for months or even years until the eye heals properly (removing the thread is quite simple and can easily be done in an ophthalmologist's office). Following surgery, eye drops to help promote healing will be needed for several months.

Corneal transplants are very common in the United States; about 40,000 are performed each year. The chances of success of this operation have risen dramatically because of technological advances, such as less irritating sutures, or threads, which are often finer than a human hair; and the surgical microscope. Corneal transplantation has restored sight to many, who a generation ago would have been blinded permanently by corneal injury, infection, or inherited corneal disease or degeneration.

What Problems Can Develop from a Corneal Transplant?

Even with a fairly high success rate, some problems can develop, such as rejection of the new cornea. Warning signs for rejection are decreased vision, increased redness of the eye, increased pain, and increased sensitivity to light. If any of these last for more than six hours, you should immediately call your ophthalmologist.

Rejection can be successfully treated if medication is administered at the first sign of symptoms. A study supported by the National Eye Institute (NEI) suggests that matching the blood type, but not tissue type, of the recipient with that of the cornea donor may improve the success rate of corneal transplants in people at high risk for graft failure. Approximately 20 percent of corneal transplant patients—between 6,000 to 8,000 a year—reject their donor corneas. The NEI-supported study, called the Collaborative Corneal Transplantation Study, found that high-risk patients may reduce the likelihood of corneal rejection if their blood types match those of the cornea donors. The study also concluded that intensive steroid treatment after transplant surgery improves the chances for a successful transplant.

Are There Alternatives to a Corneal Transplant?

Phototherapeutic keratectomy (PTK) is one of the latest advances in eye care for the treatment of corneal dystrophies, corneal scars, and certain corneal infections. Only a short time ago, people with these disorders would most likely have needed a corneal transplant. By combining the precision of the excimer laser with the control of a computer, doctors can vaporize microscopically thin layers of diseased corneal tissue and etch away the surface irregularities associated with many corneal dystrophies and scars. Surrounding areas suffer relatively little trauma. New tissue can then grow over the now-smooth surface. Recovery from the procedure takes a matter of days, rather than months as with a transplant. The return of vision can occur rapidly, especially if the cause of the problem is confined to the top layer of the cornea. Studies have shown close to an 85 percent success rate in corneal repair using PTK for well-selected patients.

The PTK procedure is especially useful for people with inherited disorders, whose scars or other corneal opacities limit vision by blocking the way images form on the retina. PTK has been approved by the U.S. Food and Drug Administration.

One of the technologies developed to treat corneal disease is the excimer laser. This device emits pulses of ultraviolet light—a laser beam—to etch away surface irregularities of corneal tissue. Because of the laser's precision, damage to healthy, adjoining tissue is reduced or eliminated.

Current Corneal Research

Vision research funded by the National Eye Institute (NEI) is leading to progress in understanding and treating corneal disease.

For example, scientists are learning how transplanting corneal cells from a patient's healthy eye to the diseased eye can treat certain conditions that previously caused blindness.

Vision researchers continue to investigate ways to enhance corneal healing and eliminate the corneal scarring that can threaten sight. Also, understanding how genes produce and maintain a healthy cornea will help in treating corneal disease.

Genetic studies in families afflicted with corneal dystrophies have yielded new insight into 13 different corneal dystrophies, including keratoconus. To identify factors that influence the severity and progression of keratoconus, the NEI is conducting a natural history study—called the Collaborative Longitudinal Evaluation of Keratoconus (CLEK)

Study—that is following more than 1200 patients with the disease. Scientists are looking for answers to how rapidly their keratoconus will progress, how bad their vision will become, and whether they will need corneal surgery to treat it. Results from the CLEK Study will enable eye care practitioners to better manage this complex disease.

The NEI also supported the Herpetic Eye Disease Study (HEDS), a group of clinical trials that studied various treatments for severe ocular herpes. HEDS researchers reported that oral acyclovir reduced by 41 percent the chance that ocular herpes, a recurrent disease, would return. The study clearly showed that acyclovir therapy can benefit people with all forms of ocular herpes. Current HEDS research is examining the role of psychological stress and other factors as triggers of ocular herpes recurrences.

About the National Eye Institute

The National Eye Institute (NEI) is one of the Federal government's National Institutes of Health. It was established by Congress in 1968 to discover safe and effective ways of preventing, diagnosing, and treating eye diseases and disorders. The NEI is the major sponsor of vision research in the U.S. This research is conducted at about 250 medical centers, hospitals, and universities across the country. Other clinical trials are conducted by NEI researchers at the National Institutes of Health campus in Bethesda, Maryland.

For more information about the NEI or NEI-sponsored clinical trials, contact the:

National Eye Institute
2020 Vision Place
Bethesda, MD 20892-3655
Phone: (301) 496-5248
E-mail: 2020@nei.nih.gov
Website: http://www.nei.nih.gov

Other Information Sources

American Academy of Ophthalmology
P.O. Box 7424
San Francisco, CA 94120-7424
Phone: (415) 561-8500
Website: http://www.aao.org

Represents ophthalmologists in the United States. Offers public information materials.

American Optometric Association
243 North Lindbergh Blvd.
St. Louis, MO 63141
Phone: (314) 991-4100
Website: http://www.aoa.org

Represents optometrists in the United States. Provides brochures on eye problems for the public.

Eye Bank Association of America
1015 Eighteenth Street NW, Suite 1010
Washington, DC 20036
Phone: (202) 775-4999
Website: http://www.restoresight.org

Establishes medical standards for evaluating and distributing eyes for corneal transplantation and research. Certifies eye banks and technicians.

U.S. Food and Drug Administration
5600 Fishers Lane (HFE-88)
Rockville, MD 20857
Toll-Free: (888) 463-6332
Website: http://www.fda.gov

Regulates food, drugs, and medical devices for use in the United States. Offers free information about refractive eye surgeries and contact lenses.

National Keratoconus Foundation
Cedars-Sinai Medical Center
8733 Beverly Blvd., Suite 201
Los Angeles, CA 90048
Toll-free: (800) 521-2524
Website: http://www.nkcf.org

Sponsors basic and clinical research on keratoconus and a public education program, including self-help groups and seminars. Provides information to patients and eye care practitioners.

Chapter 45

Dry Eye

What Is Dry Eye?

Our natural tears protect our eyes and give them moisture that is absolutely necessary for clear and comfortable vision. Some people are unable to produce enough of these tears, leaving the eyes dry and easily irritated. In this condition that affects millions of Americans, blinking no longer leaves a moist tear film to wash and soothe the eye. The irritation and discomfort that result may make a difference in one's ability to see. In rare cases, dry eye can become serious—even blinding—without proper care and treatment.

What Causes Dry Eye?

It's not clear why some people are unable to produce enough natural tears. However, one cause of dry eye is Sjögren's Syndrome, a disease involving mild to extreme dryness in both the eyes and the mouth. This disorder may be connected with menopause and arthritis. However, dry eye can also be caused by other eye disorders.

"Frequently Asked Questions about Dry Eye," reprinted with permission from Prevent Blindness America. © 2000. For additional information, call the Prevent Blindness America toll-free information line at (800) 331-2020, or visit www.preventblindness.org.

What Treatment Is Available?

Any drugstore carries over-the-counter tear replacements called artificial tears. These eyedrops may replace badly needed moisture and provide proper lubrication for normal eye functioning. Ask an eye care professional to recommend an artificial tear solution and give you instructions on how often to use it. Ointments often are used before bedtime to make sure there is enough wetness throughout the night. Due to frequent use during long periods of time, these preparations may cause allergic reactions or even toxic irritation. That's why it's important to talk with an eye care professional first.

To learn more about dry eye, please contact Prevent Blindness America or the Prevent Blindness affiliate near you.

Chapter 46

Ectropion and Entropion

Ectropion

Ectropion is the turning outward of the margin of the lower eyelid and the eyelashes. It occurs most frequently in older people, due to relaxation of the tissues as a result of aging. Other causes include skin cancer of the eyelid, trauma, eyelid scarring, and previous eyelid surgery.

The source of tear drainage is a small opening on the lower corner of the eye. As the lower lid turns outward, this opening may pull away from its normal location, disrupting the normal tear drainage process. This can lead to excessive tearing, mucous discharge, eye irritation, and chronic conjunctivitis (infection or inflammation of the inner membrane of the eyelid).

Lubricating ointments or artificial tears can be used to relieve symptoms in mild cases, but surgery is necessary to correct the problem. The procedure is usually performed under local anesthesia in an outpatient setting. During the operation, the eyelid and underlying muscles are tightened. After surgical correction, most patients no longer have symptoms.

From "Repair of Eyelid Malpositions," reprinted with permission of Healthcommunities.com, from www.visionchannel.net/ocuplasticsurgery/corrective.shtml#repair. © 2002 Healthcommunities.com, Inc.; updated September 2002. For further information, contact Nancy Gable Lucas, Editor, at nlucas@healthcommunities.com.

Entropion

Entropion is the turning inward of the upper or lower eyelid. It develops as a result of weakened structures that support the eyelid. It occurs in people of all age groups, but is most prevalent in older people. It often occurs as a result of aging, infection, or scarring inside the eyelid. Rarely, it is congenital (present at birth).

When the eyelid turns inward, the eyelashes and skin rub against the cornea, causing severe irritation, redness, and pain. If untreated, it can cause eye infections, corneal abrasions, or an eye ulcer. These conditions can threaten vision.

Surgical correction involves rotating the lid margin to a normal position and tightening the muscles. It is usually effective and is generally performed under local anesthesia in an outpatient setting.

Chapter 47

Eye Allergies and Allergic Conjunctivitis

The eyes are one of the most sensitive and vulnerable organs in the body. Airborne allergens and other particles can land directly on the surface of the eye, causing irritation and redness. Although tears constantly wash the eyes, they can't always keep out allergens like pollen or pet dander. Because of this, allergies that flare up in the eyes, also known as ocular allergies, are common.

What Are Ocular Allergies?

Eye allergies are no different than allergies that affect your sinuses, nose, or lungs. When an allergen comes in contact with your eyes, your body releases histamine—a chemical produced in reaction to a substance that the immune system can't tolerate. Special cells called mast cells make histamine. These cells are present throughout the body but are highly concentrated in the eyes.

Location of allergy symptoms depends somewhat on where the allergen has come into contact with your body. Ocular allergens tend to be airborne (as are most other allergens). The most frequent allergic triggers include:

- pollen
- pet hair or dander

- dust

- some medicines

There also are some triggers that irritate the eyes but are not true allergies, such as:

- cigarette smoke

- perfume

- diesel exhaust

What Is Allergic Conjunctivitis?

Conjunctivitis, also known as pink eye, is an inflammation of the conjunctiva (the membrane lining under the eyelids) and can be caused by allergies or infections. Allergic conjunctivitis and conjunctivitis caused by an infection can be hard to distinguish. Both have similar symptoms, such as redness, itching, and swelling in the eye area. However, when conjunctivitis is caused by allergies, both eyes are usually affected. Viral or bacterial conjunctivitis can affect either a single eye or both eyes. It is important to pinpoint whether someone has conjunctivitis because of allergies or infection since each condition has a different treatment.

Common symptoms of allergic conjunctivitis are:

- redness and itching under the eyelid

- excessive watering

- swelling of the eyeball

Common symptoms of conjunctivitis associated with infection are:

- feeling that eyelids are glued shut upon waking

- sensitivity to light

- pus on the surface of the eye

- burning sensation

Treatment

If you have ocular allergies or any other kind of allergic disease, the most effective treatment is prevention: try to avoid the allergens that trigger symptoms. For many, this is easier said than done, especially if your triggers are airborne, such as pollen.

When ocular allergies can't be controlled, there are several medications that may help relieve symptoms. Most of these treatments come in a topical form—such as eye drops or an ointment.

Eye drops, also called tear substitutes, can help in two ways: (1) by physically washing away allergens; and (2) by moistening the eye, which can become dry and red when irritated. Eye drops that contain medications to help reduce allergy symptoms also are available.

Topical Decongestants

Some eye drops contain topical decongestants that constrict small blood vessels and help reduce eye redness. These eye drops are available without a prescription. If you use eye drops with topical decongestants, be careful not to use them for prolonged periods. Overuse of topical decongestants can lead to increased swelling and redness that can last even after you stop using the drops. This is known as a rebound effect.

Topical decongestants, or any kind of eye drop containing chemicals that narrow blood vessels (called vasoconstrictors), shouldn't be used if you have glaucoma. Glaucoma is damage to the eye that results from increased pressure in the eyeball (also called intraocular pressure, or IOP). Vasoconstrictors can worsen this condition.

Topical Antihistamines

Eye drops containing antihistamines can reduce redness and swelling in the eye. Antihistamines block the effects of the chemical histamine, which is responsible for allergic symptoms like swelling, redness, and itching. Mild antihistamine eye drops are available over the counter, but stronger ones are available by prescription.

Helpful Strategies

Chilling any topical medications can help relieve redness and itching of the eyes. In addition, using cold compresses can help reduce some of the discomfort associated with conjunctivitis. A washcloth soaked in cold water works well.

Oral nonsteroidal anti-inflammatory drugs (NSAIDs), such as aspirin and ibuprofen-based medications, also can help reduce inflammation and symptoms like swelling in some patients.

407

Steroids

When topically administered medications like antihistamines and vasoconstrictors fail to help alleviate conjunctivitis symptoms, your doctor may prescribe topical steroids. Steroid eye drops can help control chronic and acute cases of conjunctivitis but should only be used as prescribed by your doctor. Steroids applied directly to the eye can cause a sharp increase in ocular pressure that can result in significant eye damage or glaucoma. Prolonged use of topical steroids in the eyes also can lead to cataracts. Cataracts form when the cornea on the surface of the eye gradually becomes opaque, causing blindness.

Because steroids can promote the growth of viruses, your doctor will want to rule out viral conjunctivitis as the cause of your eye problems before prescribing topical steroids.

Immunotherapy

Immunotherapy, also known as allergy shots, is another option for treating allergic conjunctivitis. Immunotherapy is a process that gradually desensitizes you to your allergens. Tiny amounts of the allergen are injected under the skin over the course of several years. During immunotherapy, your body will begin to develop a normal immune response to the allergen, and you won't experience red, watery eyes every time you are around pets or pollen. Although immunotherapy may take several months to produce results, it can eventually greatly diminish the need for eye drops or other medication.

When to See an Allergist

You should consult with an allergist or immunologist if you persistently have red, itchy, watery eyes. Many times, with the help of a doctor, ocular allergies and conjunctivitis can be controlled.

Chapter 48

Eye Cancer

Chapter Contents

Section 48.1

Retinoblastoma

PDQ® Cancer Information Summary. National Cancer Institute;
Bethesda, MD. Retinoblastoma: (PDQ®): Treatment – Patient.
Updated September 2002. Available at: http://cancer.gov.
Accessed September 23, 2002.

General Information

Retinoblastoma is a malignant (cancerous) tumor of the retina. The retina is the thin nerve tissue that lines the back of the eye that senses light and forms images.

Although retinoblastoma may occur at any age, it most often occurs in younger children, usually before the age of 5 years. The tumor may be in one eye only or in both eyes. Retinoblastoma is usually confined to the eye and does not spread to nearby tissue or other parts of the body. Your child's prognosis (chance of recovery and retaining sight) and choice of treatment depend on the extent of the disease within and beyond the eye.

Retinoblastoma may be hereditary (inherited) or nonhereditary. The hereditary form may be in one or both eyes, and generally affects younger children. Most retinoblastoma occurring in only one eye is not hereditary and is more often found in older children. When the disease occurs in both eyes, it is always hereditary. Because of the hereditary factor, patients and their brothers and sisters should have periodic examinations, including genetic counseling, to determine their risk for developing the disease.

A child who has hereditary retinoblastoma may also be at risk of developing a tumor in the brain while they are being treated for the eye tumor. This is called trilateral retinoblastoma, and patients should be periodically monitored by the doctor for the possible development of this rare condition during and after treatment. If your child has retinoblastoma, particularly the hereditary type, there is also an increased chance that he or she may develop other types of cancer in later years. Parents may therefore decide to continue taking their child for medical check-ups even after the cancer has been treated.

Stage Information

Stages of Retinoblastoma

Once retinoblastoma is found, more tests will be done to determine the size of the tumor and whether it has spread to surrounding tissue or to other parts of the body. This is called staging. To plan treatment, your child's doctor needs to know the stage of disease. Although there are several staging systems currently available for retinoblastoma, for the purposes of treatment retinoblastoma is categorized into intraocular and extraocular disease.

Intraocular Retinoblastoma

Cancer is found in one or both eyes, but does not extend beyond the eye into the tissues around the eye or to other parts of the body.

Extraocular Retinoblastoma

The cancer has extended beyond the eye. It may be confined to the tissues around the eye, or it may have spread to other parts of the body.

Recurrent Retinoblastoma

Recurrent disease means that the cancer has come back (recurred) or progressed (continued to grow) after it has been treated. It may recur in the eye, the tissues around the eye, or elsewhere in the body.

Treatment Option Overview

How Retinoblastoma Is Treated

There are treatments for all children with retinoblastoma, and most children can be cured. The type of treatment given depends on the extent of the disease within the eye, whether the disease is in one or both eyes, and whether the disease has spread beyond the eye. Treatment options that attempt to cure the patient and preserve vision, include the following:

- enucleation: surgery to remove the eye
- radiation therapy: radiation therapy uses high-energy radiation from x-rays and other sources to kill cancer cells and shrink

tumors. Radiation may come from a machine outside the body (external-beam radiation therapy) or may be administered by placing radioactive material into or very near the tumor (internal radiation therapy or brachytherapy).

- cryotherapy: the use of extreme cold to destroy cancer cells

- photocoagulation: the use of laser light to destroy blood vessels that supply nutrients to the tumor

- thermotherapy: the use of heat to destroy cancer cells

- chemotherapy: the use of drugs to kill cancer cells. Chemotherapy is called a systemic treatment because the drug enters the bloodstream, travels through the body, and can kill cancer cells throughout the body. In children with retinoblastoma, chemotherapy is under investigation.

Treatment by Stage

Your child may receive treatment that is considered standard based on its effectiveness in a number of patients in past studies, or you may choose to have your child take part in a clinical trial. Not all patients are cured with standard therapy and some standard treatments may have more side effects than are desired. For these reasons, clinical trials are designed to test new treatments and find better ways to treat children with cancer. Clinical trials are ongoing in many parts of the country for advanced stages of retinoblastoma. For more information, call the Cancer Information Service at 800-4-CANCER (800-422-6237); TTY at 800-332-8615.

Intraocular Retinoblastoma

Treatment depends on whether the cancer is in one or both eyes. If the cancer is in one eye, treatment may be one of the following:

- Surgery to remove the eye (enucleation) is used for large tumors when there is no expectation that useful vision can be preserved.

- External radiation therapy, photocoagulation, cryotherapy, thermotherapy, or brachytherapy may be used with smaller tumors when there is potential for preservation of sight.

If the cancer is in both eyes, treatment may be one of the following:

412

- Surgery to remove the eye with the most cancer, and/or radiation therapy to the other eye.

- Radiation therapy to both eyes if there is potential for vision in both eyes.

Clinical trials testing systemic chemotherapy with or without other types of treatment.

Extraocular Retinoblastoma

Treatment may be one of the following: radiation therapy and/or intrathecal (into the space between the lining of the spinal cord and the brain) chemotherapy.

Clinical trials are testing new combinations of chemotherapy drugs, with or without peripheral stem cell transplantation, and different ways of administrating chemotherapy drugs.

Recurrent Retinoblastoma

Treatment depends on the site and extent of the recurrence (or progression). If the cancer comes back only in the eye and is small, your child may have surgery or radiation therapy. If the cancer comes back outside of the eye, treatment will depend on many factors and individual patient needs. You may want to consider having your child participate in a clinical trial.

Section 48.2

Intraocular Melanoma

PDQ® Cancer Information Summary. National Cancer Institute;
Bethesda, MD. Intraocular (Eye) Melanoma: (PDQ®): Treatment –
Patient. Updated September 2002. Available at: http://cancer.gov.
Accessed September 23, 2002.

General Information

Intraocular melanoma, a rare cancer, is a disease in which cancer (malignant) cells are found in the part of the eye called the uvea. The uvea contains cells called melanocytes, which contain color. When these cells become cancerous, the cancer is called a melanoma. The uvea includes the iris (the colored part of the eye), the ciliary body (a muscle in the eye), and the choroid (a layer of tissue in the back of the eye). The iris opens and closes to change the amount of light entering the eye. The ciliary body changes the shape of the lens inside the eye so it can focus. The choroid layer is next to the retina, the part of the eye that makes a picture.

If there is melanoma that starts in the iris, it may look like a dark spot on the iris. If melanoma is in the ciliary body or the choroid, a person may have blurry vision or may have no symptoms, and the cancer may grow before it is noticed. Intraocular melanoma is usually found during a routine eye examination, when a doctor looks inside the eye with special lights and instruments.

The chance of recovery (prognosis) depends on the size and cell type of the cancer, where the cancer is in the eye, and whether the cancer has spread.

Stage Information

Stages of Intraocular Melanoma

Once intraocular melanoma is found (diagnosed), more tests will be done to find out exactly what kind of tumor the patient has and whether cancer cells have spread to other parts of the body. This is called staging. A doctor needs to know the stage to plan treatment. Intraocular melanoma is staged based on the area of the eye where the tumor is found and the size of the tumor.

Iris

Intraocular melanomas of the iris occur in the front colored part of the eye. Iris melanomas usually grow slowly and do not usually spread to other parts of the body.

Ciliary Body/Choroid, Small Size

Intraocular melanomas of the ciliary body and/or choroid occur in the back part of the eye. They are grouped by the size of the tumor. Small size ciliary body or choroid melanoma is 2 to 3 millimeters or less thick.

Ciliary Body/Choroid, Medium/Large Size

Intraocular melanomas of the ciliary body and/or choroid occur in the back part of the eye. They are grouped by the size of the tumor. Medium/large size ciliary body or choroid melanoma is more than 2 to 3 millimeters thick.

Extraocular Extension

The melanoma has spread outside the eye, to the nerve behind the eye (the optic nerve), or to the eye socket.

Recurrent

Recurrent disease means that the cancer has come back (recurred) after it has been treated.

Treatment Option Overview

How Intraocular Melanoma Is Treated

There are treatments for all patients with intraocular melanoma. In some cases a doctor may watch the patient carefully without treatment until the cancer begins to grow. When treatment is given, three types of treatment are commonly used:

* surgery (taking out the cancer)

- radiation therapy (using high-dose x-rays or other high-energy rays to kill cancer cells)

- photocoagulation (destroying blood vessels that feed the tumor)

Surgery is the most common treatment of intraocular melanoma. A doctor may remove the cancer using one of the following operations:

- Iridectomy removes only parts of the iris.

- Iridotrabeculectomy removes parts of the iris and the supporting tissues around the cornea, the clear layer covering the front of the eye.

- Iridocyclectomy removes parts of the iris and the ciliary body.

- Choroidectomy removes parts of the choroid.

- Enucleation removes the entire eye.

Radiation therapy uses x-rays or other high-energy rays to kill cancer cells and shrink tumors.

Radiation may come from a machine outside the body (external beam radiation therapy) or from putting materials that contain radiation (radioisotopes) in the area where the cancer cells are found (internal radiation therapy). In intraocular melanoma, internal radiation may be put next to the eye using small implants called plaques. Radiation can be used alone or in combination with surgery.

Photocoagulation is a treatment that uses a tiny beam of light, usually from a laser, to destroy blood vessels and kill the tumor.

Treatment by Stage

The choice of treatment depends on where the cancer is in the eye, how far it has spread, and the patient's general health and age.

Standard treatment may be considered because of its effectiveness in patients in past studies, or participation in a clinical trial may be considered. Not all patients are cured with standard therapy and some standard treatments may have more side effects than are desired. For these reasons, clinical trials are designed to find the best ways to treat cancer patients and are based on the most up-to-date information. A large clinical trial is ongoing in many parts of the country for patients with intraocular melanoma. To learn more about clinical trials, call the Cancer Information Service at (800) 4-CANCER [(800) 422-6237)]; TTY at (800) 332-8615.

Iris Melanoma

If the tumor is small, there are no symptoms, and the tumor is not growing, treatment may not be needed. If the tumor begins to grow or if there are symptoms, treatment may be one of the following:

1. Surgery to remove parts of the iris (iridectomy)
2. Surgery to remove parts of the iris and the supporting tissues around the cornea (iridotrabeculectomy)
3. Surgery to remove parts of the iris and the ciliary body
4. Surgery to remove the eye (enucleation)

Ciliary Body and Choroid Melanoma, Small Size

If the tumor is small, there are no symptoms, and the tumor is not growing, treatment may not be needed. If the tumor begins to grow, or if there are symptoms, treatment may be one of the following:

1. Internal radiation therapy
2. External beam radiation therapy
3. Surgery to remove the tumor and part of the iris or choroid (iridocyclectomy or choroidectomy)
4. Surgery to remove the eye (enucleation)
5. External beam radiation therapy followed by enucleation

Ciliary Body and Choroid Melanoma, Medium/Large Size

If the tumor is not growing, treatment may not be needed. If treatment is needed, it may be one of the following:

1. Internal radiation therapy
2. External beam radiation therapy
3. Surgery to remove the tumor and part of the iris or choroid (iridocyclectomy or choroidectomy)
4. Surgery to remove the eye (enucleation)
5. External beam radiation therapy followed by enucleation
6. A clinical trial. A large trial is in progress in many parts of the country comparing standard treatments. Clinical trials are also testing new treatments.

Extraocular Extension Melanoma

Treatment may be one of the following:

1. Surgery to remove the eye and other tissues in the eye socket (orbital exenteration) with or without radiation therapy

2. Surgery to remove the eye (enucleation) with or without radiation therapy

Recurrent Intraocular Melanoma

Treatment will depend on the treatment the patient received before, the patient's age and health, where the cancer came back, and how far the cancer has spread. The patient may want to take part in a clinical trial.

To Learn More

Call

For more information, U.S. residents may call the National Cancer Institute's (NCI's) Cancer Information Service toll-free at (800) 4-CANCER [(800) 422-6237] Monday through Friday from 9:00 a.m. to 4:30 p.m. Deaf and hard-of-hearing callers with TTY equipment may call (800) 332-8615. The call is free and a trained Cancer Information Specialist is available to answer your questions.

Websites and Organizations

The NCI's Cancer.gov website (http://cancer.gov) provides online access to information on cancer, clinical trials, and other websites and organizations that offer support and resources for cancer patients and their families. There are also many other places where people can get materials and information about cancer treatment and services. Local hospitals may have information on local and regional agencies that offer information about finances, getting to and from treatment, receiving care at home, and dealing with problems associated with cancer treatment.

Publications

The NCI has booklets and other materials for patients, health professionals, and the public.

These publications discuss types of cancer, methods of cancer treatment, coping with cancer, and clinical trials. Some publications provide information on tests for cancer, cancer causes and prevention, cancer statistics, and NCI research activities. NCI materials on these and other topics may be ordered online or printed directly from the NCI Publications Locator (http://cissecure.nci.nih.gov/ncipubs). These materials can also be ordered by telephone from the Cancer Information Service toll-free at (800) 4-CANCER [(800) 422-6237]; TTY at (800) 332-8615.

LiveHelp

The NCI's LiveHelp service, a program available on several of the Institute's websites, provides Internet users with the ability to chat online with an Information Specialist. The service is available from 9:00 a.m. to 7:30 p.m. Eastern time, Monday through Friday. Information Specialists can help Internet users find information on NCI Web sites and answer questions about cancer.

Write

For more information from the NCI, please write to this address: National Cancer Institute Office of Communications, 31 Center Drive, MSC, 2580 Bethesda, MD 20892-2580.

Chapter 49

Eyelid Surgery

Eyelid surgery (technically called blepharoplasty) is a procedure to remove fat—usually along with excess skin and muscle—from the upper and lower eyelids. Eyelid surgery can correct drooping upper lids and puffy bags below your eyes—features that make you look older and more tired than you feel, and may even interfere with your vision. However, it won't remove crow's feet or other wrinkles, eliminate dark circles under your eyes, or lift sagging eyebrows. While it can add an upper eyelid crease to Asian eyes, it will not erase evidence of your ethnic or racial heritage. Blepharoplasty can be done alone, or in conjunction with other facial surgery procedures such as a facelift or browlift.

If you're considering eyelid surgery, this chapter will give you a basic understanding of the procedure—when it can help, how it's performed, and what results you can expect. It can't answer all of your questions, since a lot depends on the individual patient and the surgeon. Please ask your surgeon about anything you don't understand.

The Best Candidates for Eyelid Surgery

Blepharoplasty can enhance your appearance and your self-confidence, but it won't necessarily change your looks to match your ideal, or cause other people to treat you differently. Before you decide

From "Blepharoplasty: Eyelid Surgery." © 1993 American Society of Plastic Surgeons, www.plasticsurgery.org, (888) 475-2784. Reprinted with permission. Reviewed by David A. Cooke, M.D., on September 15, 2002.

to have surgery, think carefully about your expectations and discuss them with your surgeon.

The best candidates for eyelid surgery are men and women who are physically healthy, psychologically stable, and realistic in their expectations. Most are 35 or older, but if droopy, baggy eyelids run in your family, you may decide to have eyelid surgery at a younger age.

A few medical conditions make blepharoplasty more risky. They include thyroid problems such as hypothyroidism and Graves' disease, dry eye or lack of sufficient tears, high blood pressure or other circulatory disorders, cardiovascular disease, and diabetes. A detached retina or glaucoma is also reason for caution; check with your ophthalmologist before you have surgery.

All Surgery Carries Some Uncertainty and Risk

When eyelid surgery is performed by a qualified plastic surgeon, complications are infrequent and usually minor. Nevertheless, there is always a possibility of complications, including infection or a reaction to the anesthesia. You can reduce your risks by closely following your surgeon's instructions both before and after surgery.

The minor complications that occasionally follow blepharoplasty include double or blurred vision for a few days; temporary swelling at the corner of the eyelids; and a slight asymmetry in healing or scarring. Tiny whiteheads may appear after your stitches are taken out; your surgeon can remove them easily with a very fine needle.

Following surgery, some patients may have difficulty closing their eyes when they sleep; in rare cases this condition may be permanent. Another very rare complication is ectropion, a pulling down of the lower lids. In this case, further surgery may be required.

Planning Your Surgery

The surgeon closes the incisions with fine sutures, which will leave nearly invisible scars. The initial consultation with your surgeon is very important. The surgeon will need your complete medical history, so check your own records ahead of time and be ready to provide this information. Be sure to inform your surgeon if you have any allergies; if you're taking any vitamins, medications (prescription or over the counter), or other drugs; and if you smoke.

In this consultation, your surgeon or a nurse will test your vision and assess your tear production. You should also provide any relevant information from your ophthalmologist or the record of your most recent eye exam. If you wear glasses or contact lenses, be sure to bring them along.

You and your surgeon should carefully discuss your goals and expectations for this surgery. You'll need to discuss whether to do all four eyelids or just the upper or lower ones, whether skin as well as fat will be removed, and whether any additional procedures are appropriate.

Your surgeon will explain the techniques and anesthesia he or she will use, the type of facility where the surgery will be performed, and the risks and costs involved. (Note: Most insurance policies don't cover eyelid surgery, unless you can prove that drooping upper lids interfere with your vision. Check with your insurer.)

Don't hesitate to ask your doctor any questions you may have, especially those regarding your expectations and concerns about the results.

Preparing for Your Surgery

Your surgeon will give you specific instructions on how to prepare for surgery, including guidelines on eating and drinking, smoking, and taking or avoiding certain vitamins and medications. Carefully following these instructions will help your surgery go more smoothly.

While you're making preparations, be sure to arrange for someone to drive you home after your surgery, and to help you out for a few days if needed.

Where Your Surgery Will Be Performed

Eyelid surgery may be performed in a surgeon's office-based facility, an outpatient surgery center, or a hospital. It's usually done on an outpatient basis; rarely does it require an inpatient stay.

Types of Anesthesia

Eyelid surgery is usually performed under local anesthesia—which numbs the area around your eyes—along with oral or intravenous sedatives. You'll be awake during the surgery, but relaxed and insensitive to pain. (However, you may feel some tugging or occasional discomfort.) Some surgeons prefer to use general anesthesia; in that case, you'll sleep through the operation.

The Surgery

Blepharoplasty usually takes one to three hours, depending on the extent of the surgery. If you're having all four eyelids done, the surgeon will probably work on the upper lids first, then the lower ones.

In a typical procedure, the surgeon makes incisions following the natural lines of your eyelids; in the creases of your upper lids, and just below the lashes in the lower lids. The incisions may extend into the crow's feet or laugh lines at the outer corners of your eyes. Working through these incisions, the surgeon separates the skin from underlying fatty tissue and muscle, removes excess fat, and often trims sagging skin and muscle. The incisions are then closed with very fine sutures.

If you have a pocket of fat beneath your lower eyelids but don't need to have any skin removed, your surgeon may perform a transconjunctival blepharoplasty. In this procedure the incision is made inside your lower eyelid, leaving no visible scar. It is usually performed on younger patients with thicker, more elastic skin.

After Your Surgery

After surgery, the surgeon will probably lubricate your eyes with ointment and may apply a bandage. Your eyelids may feel tight and sore as the anesthesia wears off, but you can control any discomfort with the pain medication prescribed by your surgeon. If you feel any severe pain, call your surgeon immediately.

Your surgeon will instruct you to keep your head elevated for several days, and to use cold compresses to reduce swelling and bruising. (Bruising varies from person to person: it reaches its peak during the first week, and generally lasts anywhere from two weeks to a month.) You'll be shown how to clean your eyes, which may be gummy for a week or so. Many doctors recommend eye drops, since your eyelids may feel dry at first and your eyes may burn or itch. For the first few weeks you may also experience excessive tearing, sensitivity to light, and temporary changes in your eyesight, such as blurring or double vision.

Your surgeon will follow your progress very closely for the first week or two. The stitches will be removed two days to a week after surgery. Once they're out, the swelling and discoloration around your eyes will gradually subside, and you'll start to look and feel much better.

Getting Back to Normal

After surgery, the upper eyelids no longer droop and the skin under the eyes is smooth and firm. You should be able to read or watch television after two or three days. However, you won't be able to wear contact lenses for about two weeks, and even then they may feel uncomfortable for a while.

Most people feel ready to go out in public (and back to work) in a week to 10 days. By then, depending on your rate of healing and your doctor's instructions, you'll probably be able to wear makeup to hide the bruising that remains. You may be sensitive to sunlight, wind, and other irritants for several weeks, so you should wear sunglasses and a special sunblock made for eyelids when you go out.

Your surgeon will probably tell you to keep your activities to a minimum for three to five days, and to avoid more strenuous activities for about three weeks. It's especially important to avoid activities that raise your blood pressure, including bending, lifting, and rigorous sports. You may also be told to avoid alcohol, since it causes fluid retention.

Your New Look

Healing is a gradual process, and your scars may remain slightly pink for six months or more after surgery. Eventually, though, they'll fade to a thin, nearly invisible white line.

On the other hand, the positive results of your eyelid surgery—the more alert and youthful look—will last for years. For many people, these results are permanent.

Chapter 50

Macular Hole

The information provided in this chapter was developed by the National Eye Institute (NEI) to help patients and their families search for general information about macular hole. An eye care professional who has examined the patient's eyes and is familiar with his or her medical history is the best person to answer specific questions.

What Is a Macular Hole?

The macula is a tiny oval area made up of millions of nerve cells located at the center of the retina. The retina is the light-sensitive tissue at the back of the eye. The macula is responsible for sharp, central vision. A macular hole is just that: a hole in the macula.

What Causes a Macular Hole?

The eye contains a jelly-like substance called the vitreous. Shrinking of the vitreous usually causes the hole. As a person ages, the vitreous becomes thicker and stringier and begins to pull away from the retina. If the vitreous is firmly attached to the retina when it pulls away, a hole can result.

"Macular Hole Resource Guide," National Eye Institute, available online at http://www.nei.nih.gov, April 2002.

What Are the Symptoms of a Macular Hole?

The size of the hole and its location on the retina determine how much it will affect vision. Generally, people notice a slight distortion or reduction in their eyesight. However, if the hole goes all the way through the macula, you can lose a lot of your central and detailed vision.

Is a Macular Hole the Same as Macular Degeneration?

No, they are two different diseases even though they have similar symptoms. An eye care professional will know the difference.

How Is a Macular Hole Treated?

A surgical procedure called vitrectomy is often used to treat holes that go all the way through the macula. The vitreous is removed to prevent it from pulling on the retina. It is replaced with a gas bubble that eventually fills with natural fluids.

Following surgery, patients must usually keep their faces down for two or three weeks. This position allows the bubble to press against the macula and seal the hole.

Vitrectomy can lead to complications, most commonly an increase in how fast cataracts develop. Other less common complications include infection and retinal detachment either during surgery or afterward.

How Successful Is This Surgery?

The surgery is about 90 percent effective in closing the hole. However, improvement in people's vision is more variable. More than half of those who have the surgery can expect an improvement of two lines or more on the vision chart.

Is My Other Eye at Risk?

Very few people get a macular hole in the second eye. Your eye care professional will be able to talk to you about your risk.

Research

Research studies are being conducted to determine other treatments for macular holes. Currently the research is looking at using silicon oil to close the macular hole instead of the gas bubble that is being used now. No definite conclusions have been reached at this time.

Other Resources

The following organization may be able to provide additional information on macular holes:

American Academy of Ophthalmology
P.O. Box 7424
San Francisco, CA 94120-7424
Phone: (415) 561-8500

For additional information, you may also wish to contact a local library.

Medical Literature

Below is a sample of the citations available in MEDLINE, a comprehensive medical literature database coordinated by the National Library of Medicine (NLM). MEDLINE contains information on medical journal articles published from 1966 to the present. You can conduct your own free literature search by accessing MEDLINE through the Internet at http://medlineplus.nlm.nih.gov. You can also get assistance with a literature search at a local library.

To obtain copies of any of the articles listed below, contact a local community, university, or medical library. If the library you visit does not have a copy of a particular article, you may usually obtain it through an inter-library loan.

Please keep in mind that articles in the medical literature are usually written in technical language. We encourage you to share any articles you order with a health care professional who can help you understand them.

Surgical Management of Macular Holes: A Report by the American Academy of Ophthalmology

Benson WE, Cruickshanks KC, Fong DS, Williams GA, Bloome MA, Frambach DA, Kreiger AE, Murphy RP. *Ophthalmology* 2001; 108(7):1328-1335.

This document describes macular hole surgery and examines the available evidence to address questions about the effectiveness of the procedure for different stages of macular hole, complications during and after surgery, and modifications to the technique. The evidence does not support surgery for patients with stage 1 holes.

Properly conducted, well-designed randomized trials support surgery for stage 2 holes to prevent progression to later stages of the disease and further visual loss. Additional evidence shows that surgery improves the vision in a majority of patients with stage 3 and stage 4 holes. There is no strong evidence that adding another form of therapy at the time of surgery results in improved surgical outcomes. Patient inconvenience, patient preference, and quality of life issues have not been studied.

Macular Hole Surgery in 2000

Margherio AR. Michigan State University College of Human Medicine, Grand Rapids, MI. *Current Opinion in Ophthalmology* 2000; 11(3):186-90.

This article begins by describing possible causes of macular holes. It then discusses the different stages of macular holes, the surgeries being used to close the holes, and different procedures that combined with surgery can get the best possible results.

Complications of Macular Hole Surgery

Javid CG; Lou PL. Massachusetts Eye and Ear Infirmary, Boston, MA. *International Ophthalmology Clinics* 2000; 40(1):225-32.

This article begins with a brief overview of macular holes. The article discusses why macular holes form, conditions that can be mistaken for macular holes, and the different stages of macular holes. The article continues on to describe how a vitrectomy is done and talks about the different complications that can follow vitrectomy. Six possible complications are discussed in detail.

Possible reasons for complications are mentioned, as well as how common each complication is.

Macular Hole

University of Pennsylvania Scheie Eye Institute, Retina Service, Philadelphia, PA. *Survey of Ophthalmology* 1998; 42(5):393-416.

This article reports on different theories that have been proposed over the years to explain the development of macular holes and then describes the current theory. The different stages of macular holes are explained, along with different diagnostic tests for detecting them. The article then lists various diseases that can be confused with a macular hole and details how macular holes progress. Risk factors for developing a hole in the unaffected eye are also noted.

The article ends with a discussion of the success of different treatments used to manage macular holes and describes the complications that can result from these treatments.

The National Eye Institute (NEI), part of the National Institutes of Health (NIH), is the Federal government's principal agency for conducting and supporting vision research. Inclusion of an item in this chapter does not imply the endorsement of the NEI or the NIH.

Chapter 51

Macular Pucker

The information provided in this chapter was developed by the National Eye Institute to help patients and their families search for general information about macular pucker. An eye care professional who has examined the patient's eyes and is familiar with his or her medical history is the best person to answer specific questions.

What Is a Macular Pucker?

The macula is a tiny oval area made up of millions of nerve cells located at the center of the retina. The retina is the light-sensitive tissue at the back of the eye that sends visual signals to the brain through the optic nerve. The macula is responsible for sharp, central vision. A macular pucker or epiretinal membrane is scar tissue that has formed on the retina.

What Causes a Macular Pucker?

As we age, the vitreous, the jelly-like substance inside the eye that makes the eye round, changes consistency and starts to shrink. This shrinking causes the vitreous to pull away from the retina and scar tissue may develop. If this scar tissue contracts, it causes the retina to wrinkle. Other causes of macular pucker include trauma (from

"Macular Pucker Resource Guide," National Eye Institute, available online at http://www.nei.nih.gov, April 2002.

either surgery or an eye injury), retinal detachment, inflammation, and problems with the retinal blood vessels.

What Are the Symptoms of a Macular Pucker?

If the retinal wrinkling happens in the macula, patients may notice that their vision is blurry or mildly distorted and straight lines can appear wavy.

How Is a Macular Pucker Treated?

The only treatment for this condition is surgery. Since surgery always involves risks, it is recommended only for patients whose vision is significantly affected. In most cases, treatment is not recommended. Patients should talk with their eye care professional about whether treatment is appropriate.

Surgery consists of a vitrectomy combined with peeling away of the scar tissue. During a vitrectomy, the vitreous and scar tissue are removed. The surgeon then replaces the vitreous with salt solution.

Most patients recover about half of their lost vision, and distortion is significantly reduced. The most common complication of vitrectomy is an increase in the rate of cataract development.

Cataract surgery may be needed within a few years after the vitrectomy. Other, less common complications are retinal detachment either during or after surgery and infection after surgery. The macular pucker may grow back, but this is a rare occurrence.

Research

Research studies are being conducted to determine other treatments for macular pucker. Please note that both of the procedures described below need additional clinical testing. We suggest you share this information with your eye care professional.

Some physicians are researching the use of a surgical procedure in which scar tissue is peeled off without performing the vitrectomy.

Other doctors are researching a new surgical technique to remove the internal limiting membrane (a layer of the retina) for patients with both macular pucker and macular hole. This surgical technique is called Fluidic Internal Limiting Membrane Separation (FILMS). After a vitrectomy, fluid is injected between the membrane and the retina that causes the membrane, along with the scar tissue, to lift away. It is then removed with forceps.

Resources

The following organizations may be able to provide additional information on macular pucker:

National Eye Institute
2020 Vision Place
Bethesda, MD 20892-3655
Phone: (301) 496-5248
Website: http://www.nei.nih.gov

American Academy of Ophthalmology
P.O. Box 7424
San Francisco, CA 94120-7424
Phone: (415) 561-8500

For additional information, you may wish to contact a local library.

Medical Literature

Below is a sample of the citations available through MEDLINE/PubMed, a service of the National Library of Medicine. MEDLINE/PubMed provides access to over 11 million medical literature citations from 1966 to the present and includes links to many sites providing full text articles and other related resources. You can conduct your own free literature search by accessing MEDLINE through the Internet at http://medlineplus.nlm.nih.gov/hinfo.html. You can also get assistance with a literature search at a local library.

To obtain copies of any of the articles listed below, contact a local community, university, or medical library. If the library you visit does not have a copy of a desired article, you may usually obtain it through an inter-library loan.

Please keep in mind that articles in the medical literature are usually written in technical language. We encourage you to share any articles you order with a health care professional who can help you understand them.

Postoperative Complications of Epiretinal Membrane Surgery

Graham K, D'Amico DJ. Retina Service, Massachusetts Eye and Ear Infirmary, Boston 02114, USA. *International Ophthalmology Clinics* 40(1):215-223, Winter 2000.

Since the initial description by Machemer, surgical removal of an epiretinal membrane (ERM) in nondiabetic eyes has become a routine procedure after which the majority of patients experience visual improvement. Of patients undergoing ERM surgery, 74 percent to 87 percent can expect visual improvement of at least two lines on the Snellen chart. In general, surgical removal of ERMs that are idiopathic (no known cause) is more successful than removal of membranes that are secondary to retinal tears or detachments. Poor visual outcome from ERM surgery is most commonly due to cataract development, retinal breaks, and retinal detachments. Other postoperative complications include cystoid macular edema (CME), retinal phototoxicity, endophthalmitis, subretinal neovascularization, and recurrent ERMs. These complications should be considered when evaluating a patient with poor vision after ERM surgery.

Macular Epiretinal Membranes

Pournaras CJ, Donati G, Brazitikos PD, Kapetanios AD, Dereklis DL, Stangos NT. Department of Clinical Neurosciences, University Hospitals of Geneva, Geneva, Switzerland. *Seminars in Ophthalmology* 15(2):100-107, June 2000.

Epiretinal membranes (ERM) are a common finding in older patients. Although they may be associated with numerous clinical conditions, most epiretinal membranes occur in the absence of ocular pathology (disease). Patients' symptoms range from asymptotic to complaints of severe vision loss and metamorphopsia (distortion). Pars plana vitrectomy has been found to be effective in removing ERM from the macula, improving the visual acuity and decreasing metamorphopsia.

Both idiopathic and secondary ERMs do well after surgery, although secondary ERMs showed a greater amount of improvement than idiopathic ones. Complications are frequent including accelerated postoperative nuclear sclerosis (cataracts), retinal breaks and retinal detachment (RD), macular edema, retinal pigment epithelium (RPE) changes, and, occasionally, macular hole and hypotony (low eye pressure). However, only RD involving the macula has a worsening prognosis on final outcome.

Epiretinal Membranes

Jacobsen CH. School of Optometry, University of California-Berkeley. *Optometry Clinics* 5(1):77-94, 1996.

Epiretinal membranes are a common finding in older patients but are rare in young patients. Although they may be associated with other ocular conditions, most epiretinal membranes occur in the absence of ocular disease. Patient symptoms range from asymptomatic to complaints of severe vision loss and distortion. Epiretinal membranes are commonly classified according to their density and contractile characteristics. In this review, cellophane maculopathy refers to thin, glistening membrane, surface wrinkling maculopathy is characterized by fine, superficial retinal folds and macular pucker is associated with a dense, grayish-white membrane causing a characteristic pattern of severe retinal distortion. With sufficient visual disturbance, epiretinal membranes may be treated by pars plana posterior vitrectomy and epiretinal membrane peeling.

The National Eye Institute (NEI), part of the National Institutes of Health (NIH), is the Federal government's principal agency for conducting and supporting vision research. Inclusion of an item in this chapter does not imply the endorsement of the NEI or the NIH.

Chapter 52

Retinal Detachment

The information provided in this chapter was developed by the National Eye Institute (NEI) to help patients and their families in searching for general information about retinal detachment. An eye care professional who has examined the patient's eyes and is familiar with his or her medical history is the best person to answer specific questions.

What Is Retinal Detachment?

The retina is the light-sensitive layer of tissue that lines the inside of the eye and sends visual messages through the optic nerve to the brain. When the retina detaches, it is lifted or pulled from its normal position. If not promptly treated, retinal detachment can cause permanent vision loss.

In some cases there may be small areas of the retina that are torn. These areas, called retinal tears or retinal breaks, can lead to retinal detachment.

What Are the Symptoms of Retinal Detachment?

Symptoms include a sudden or gradual increase in the number of floaters and/or light flashes in the eye or the appearance of a curtain over the field of vision. A retinal detachment is a medical emergency.

"Retinal Detachment Resource Guide," National Eye Institute, available online at http://www.nei.nih.gov, August 2002.

Anyone experiencing the symptoms of a retinal detachment should see an eye care professional immediately.

What Are the Different Types of Retinal Detachment?

There are three different types of retinal detachment:

- Rhegmatogenous—A tear or break in the retina causes it to separate from the retinal pigment epithelium (RPE), the pigmented cell layer that nourishes the retina, and fill with fluid. These types of retinal detachments are the most common.

- Tractional—In this type of detachment, scar tissue on the retina's surface contracts and causes it to separate from the RPE. This type of detachment is less common.

- Exudative—Frequently caused by retinal diseases, including inflammatory disorders and injury/trauma to the eye. In this type, fluid leaks into the area underneath the retina (subretina).

Who Is at Risk for Retinal Detachment?

Although anyone can experience a retinal detachment, people with certain eye conditions are at increased risk. Some examples of these conditions include posterior vitreous detachment, lattice degeneration, x-linked retinoschisis, degenerative myopia, and uveitis. Injuries to the eye or head can also cause retinal detachment.

How Is Retinal Detachment Treated?

Small holes and tears are treated with laser surgery or a freeze treatment called cryopexy. These procedures are usually performed in the doctor's office. During laser surgery tiny burns are made around the hole to weld the retina back to into place. Cryopexy is a similar procedure that freezes the area around the hole.

Retinal detachments are treated with surgery that may require the patient to stay in the hospital. In some cases a scleral buckle, a tiny synthetic band, is attached to the outside of the eyeball to gently push the wall of the eye against the detached retina. If necessary, a vitrectomy may also be performed to treat more severe cases. During a vitrectomy, the doctor makes a tiny incision in the sclera (white of the eye). Next, a small instrument is placed into the eye to remove the vitreous. Salt solution is then injected to into the eye to replace the vitreous.

Early treatment can usually improve the vision of most patients with retinal detachment. Some patients, however, will need more than one procedure to repair the damage.

National Eye Institute-Supported Research

The NEI supported The Silicone Study, a nationwide clinical trial that compared the use of silicone oil and long-acting intraocular gas for repairing retinal detachment complicated by proliferative vitreoretinopathy (PVR). Results indicate that silicone is slightly more effective than gas in reattaching retinas with no previous vitrectomy (surgical removal of the vitreous gel).

Other Resources

The following organization may be able to provide additional information on retinal detachment:

American Academy of Ophthalmology
P.O. Box 7424
San Francisco, CA 94120-7424
Phone: (415) 561-8500
Website: http://www.aao.org

For additional information, you may also wish to contact a local library.

Medical Literature

Below is a sample of the citations available in MEDLINE, a comprehensive medical literature database coordinated by the National Library of Medicine (NLM). MEDLINE contains information on medical journal articles published from 1966 to the present. You can conduct your own free literature search by accessing MEDLINE through the Internet at http://medlineplus.nlm.nih.gov. You can also get assistance with a literature search at a local library.

To obtain copies of any of the articles listed below, contact a local community, university, or medical library. If the library you visit does not have a copy of a desired article, you may usually obtain it through an inter-library loan.

Please keep in mind that articles in the medical literature are usually written in technical language. We encourage you to share any articles you order with a health care professional who can help you understand them.

441

The Repair of Rhegmatogenous Retinal Detachments

American Academy of Ophthalmology. *Ophthalmology* 103(8):1313-24, August 1996.

Retinal detachments are the result of separation of the sensory retina from the retinal pigment epithelium (RPE), and they generally lead to severe visual loss if not successfully treated. There are four major types of retinal detachments: (1) rhegmatogenous, (2) traction, (3) exudative, and (4) combined mechanism. Rhegmatogenous retinal detachments occur in approximately 1 in 10,000 persons each year. In more than half of these eyes, the detachment occurs spontaneously, with no history of surgical or non-surgical trauma.

Various treatments are used to repair most detachments, including retinal reattachment using cryopexy, diathermy, or laser in conjunction with indentation of the sclera with a scleral buckle, or retinal reattachment surgery using pars plana vitrectomy or pneumatic retinopexy with or without a scleral buckle.

Vitrectomy for the Management of Recurrent Retinal Detachments

Holekamp NM, Grand MG. *Current Opinion in Ophthalmology* 8(3):44-9, June 1997.

Repair of rhegmatogenous retinal detachment is successful in approximately 90 percent of cases. Assuming all retinal breaks are identified and closed, the most common reason for eventual failure of surgery is the development of proliferative vitreoretinopathy, accounting for the failure of 7 percent to 10 percent of primary repairs and an increased proportion of secondary procedures. Recurrent retinal detachment complicated by proliferative vitreoretinopathy is now most frequently treated by pars plana vitrectomy with intraoperative peeling of membranes. This article reviews the latest developments in vitreous surgery to repair recurrent retinal detachments due to proliferative vitreoretinopathy, focusing on the most recent reports in the literature.

The National Eye Institute, part of the National Institutes of Health, is the Federal government's principal agency for conducting and supporting vision research. Inclusion of an item in this chapter does not imply the endorsement by the National Eye Institute or the National Institutes of Health.

Chapter 53

Spots and Floaters

What Are Floaters?

The small spots you may see occasionally in your field of vision are called muscae volitantes, commonly known as floaters. A clear, gel-like fluid, called the vitreous body, fills the inside cavity of the eye. If some of this gel clumps, floaters can result. Floaters can also occur from small flecks of protein or other material that were trapped in the vitreous during the eye's formation.

What Causes Floaters?

Over time, the vitreous gel shrinks and detaches from the retina; the pulling can cause small amounts of bleeding. This is a common cause of floaters in people who are nearsighted or who have had a cataract operation. Less frequently, floaters may result from eye disease, eye injury, or crystal-like deposits that form in the vitreous.

Can Anything Be Done about Floaters?

Most people sometimes see spots, although they can become more noticeable with age. While floaters are generally not treated, there

"Frequently Asked Questions about Floaters," reprinted with permission from Prevent Blindness America. © 2000. For additional information, call the Prevent Blindness America toll-free information line at (800) 331-2020, or visit www.preventblindness.org.

are ways of coping with them. If a floater appears in your line of vision, move your eye around. This causes the fluid inside the eye to shift and allows the floaters to move out of the way. Since we usually move our eyes from side to side, looking up and down may be more effective in removing floaters from your line of sight.

A few floaters generally do not indicate serious eye problems. However, if a large number suddenly appear, or they seem to worsen over time, it's wise to get an eye examination. If the floaters appear simultaneously with flashes of light or a curtain or veil over some of the vision, they might be a sign of serious conditions such as retinal weakness or tears, hemorrhaging due to diabetes, or high blood pressure. Retinal tears and hemorrhaging demand immediate medical attention.

To learn more about floaters, please contact Prevent Blindness America or the Prevent Blindness affiliate near you.

Part Seven

Current Research and Clinical Trials

Chapter 54

Facts about Clinical Trials in Vision Research

If you or someone you know is thinking about taking part in a clinical trial, this chapter can answer some of your questions. The National Eye Institute (NEI) conducts or sponsors clinical trials to find new ways to treat or prevent eye disease and vision loss. Clinical trials in vision research have led to new medicines and surgeries that have saved or improved sight for thousands of people.

What Is a Clinical Trial?

Clinical trials involve medical research with people. Most medical research begins with studies in test tubes and in animals. Treatments that show promise in these early studies may then be tried with people. The only sure way to find out whether a new treatment is safe, effective, and better than other treatments is to try it on patients in a clinical trial.

What Kinds of Clinical Trials Are There?

Clinical trials are carried out in three parts, or phases.

- Phase I. Researchers first conduct Phase I trials in small numbers of patients and healthy volunteers. If the new treatment is a medicine, researchers also want to find out how much of it can be given safely.

National Eye Institute, National Institutes of Health, NIH Publication No. 99-4124, available online at http://www.nei.nih.gov, April 2000.

- Phase II. Researchers conduct Phase II trials in small numbers of patients to find out the effect of a new treatment on an eye disease or disorder.

- Phase III. Finally, researchers conduct Phase III trials to find out whether the new treatments work better, the same, or not as well as the standard treatments already being used. Phase III trials also help to determine if new treatments have any side effects. These trials—which may involve hundreds, perhaps thousands, of people around the country—can also compare new treatments with no treatment.

Where Do Clinical Trials Take Place?

The NEI supports clinical trials at about 250 medical centers, hospitals, universities, and doctors' offices across the country. NEI researchers conduct other clinical trials at the National Institutes of Health in Bethesda, Maryland.

How Is a Clinical Trial Conducted?

At each facility taking part in the clinical trial, the principal investigator is the researcher in charge of the study. Most of the people who conduct clinical trials in eye disease are ophthalmologists or optometrists. The clinic coordinator knows all about how the study works and makes all the arrangements for your visits.

All doctors who take part in the study carefully follow a detailed treatment plan called a protocol. This plan fully explains how the doctors will treat you in the study. The protocol ensures that all patients are treated in the same way, no matter where they receive care.

- Clinical trials are controlled. This means that researchers compare the effects of the new treatment with those of the standard treatment. In some cases, when no standard treatment exists, the new treatment is compared with no treatment.

- Patients who get the new treatment are in the treatment group.

- Patients who get the standard treatment or no treatment are in the control group.

- In some clinical trials, patients in the treatment group get a new medicine and patients in the control group get a placebo. A placebo is a harmless substance—a dummy pill—that looks like the real treatment but has no effect on the eye disease or disorder. In other clinical trials, where a new surgery or device (not a medicine) is being tested, patients in the control group may receive a sham treatment. This treatment, like a placebo, has no effect on the eye disease or disorder and does not harm patients.

- Researchers assign patients randomly to the treatment or control group. This is like flipping a coin to decide which patients are in each group. Patients do not know ahead of time which group that is. The chance of any patient getting the new treatment is about 50 percent. Patients cannot request to receive the new treatment instead of the placebo or sham treatment. In some clinical trials, where the disease or disorder affects both eyes, one eye may be in the treatment group, and the other eye may be in the control group.

- Patients often do not know until the study is over whether they are in the treatment group or the control group. This is called a masked study. In some trials, neither doctors nor patients know who is getting what treatment. This is called a double masked study. These types of trials help to ensure that what patients or doctors might think about the treatment will not affect the study results.

What Is Expected of Patients in a Clinical Trial?

Patients in a clinical trial are expected to have eye exams and other tests. You may also need to take medications and/or undergo surgery. Depending upon the treatment and the examination procedure, you may need a hospital stay.

You may have to go back to the medical facility later for follow-up examinations. These exams help find out how well the treatment is working. Follow-up studies can take months or years. However, the success of the clinical trial often depends on learning what happens to patients over a long period of time. Only patients who continue to return for follow-up examinations can provide this important long-term information.

What Are the Benefits of Participating in a Clinical Trial?

Participating in a clinical trial can bring many benefits:

- There is the hope that a new treatment will be more effective than the current treatment for an eye disease or disorder. Only about half of the people in a clinical trial get the new treatment. If the new treatment is effective and safer than the current treatment, those patients who do not receive the new treatment during the clinical trial may be among the first to benefit from the new treatment when the study is over.

- If the treatment is effective, it may help to improve vision and control or prevent eye disease or disorder.

- Clinical trial patients receive the highest quality medical care. Experts watch them closely during the study and may continue to follow them after the study is over.

- People who take part in these trials contribute to new knowledge that may help other people with the same eye problems. In cases where certain eye diseases or disorders run in families, your participation may lead to better care for family members.

Once you agree to take part in a clinical trial, you will be asked to sign an informed consent. This document explains a clinical trial's risks and benefits, what researchers expect of you, and your rights as a patient.

What Are the Risks?

Clinical trials may involve risks as well as possible benefits.

- Whether or not a new treatment will work cannot be known ahead of time. There is always a chance that a new treatment may not work better than a standard treatment, may not work at all, or may be harmful.

- The treatment you receive may cause side effects that are serious enough to require medical attention.

How Is Patient Safety Protected?

Clinical trials can raise fears of the unknown. Understanding the safeguards that protect patients can ease some of these fears.

- Before a clinical trial begins, researchers must get approval from their hospital's Institutional Review Board (IRB), an advisory group that makes sure a clinical trial is designed to protect patient safety.

- During a clinical trial, doctors will closely watch you to see if the treatment is working and if you are having any side effects. All the results are carefully recorded and reviewed.

- A group of experts—the Data and Safety Monitoring Committee— carefully watches each clinical trial supported by the NEI. This group can recommend that a study be stopped at any time.

- Patients are asked to take part in a clinical trial only if they volunteer and understand the risks and benefits.

What Are a Patient's Rights in a Clinical Trial?

Patients who are eligible for a clinical trial will be given information to help them decide whether to take part. As a patient, you have the right to:

- Be told about all known risks and benefits of treatments involved in the study.

- Know how the researchers plan to carry out the study, for how long, and where.

- Know what is expected of you.

- Know any costs involved for you or your insurers.

- Be informed about any medical or personal information that may be shared with other researchers directly involved in the clinical trial.

- Talk openly with doctors and ask any questions.

After you join a clinical trial, you have the right to:

- Leave the study at any time. Participation is strictly voluntary. However, you should not enroll if you do not plan to complete the study.

- Receive any new information about the new treatment.

- Continue to ask questions and get answers.

- Maintain your privacy. Your name will not appear in any reports based on the study.

- Be informed of your treatment assignment once the study is completed.

What about Costs?

In some clinical trials, the medical facility conducting the research pays for treatment costs and some other expenses. You or your health insurance may have to pay for some things that are considered part of standard care. These things may include hospital stays, laboratory and other tests, and medical procedures. You also may need to pay for travel between your home and the clinic. For clinical trials conducted at the NEI's medical facility in Bethesda, Maryland, medical care is provided at no cost to patients. You should find out about costs ahead of time. If you have health insurance, find out exactly what it will cover. If you don't have health insurance, or if your insurance company will not cover your costs, talk to the clinic staff about other options for covering the cost of your care.

What Questions Should You Ask before Deciding to Join a Clinical Trial?

Questions you should ask when thinking about joining a clinical trial include the following:

- What is the purpose of the clinical trial?

- What are the standard treatments for my disease or condition? Why do researchers think the new treatment may be better? What is likely to happen to me with or without the new treatment?

- What tests and treatments will I need? Will I need surgery? Medicines? Hospitalization?

- How long will the treatment last? How often will I have to come back for follow-up exams?

- What are the treatment's possible benefits to my condition? What are the short- and long-term risks? What are the possible side effects?

- Will the treatment be uncomfortable? Will it make me feel sick? If so, for how long?

- How will my health be monitored?

- Where will I need to go for the clinical trial? How will I get there?

- How much will it cost me to be in the study? What costs are covered by the study? How much will my health insurance cover?

- Will I be able to see my own doctor? Who will be in charge of my care?

- Will taking part in the study affect my daily life? Will I have the time to be in it?

- How do I feel about taking part in a clinical trial? Are there family members or friends who may benefit from my contributions to new medical knowledge?

What Clinical Trials Are Being Held? Who Can Take Part in Them?

The NEI conducts or sponsors research on many eye diseases and disorders. Because funding for eye research goes to the medical areas that show promising research opportunities, it is not possible for the NEI to sponsor clinical trials in every eye disease and disorder at all times.

Not everyone can take part in a clinical trial for a specific eye disease or disorder. Each study enrolls patients with certain features, or eligibility criteria. These criteria may include the type and stage of disease or disorder, as well as the age and previous treatment history of the patient.

You or your doctor can contact the NEI to find out more about specific clinical trials and their eligibility criteria. If you are interested in joining a clinical trial, your doctor must contact one of the trial's investigators and provide details about your diagnosis and medical history.

The NEI's website lists the clinical trials the NEI is helping to support. Each trial description includes information on its background and purpose, as well as patient eligibility. There is information on how to participate in a trial and how to refer a patient to a trial.

Chapter 55

Oxygen Restrictions Can Be Eased for Premature Infants with Blinding Eye Disease

Modest supplemental oxygen given to premature infants with moderate cases of retinopathy of prematurity (ROP), a potentially blinding eye disorder, may not significantly improve ROP, but definitely does not make it worse, according to researchers funded by the Federal government's National Institutes of Health (NIH). The results mean that clinicians do not have to be as restrictive as they have been when giving supplemental oxygen to infants who have already developed moderate ROP. These findings appear in a scientific paper published in the February [2002] issue of *Pediatrics*.

"Up to now, there have been tight restrictions on the amount of oxygen low birthweight infants were permitted to have," said Carl Kupfer, M.D., director of the National Eye Institute (NEI), which funded the study in collaboration with the National Institute of Child Health and Human Development (NICHD) and the National Institute of Nursing Research (NINR). "This is because doctors have been concerned about a possible adverse effect of supplemental oxygen on the eyes of infants with ROP. While the benefits and risks of supplemental oxygen must be individually considered for each infant, doctors need no longer worry that supplemental oxygen, as used in this study, will harm eyes with moderate ROP."

Many premature infants need supplemental oxygen soon after birth because their lungs are not sufficiently mature to efficiently

"Oxygen Restrictions Can Be Eased for Premature Infants with Blinding Eye Disease," National Institutes of Health, National Eye Institute, http://www.nei.nih.gov, February 7, 2000.

455

transfer oxygen into their bodies. Doctors have long known that supplemental oxygen, while helping infants survive, might increase cases of ROP. They have also been concerned that it might allow the disease to progress from a moderate stage, when surgery is not needed, to a severe stage, which usually requires surgery and sometimes permanently damages sight. However, recent research had suggested that controlled amounts of supplemental oxygen might actually keep ROP from progressing from moderate to severe. If controlled amounts of supplemental oxygen could help prevent the progression of ROP, then infants could avoid this threat to their sight and consequently the invasive surgery for severe ROP, with its possible long-term side effects.

Retinopathy of prematurity develops when abnormal blood vessels grow and spread throughout the retina, the nerve tissue that lines the back of the eye. The scarring and bleeding caused by the excess growth of these blood vessels can lead to retinal detachment, resulting in vision loss. ROP develops in about 14,000 to 16,000 infants each year who weigh less than 2 3/4 pounds (1250 grams) at birth. In most cases (80 percent), the disease improves and leaves no permanent damage. However, about 1,100 to 1,500 infants annually develop ROP that is severe enough to require surgical treatment.

The most effective proven treatments for severe ROP are cryotherapy and laser therapy, which usually will stop the growth of abnormal blood vessels and prevent retinal detachment. The effectiveness of cryotherapy—a freezing treatment—was demonstrated several years ago through another NEI-sponsored clinical trial. However, even with these therapies, about 400 to 600 infants with ROP become legally blind each year. Cryotherapy and laser therapy are considered invasive surgeries on the eye, and doctors don't know their long-term side effects.

"Of the infants in the study with moderate ROP who received the supplemental oxygen, 41 percent progressed to severe ROP," said study chair Dale Phelps, M.D., professor of Pediatrics and Ophthalmology at Children's Hospital at Strong at the University of Rochester School of Medicine and Dentistry. "Of the infants with moderate ROP who did not receive the supplemental oxygen, 48 percent progressed to severe ROP. Statistically, there is no difference.

"However, we found something we did not expect," Dr. Phelps said. "The infants in the study fell into two groups—those whose moderate ROP was complicated with dilated eye blood vessels, and those whose blood vessels were not dilated. Modest supplemental oxygen significantly reduced the need for surgery in the second group. This finding needs to be confirmed with additional research before we can recommend modest supplemental oxygen as a treatment for infants with moderate ROP without dilated blood vessels."

Dr. Phelps said there were side effects in some infants who received the supplemental oxygen, including a temporary worsening of their chronic lung disease. "In addition, we examined the infants three months after their due dates, when they were no longer on the treatment," Dr. Phelps said. "We found, at the three-month exam, that the children who received the supplemental oxygen were more likely than those who did not receive the extra oxygen to be either in the hospital, on oxygen, and/or on medications for chronic lung disease. However, these side effects themselves are not life-threatening, and are acceptable risks for infants who require extra oxygen for cardiopulmonary reasons."

The clinical trial, called the Supplemental Therapeutic Oxygen for Prethreshold ROP (STOP-ROP) study, initially enrolled 649 infants; 597 completed the study. The clinical trial was conducted at 30 study centers involving 71 hospitals across the United States.

The NEI, NICHD, and NINR are part of the National Institutes of Health, an agency of the U.S. Department of Health and Human Services.

Chapter 56

A Leading Cause of Blindness May Be Controlled by a Simple Course of Oral Antibiotic

A study published in the August 21 [1999] issue of *Lancet* provides evidence that treating entire communities with a short course of the oral antibiotic azithromycin is more effective than the standard six-week course of daily tetracycline ointment in controlling development of trachoma. Children are particularly vulnerable to infection by the bacterium *Chlamydia trachomatis*, which results in trachoma, a leading cause of preventable blindness in the world.

"We have known for decades that we had the antibiotics to successfully treat this disease when cases developed, but we didn't seem to have the right drug delivery method to control the infection over time. Now we know that we do, and we are very excited at the promise of these results," says Julius Schachter, Ph.D., professor of laboratory medicine at the University of California at San Francisco (UCSF) and lead investigator of the study.

Trachoma affects the inner eyelid. Of the nearly 600 million people living in trachoma endemic areas, 150 million have active disease as conjunctivitis. After repeated episodes, which begin in childhood, scarring occurs, and the eyelids turn inward causing damage to the cornea. Total blindness occurs in middle to late life. In endemic communities, 25 percent of individuals age 50 to 60 may become blind. Blind adults may not be able to earn a living and can be an economic burden to families and communities.

National Institutes of Health, National Institute of Allergy and Infectious Diseases, http://www.nih.gov/news/pr/aug99/niaid-19a.htm, August 1999.

459

"Six million people around the world are blind or severely disabled due to this disease," says Anthony S. Fauci, M.D., director of the National Institute of Allergy and Infectious Diseases (NIAID). "Treatment of trachoma with azithromycin provides long-term benefits not usually available for people in developing countries." Thomas C. Quinn, M.D., of National Institute of Allergy and Infectious Diseases (NIAID) and Johns Hopkins University, is a co-author of the study. NIAID, the Edna McConnell Clark Foundation, Abbott Laboratories, and Pfizer Inc. supported the study.

Since the 1950s, the standard treatment for trachoma has been daily application of tetracycline ointment in the inflamed eye for six weeks. In the UCSF study, researchers compared the effect of the two antibiotic regimens on infection rates in villages located in trachoma endemic areas where transmission of infection is high. The villages were in the African countries of Egypt, The Gambia, and Tanzania. Village-by-village comparison of treatments showed that three doses of oral azithromycin at one-week intervals reduced levels of chlamydial infection significantly more than the standard tetracycline regimen delivered by health providers. Furthermore, village-wide treatment with azithromycin resulted in a 60 to 90 percent decrease in infection rates a year later.

The authors conclude that the effective reduction of chlamydial infection, coupled with the ease of administration, make azithromycin an important component of trachoma control programs. Although azithromycin costs more than tetracycline ointment, the expense may be offset by the higher costs of distributing and administering multiple doses of the ointment.

Treatment with antibiotics is one of several steps in a comprehensive trachoma control strategy called SAFE: Surgery for advanced disease; Antibiotics to treat and prevent infections; Face washing and good personal hygiene; and Environmental improvements, such as better access to clean water and sanitation and health education. The strategies of SAFE, including treatment with azithromycin, may provide substantial benefit to people in endemic areas by reducing both individual infections and persistence of infection in low-prevalence areas.

"Last November [1998], as a result of these research findings, Pfizer and the Edna McConnell Clark Foundation pledged $66 million to eliminate blinding trachoma. A key component is Pfizer's donation of Zithromax®, their trade name for azithromycin, which the World Health Organization (WHO) now recommends for the treatment of trachoma," says Penny Hitchcock, D.V.M., chief of the sexually transmitted diseases branch of the NIAID. Pfizer and the Edna McConnell

Clark Foundation founded the International Trachoma Initiative, an independent agency using azithromycin in the SAFE strategy to control trachoma in Tanzania, Morocco, Mali, Ghana, and Vietnam.

C. trachomatis infects not only the eyes, but the nose, throat, genital tract, and rectum as well. The eye infection is transmitted easily from person to person by hand-to-eye contact, possibly aided by flies attracted to the sticky discharge from the eyes. In earlier studies in Tanzania and The Gambia, many children who had been treated with topical tetracycline showed evidence of recurring infection within weeks of treatment. The ointment treats only eye infections and is very short-acting. Oral antibiotics that work throughout the body are more effective for treating trachoma than antibiotic ointment. Although short-acting oral antibiotics also can be used to treat the infection, the need for repeated doses makes them less effective compared with fewer doses of a longer-acting oral antibiotic.

According to the *Lancet* report, short-course azithromycin proved to be an efficient and effective way to treat many people. "In our study, the advantage of oral azithromycin will be even greater because of the good compliance that can be achieved," says Dr. Schachter. "In these studies, health care workers made extraordinary efforts to administer topical tetracycline. In most treatment programs for endemic trachoma, eye ointment is provided to families for treatment, so topical drug delivery is probably lower than in this study."

As the study designers expected, at all sites the prevalence of trachoma was highest in children—greater than 30 percent in children younger than 10 years old. Traditionally, children have been targeted for intervention, but an appreciable number of older individuals also tested positive for the bacterium.

"A goal for this study was to assess control of trachoma through treatment of entire communities," Dr. Schachter explains. "This study not only shows that a short course of oral antibiotic achieves greater patient compliance than the longer term traditional treatment, but that control of this disease can be achieved through treatment of all individuals within a community. The results indicate that with azithromycin, trachoma control is an attainable goal."

NIAID is a component of the National Institutes of Health (NIH). NIAID conducts and supports research to prevent, diagnose, and treat illnesses such as HIV disease and other sexually transmitted diseases, tuberculosis, malaria, asthma, and allergies. NIH is an agency of the U.S. Department of Health and Human Services. Press releases, fact sheets, and other NIAID-related materials are available on the NIAID website at http://www.niaid.nih.gov.

Reference

J. Schachter, et al. Azithromycin in control of trachoma. *Lancet* 1999; 354:630-663.

Chapter 57

Antiviral Drug Sharply Reduces Return of Herpes of the Eye

Researchers have found that an antiviral drug, often used to suppress genital herpes, also decreases the recurrence of herpes of the eye. A paper detailing these findings is published in the July 30, 1998 issue of *The New England Journal of Medicine*.

Scientists found that the drug acyclovir, taken by mouth, reduced by 41 percent the probability that any form of herpes of the eye would return in patients who had the infection in the previous year. Importantly, researchers noted a 50 percent reduction in the rate of return of the more severe form of the disease—stromal keratitis—among patients who had this infection during the past year. Stromal keratitis causes scarring of the cornea, which can lead to loss of vision and possibly blindness. Recurring episodes of stromal keratitis can often result in the need for a corneal transplant.

"This drug is the first treatment that helps prevent herpes of the eye from returning," said Dr. Carl Kupfer, director of the National Eye Institute (NEI), part of the Federal government's National Institutes of Health (NIH) and the agency that supported the clinical trial. "The results of this study should change medical practice."

Herpes of the eye, or ocular herpes, is caused by the herpes simplex virus. This infection can produce a painful sore on the eyelid or surface of the eye and cause inflammation of the cornea, the transparent tissue that covers the front of the eye. The less severe forms of ocular herpes include blepharitis, conjunctivitis, and epithelial

"Antiviral Drug Sharply Reduces Return of Herpes of the Eye," National Institutes of Health, http://www.nih.gov, July 29, 1998.

keratitis. The more severe form of ocular herpes is stromal keratitis, which causes the body's immune system to attack and destroy an inner layer of the cornea. Stromal keratitis is more difficult to treat than less severe ocular herpes infections.

An estimated 400,000 Americans have had some form of ocular herpes. Previous studies show that once people develop ocular herpes, they have up to a 50 percent chance of having a recurrence. This second flare-up could come weeks or even years after the initial occurrence. Each year, nearly 50,000 new and recurring cases are diagnosed in the United States, with the more serious stromal keratitis accounting for about 25 percent.

The clinical trial—called the Acyclovir Prevention Trial (APT)—followed 703 patients who had herpes of the eye during the preceding year, but did not currently have an active case of the disease. Of this number, 357 received acyclovir by mouth, and 346 received a placebo. Researchers discovered that the probability of a recurrence of any form of ocular herpes during the treatment period was significantly lower in the acyclovir group (19 percent) than in the placebo group (32 percent). This represents a reduction by 41 percent between the two groups.

Among the 703 patients, researchers examined 337 patients with a prior history of the more serious stromal keratitis. Acyclovir reduced the rate of recurrences of stromal keratitis from 28 percent to 14 percent, a difference of 50 percent between the two groups. The study medication caused no serious side effects.

"The study clearly shows that acyclovir therapy can benefit people with all forms of ocular herpes," said Dr. Kirk Wilhelmus, professor in the Department of Ophthalmology at the Baylor College of Medicine and chairman of the APT clinical trial. "Ocular herpes can be painful, chronic, and disabling. This new treatment will improve people's quality of life. Those who have had the more serious stromal keratitis will benefit the most."

Dr. Wilhelmus noted that not all patients had the same benefit from taking acyclovir. "Patients should consult with their eye care professionals to see if prolonged use of acyclovir is right for them," he said.

Researchers also found that oral acyclovir reduced the risk of herpes infections in other parts of the body, particularly the mouth and face, by 43 percent. During the 12-month treatment period, 20 percent of patients in the group receiving acyclovir had at least one herpes infection affecting the mouth or face, as compared with 35 percent of patients in the placebo group.

Once treatment stopped, the rate of ocular herpes or herpes affecting the mouth and face did not increase, according to Dr. Wilhelmus.

"During the six months after treatment ended, the percentages of herpes recurrences affecting the eye or the mouth and face was the same in both the treatment and placebo groups," he said.

The Acyclovir Prevention Trial is part of a larger study—called the Herpetic Eye Disease Study—that is supported through cooperative agreements with the NEI. The APT was conducted at 74 university and community-based clinical sites nationwide, reporting to eight regional centers.

Background

The Acyclovir Prevention Trial: Ocular Herpes

Like other herpetic infections, herpes of the eye remains a controllable, but incurable, problem. In one large, unrelated study, researchers found that recurrence rate of ocular herpes was 10 percent within one year, 23 percent within two years, and 63 percent within 20 years. Some factors believed to be associated with recurrence include fever, stress, sunlight, and eye injury.

The less severe forms of ocular herpes include epithelial keratitis, conjunctivitis, and blepharitis. The more severe form of ocular herpes—stromal keratitis—can lead to corneal scarring and can be associated with secondary glaucoma and cataract. Standard treatment with antiviral eye drops or ointment helps to stop the herpes virus from multiplying. However, until the APT, there was still no known effective method for reducing the frequency of ocular herpes recurrence.

The APT Protocol

The Acyclovir Prevention Trial (APT) is a multicenter randomized clinical trial designed to determine if the antiviral drug acyclovir, given orally, would prevent herpes simplex virus infection from recurring in the eyes of patients who had the infection in the past.

To be eligible for participation, patients must have experienced a form of ocular herpes in one or both eyes during the preceding year. This infection had to be inactive and untreated for at least the previous 30 days before enrollment. About 29 percent of the enrolled patients had experienced one previous episode of ocular herpes; 71 percent experienced multiple previous recurrences. The most common types of prior ocular herpes were epithelial keratitis (47 percent), stromal keratitis (16 percent), and both epithelial keratitis and stromal

465

keratitis (32 percent). About 49 percent of patients had a history of fever blisters or other previous symptoms of herpes of the mouth and/or face.

Of the 703 patients, 357 were randomly assigned to the acyclovir group, and 346 to the placebo group. All patients were followed for all forms of ocular and nonocular recurrences during a 12-month treatment period, followed by a six-month observation period. The acyclovir group received oral acyclovir 400 mg twice daily for 12 months. The other group received placebo capsules that were identical in appearance and taste to the acyclovir capsules. Study medication (acyclovir or placebo) was continued for the full 12 months regardless of whether a recurrence occurred.

Herpes recurrences were classified as either superficial ocular infections (blepharitis, conjunctivitis, and/or epithelial keratitis); stromal keratitis; or iritis. When patients had a recurrence of ocular herpes, they were treated with standard topical medication, but continued to receive the oral acyclovir or placebo for the entire 365-day period.

Only four percent of patients in the acyclovir group and five percent in the placebo group stopped treatment because of side effects. One-half of these side effects were due to gastrointestinal upset; some patients may have had intolerance to the lactose contained in the study capsules (Treatment medication that does not contain lactose is now available). Glaxo Wellcome supplied to APT investigators over a half million free capsules of its brand name acyclovir, called Zovirax®.

Secondary Findings

In addition to the main findings, doctors also noted that:

- During the 12 months of treatment, oral acyclovir reduced the incidence of epithelial keratitis from 11 percent to nine percent, and the incidence of stromal keratitis from 13 percent to eight percent.

- During the 12-month treatment period, four percent of patients in the acyclovir group and nine percent in the placebo group had more than one recurrence.

Chapter 58

Studies of Ocular Complications of AIDS (SOCA): The HPMPC Peripheral CMV Retinitis Trial (HPCRT)

Purpose

To test and evaluate the efficacy and safety of intravenous cidofovir (Vistide®, previously known as HPMPC) for the treatment of retinitis.

Background

CMV retinitis is the most common intraocular infection in patients with AIDS and is estimated to affect 35 percent to 40 percent of patients with AIDS. Untreated CMV retinitis is a progressive disorder, the end result of which is total retinal destruction and blindness. As of September 1997, drugs approved by the U.S. Food and Drug Administration (FDA) for the treatment of CMV retinitis were ganciclovir (Cytovene®), foscarnet (Foscavir®), and cidofovir (Vistide®). Cidofovir has a prolonged duration of effect permitting intermittent administration. All systemically administered anti-CMV drugs are given in a similar fashion consisting of initial 2-week high-dose treatment (induction) to control the infection followed by long-term lower dose treatment (maintenance) to prevent relapse. Cidofovir is administered as an intravenous infusion once weekly for induction therapy and once

"Clinical Studies—Studies of the Ocular Complications of AIDS (SOCA)—HPMPC Peripheral CMV Retinitis Trial (HPCRT)," National Eye Institute, available online at http://www.nei.nih.gov, October 1999.

every two weeks as maintenance therapy. The HPCRT evaluated the efficacy and safety of cidofovir therapy.

Description

The HPCRT was a multicenter, randomized, controlled clinical trial of cidofovir for the treatment of CMV retinitis. Patients with small peripheral CMV retinitis lesions (i.e., not at risk of immediate loss of visual acuity) were randomized to immediate treatment with cidofovir or deferred therapy until the retinitis had progressed 750 μm. Patients randomized to immediate therapy received either 1) low-dose cidofovir at 5 mg/kg once weekly induction for 2 weeks, followed by 3 mg/kg once every 2 weeks for maintenance or 2) high-dose cidofovir at 5 mg/kg once weekly induction for 2 weeks followed by 5 mg/kg once every 2 weeks for maintenance. Patients whose retinitis progressed were given treatment according to best medical judgment, and those assigned to deferral were generally treated with cidofovir.

Outcomes in this trial included retinitis progression, loss of retinal area, and morbidity.

Patient Eligibility

Patients were age 13 years or older with diagnoses of AIDS, according to current Centers for Disease Control and Prevention (CDC) definition, and small peripheral CMV retinitis. Retinitis lesion(s) must have been confined to less than 25 percent of the total area of the retina and confined to the periphery of the retina. Peripheral lesions were those located at least 1,500 μm from the margin of the optic disc and 3,000 mm from the center of the fovea (entirely in zone 2 or 3). Patients must have had at least one lesion 750 μm or greater in size that could be photographed and the ability to read three or more lines on ETDRS chart at 1 meter (Snellen equivalent of 8/200 or greater) in at least one eye diagnosed with CMV retinitis.

Results

The HPCRT demonstrated that cidofovir (HPMPC) was effective for controlling CMV retinitis. When compared with deferral of therapy, both low-dose and high-dose cidofovir significantly prolonged the time to progression and reduced the rate of loss of retinal area. The most common side effect of cidofovir was nephrotoxicity [impairment of kidney function], which generally was reversible with discontinuing cidofovir therapy.

Publications

The Studies of Ocular Complications of AIDS Research Group in collaboration with the AIDS Clinical Trials Group: Cidofovir (HPMPC) for the treatment of cytomegalovirus retinitis in patients with AIDS: The HPMPC Peripheral Cytomegalovirus Retinitis Trial. *Ann Intern Med* 126: 264-274, 1997.

Chapter 59

Lutein and Eye Disease Prevention

Claims made about an association between lutein and eye health are speculative and should be viewed with caution. The possible benefits of lutein for the eye remain uncertain.

Certain foods contain antioxidants—molecules that can help maintain healthy cells and tissues in the eye. One category of these antioxidants, called carotenoids, may play a role in maintaining eye health as well as overall health. One of these carotenoids—lutein—is concentrated in the retina and lens of the eye.

There is little definitive scientific evidence at this time to support claims that taking supplements containing lutein can decrease the risk of developing advanced age-related macular degeneration (AMD), a blinding eye disease, or cataract. However, a number of studies intended to examine trends in a population—and not hard medical evidence— suggest a link between lutein and decreased risk of eye disease:

- In 1994, a National Eye Institute (NEI)-supported study indicated that consumption of foods rich in carotenoids—particularly green, leafy vegetables such as collard greens, kale, and spinach—was associated with a reduced risk of developing AMD.[1]

- In 1999, data from the Nurses Health Study showed a reduced likelihood of cataract surgery with increasing intakes of lutein and another carotenoid—zeaxanthin.[2]

"Lutein and Its Role in Eye Disease Prevention," National Institutes of Health, National Eye Institute, http://www.nei.nih.gov, July 2002.

- In 1999, the Health Professionals Follow-up Study found a trend toward a lower risk of cataract extraction with higher intakes of lutein and zeaxanthin.[3]

- In 1999, a follow-up to an NEI-supported population-based study—called the Beaver Dam Study—concluded that people with diets higher in lutein and zeaxanthin had a lower risk of developing cataract.[4]

- In 2001, data from the Third National Health and Nutrition Examination Survey reported that higher intakes of lutein and zeaxanthin among people ages 40-59 may be associated with a reduced risk of advanced AMD.[5]

Conversely, in 1998, the Beaver Dam Study found no significant association between the risk of either early or advanced AMD in groups that had either the highest intakes of lutein and zeaxanthin or the lowest intakes of lutein and zeaxanthin. The study researchers caution that generally, the consumption of lutein and zeaxanthin in this population may have been too low to have had an impact on the risk of AMD.[6-7]

These conflicting data make it clear that the relationship between lutein and eye health needs to be examined more closely before conclusions can be drawn.

What's Next for Lutein?

The NEI is investigating the role of nutrition—including the effects of lutein—in eye disease.

Specifically, the NEI is:

- Conducting a pilot study to see how well lutein is absorbed into the bloodstream in people over age 60. This is a first step in testing this substance as a possible treatment for AMD. The pilot study is not designed to treat AMD; its purpose is to help determine the best dose of lutein oral supplements in people over age 60. This dose of lutein can then be separately tested in humans as a possible treatment for AMD.

- Supporting a study that compares the intake of lutein and zeaxanthin with the likelihood of developing AMD and/or cataract. Researchers explain that results from this study—called the Carotenoids and Age-Related Eye Disease in Women's Health

Study—will help health professionals make dietary recommendations regarding the benefit of eating diets rich in lutein and zeaxanthin. Study results will also provide information needed to conduct clinical trials that can evaluate the effectiveness of lutein and zeaxanthin supplements on the progression of age-related eye disease.

The Role of Nutrition in Eye Disease Prevention

In October 2001, the NEI published the results of a seven-year study—called the Age-Related Eye Disease Study (AREDS)—that showed that a high-dose combination of vitamin C, vitamin E, beta-carotene, and zinc significantly reduces the risk of developing advanced stages of AMD by about 25 percent. These high levels of antioxidants and zinc are the first effective treatment to slow the progression of AMD. The nutrients are not a cure for AMD, nor will they restore vision already lost from the disease. But they are playing a vital role in helping people at high risk for developing advanced AMD keep their vision. In the same study, the antioxidant and zinc combination showed no significant effect on the development or progression of cataract.

Lutein was not part of this study because during the AREDS planning stages in the early 1990s, lutein and zeaxanthin were not commercially available.

References

1. Seddon, Johanna M., MD, et al, "Dietary Carotenoids, Vitamins A, C, and E, and Advanced Age-Related Macular Degeneration," *JAMA*, Vol. 272, No. 18, November 1994, pgs. 1413-1420.

2. Chasen-Taber et al., "A Prospective Study of Carotenoid and Vitamin A Intakes and Risk of Cataract Extraction in US Women," *American Journal of Clinical Nutrition*, 1999, Vol. 70, pgs. 509-516.

3. Brown et al., "A Prospective Study of Carotenoid Intake and Risk of Cataract Extraction in US Men," *American Journal of Clinical Nutrition*, 1999, Vol. 70, pgs. 517-524.

4. Lyle et al., "Serum Carotenoids and Tocopherols and Incidence of Age-Related Nuclear Cataract," *American Journal of Clinical Nutrition*, 1999, Vol. 69, pgs. 272-277.

5. Mares-Perlman et al., "Lutein and Zeaxanthin in the Diet and Serum and Their Relation to Age-Related Maculopathy in the Third National Health and Nutrition Examination Survey," *American Journal of Epidemiology*, 2001, Vol. 153, No. 5, pgs. 424-432.

6. Mares-Perlman et al., "Association of Zinc and Antioxidant Nutrients With Age-Related Maculopathy," *Archives of Ophthalmology*, 1996, Vol. 114, No. 8, pgs. 991-997.

7. VandenLangenberg et al., "Associations Between Antioxidant and Zinc Intake and the 50-Year Incidence of early Age-Related Maculopathy in the Beaver Dam Eye Study," *American Journal of Epidemiology*, 1998, Vol. 148, No. 2, pgs. 204-14.

Chapter 60

The Effect of Antioxidant Vitamins and Zinc on Age-Related Macular Degeneration and Cataract

High levels of antioxidants and zinc significantly reduce the risk of advanced age-related macular degeneration (AMD) by about 25 percent. These same nutrients also reduce the risk of vision loss caused by advanced AMD by about 19 percent. They have no significant effect on the development or progression of cataract.

These results are from the Age-Related Eye Disease Study (AREDS), a major clinical trial sponsored by the National Eye Institute, one of the Federal government's National Institutes of Health. The nutrients are not a cure for AMD, nor will they restore vision already lost from the disease. However, they may play a key role in helping people at high risk for developing advanced AMD keep their vision.

Who Should Take the Nutrients?

People who are at high risk for developing advanced AMD should consider taking the formulation used in the study. Your eye care professional can tell you if you have AMD and if you are at risk for developing the advanced form of the disease. The doctor should give you a dilated eye exam in which drops are placed in your eyes. This allows for a careful examination of the inside of the eye to look for signs of AMD. If you are already taking daily multivitamins and your doctor

"Results—Age-Related Eye Disease Study: The Effect of Antioxidant Vitamins and Zinc on Age-related Macular Degeneration and Cataract," National Institutes of Health, National Eye Institute, http://www.nei.nih.gov, October 2001.

475

suggests you take the formulation used in the AREDS, review all the supplements with your doctor.

What Is the Dosage of the Nutrients Used in the Study?

The specific daily amounts of antioxidants and minerals used by the study researchers were 500 milligrams of vitamin C; 400 international units of vitamin E; 15 milligrams of beta carotene; 80 milligrams of zinc as zinc oxide; and two milligrams of copper as cupric oxide. Copper was added to the AREDS formulations containing zinc to prevent copper deficiency, which may be associated with high levels of zinc supplementation.

Where Can I Obtain the Formulation Used in the Study?

Bausch and Lomb, an eye care company, was a collaborator in the AREDS and provided the study nutrients. The company markets the formulation used in the AREDS; other companies may provide similar formulations. Antioxidant vitamins and zinc can also be purchased separately; however, consumers should discuss the use of these high levels of nutrients with their doctors, and be certain to include copper whenever taking high levels of zinc.

Are There Any Side Effects from the Nutrients?

The AREDS participants reported few side effects from the treatments. About 7.5 percent of participants assigned to the zinc treatments—compared with five percent who did not have zinc in their assigned treatment—had urinary tract problems that required hospitalization. Participants in the two groups that took zinc also reported anemia at a slightly higher rate; however, testing of all patients for this disorder showed no difference among treatment groups. Yellowing of the skin, a well-known side effect of large doses of beta carotene, was reported slightly more often by participants taking antioxidants. In two large clinical trials sponsored by the National Cancer Institute, beta carotene was shown to significantly increase the risk of lung cancer among smokers.

Where Can I Obtain More Information?

For more information, contact your eye care professional or the National Eye Institute at (301) 496-5248.

Part Eight

Additional Help and Information

Chapter 61

Eye-Related Terms

Age-related macular degeneration (ARMD): A common macular degeneration beginning with drusen of the macula and pigment disruption and sometimes leading to severe loss of central vision.[1]

Amblyopia: Poor vision caused by abnormal development of visual areas of the brain in response to abnormal visual stimulation during early development.[1]

Amsler grid: A grid pattern that looks like a checkerboard. People who experience early changes in vision due to conditions such as age-related macular degeneration will find the grid appears distorted because of loss of central vision.[2]

Anophthalmia: The absence of one or both eyes.[2]

Anterior chamber: A space in the front of the eye from which clear fluid flows continuously in and out and nourishes nearby tissues.[2]

Anterior uveitis: Inflammation involving the ciliary body and iris.[1]

Astigmatism: Astigmatism is a condition in which the uneven curvature of the cornea blurs and distorts both distant and near objects. A normal cornea is round, with even curves from side to side and top

Definitions in this chapter were compiled from several sources. Terms marked 1 are from *Stedman's Medical Dictionary, 27th Edition.* © 2000, Lippincott Williams & Wilkins. All rights reserved. Terms marked 2 are from various publications produced by the National Eye Institute.

to bottom. With astigmatism, the cornea is shaped more like the back of a spoon, curved more in one direction than in another. This causes light rays to have more than one focal point and focus on two separate areas of the retina, distorting the visual image. [2]

Behçet's disease: A syndrome characterized by simultaneously or successively occurring recurrent attacks of genital and oral ulcerations; a phase of a generalized disorder, occurring more often in men than in women, with variable manifestations.[1]

Blepharitis: Inflammation of the eyelids.[1]

Blepharospasm: An abnormal, involuntary blinking or spasm of the eyelids.[2]

Cataract: A clouding of the lens. People with cataracts see through a haze. In a usually safe and successful surgery, the cloudy lens can be replaced with a plastic lens.[2]

Choroid: A layer of blood vessels that feeds the retina.[2]

Ciliary body: A thickened portion of the vascular tunic of the eye between the choroid and the iris; it consists of three parts or zones.[1]

Color blindness: Misleading term for anomalous or deficient color vision; complete color blindness is the absence of one of the primary cone pigments of the retina.[1]

Conjunctivitis: Inflammation of the conjunctiva, the mucous membrane on the surface of the eyeball and the surface of the lids.[1]

Cornea: The cornea is the eye's outermost layer. It is the clear, dome-shaped surface that covers the front of the eye and refracts light for vision.[2]

Diabetic retinopathy: Retinal changes occurring in diabetes mellitus.[1]

Ectropion: A rolling outward of the margin of an eyelid.[1]

Endothelium: The extremely thin, innermost layer of the cornea. Endothelial cells are essential in keeping the cornea clear.[2]

Entropion: The infolding of the margin of an eyelid.[1]

Epithelium: The epithelium is the cornea's outermost region, comprising about 10 percent of the tissue's thickness. The epithelium functions primarily to block the passage of foreign material, such as dust, water, and bacteria, into the eye and other layers of the cornea; and provide a smooth surface that absorbs oxygen and cell nutrients from tears, then distributes these nutrients to the rest of the cornea.[2]

Eye: The organ of vision that consists of the eyeball and the optic nerve.[1]

Floaters: An object in the field of vision that originates in the vitreous body.[1]

Fovea: The center of the macula; gives the sharpest vision.[2]

Glaucoma: An eye disease, related to high pressure inside the eye, that damages the optic nerve and leads to vision loss. Glaucoma affects peripheral, or side, vision.[2]

Histoplasmosis: A widely distributed infectious disease caused by *Histoplasma capsulatum* and occurring occasionally in outbreaks; usually acquired by inhalation of spores of the fungus in soil dust and manifested by a self-limited pneumonia.[1]

Hyperopia: Hyperopia, or farsightedness, is the opposite of myopia. Distant objects are clear, and close-up objects appear blurry. With hyperopia, images focus on a point beyond the retina. Hyperopia results from an eye that is too short.[2]

Iris: The colored part of the eye; regulates the amount of light entering the eye.[2]

Lacrimal gland: The gland that secretes tears.[1]

Laser trabeculoplasty: Laser surgery to treat glaucoma.[2]

Laser-assisted in situ keratomileusis (LASIK): A refractive procedure to correct myopia by which a flap of cornea is made, excimer laser ablation of corneal stoma is performed, and the flap laid back in position.[1]

Lens: The clear part of the eye behind the iris that helps to focus light on the retina. Allows the eye to focus on both far and near objects.[2]

Low vision: A visual impairment, not corrected by standard eyeglasses, contact lenses, medication, or surgery, that interferes with the ability to perform everyday activities.[2]

Macula: The small sensitive area of retina that gives central vision; contains the fovea.[2]

Macular hole: A hole in the macula.[2]

Macular pucker: Scar tissue that has formed on the retina.[2]

Microphthalmia: A disorder in which one or both eyes are abnormally small.[2]

Myopia: When the cornea is curved too much, or if the eye is too long, faraway objects will appear blurry because they are focused in front of the retina. This condition is also called nearsightedness.[2]

Ophthalmologist: A medical doctor who diagnoses and treats all diseases and disorders of the eye and can prescribe glasses and contact lenses.[2]

Ophthalmology: The medical specialty concerned with the eye, its diseases, and refractive errors.[1]

Optic nerve: A bundle of more than 1 million nerve fibers. It connects the retina, the light-sensitive layer of tissue at the back of the eye, with the brain. A healthy optic nerve is necessary for good vision.[2]

Optician: A trained professional who grinds, fits, and dispenses glasses by prescription from an optometrist or ophthalmologist.[2]

Optometrist: A primary eye care provider who prescribes glasses and contact lenses and diagnoses and treats certain conditions and diseases of the eye.[2]

Optometry: The profession concerned with the examination of the eyes and related structures to determine the presence of vision problems and eye disorders and with the prescription and adaptation of lenses and other optical aids or the use of visual training for maximum visual efficiency.[1]

Photorefractive keratectomy (PRK): Removal of part of the cornea with a laser to change its shape, and thus to modify the refractive error of the eye (reduce its myopia, for example).[1]

Presbyopia: The physiologic loss of accommodation in the eyes in advancing age.[1]

Pupil: The opening at the center of the iris. The iris adjusts the size of the pupil and controls the amount of light that can enter the eye.[2]

Radial keratotomy (RK): A keratotomy with radial incisions around a clear central zone. A form of refractive keratoplasty used in the treatment of myopia.[1]

Refractive errors: Refractive errors occur when the curve of the cornea is irregularly shaped (too steep or too flat). When the cornea is of normal shape and curvature, it bends, or refracts, light on the retina with precision. However, when the curve of the cornea is irregularly shaped, the cornea bends light imperfectly on the retina. This affects good vision.[2]

Retina: The retina is the light-sensitive layer of tissue that lines the inside of the eye and sends visual messages through the optic nerve to the brain.[2]

Retinal detachment: When the retina detaches, it is lifted or pulled from its normal position.[2]

Retinitis pigmentosa: A progressive retinal degeneration characterized by bilateral nyctalopia, constricted visual fields, electroretinogram abnormalities, and pigmentary infiltration of the inner retinal layers.[1]

Sclera: The tough, white outer coat of the eye.[2]

Sjögren's syndrome: Keratoconjunctivitis sicca, dryness of mucous membranes, telangiectasias or purpuric spots on the face, and bilateral parotid enlargement; seen in menopausal women and often associated with rheumatoid arthritis, Raynaud phenomenon, and dental caries; there are changes in the lacrimal and salivary glands resembling those of Mikulicz disease.[1]

Strasbismus: An imbalance in the positioning of the two eyes. Strabismus can cause the eyes to cross in (esotropia) or turn out (exotropia).[2]

Stye: An inflammation of a gland of the eyelid.[1]

Usher syndrome: Autosomal recessive inheritance with genetic heterogeneity; the three forms are distinguishable by linkage data: type 1 causes sensorineural hearing loss, loss of vestibular function, and retinitis pigmentosa; types 2 and 3 are characterized by hearing loss and retinitis pigmentosa.[1]

Vitreous humor: The clear gel filling the inside of the eye.[2]

Chapter 62

Directory of Eye Care Organizations

Government Organizations

Administration on Aging/ Department of Health and Human Services
330 Independence Avenue, SW
Washington, DC 20201
Toll-Free: (800) 677-1116
Phone: (202) 619-7501
Fax: (202) 260-1012
E-mail: AoAInfo@aoa.gov
Website: http:// www.aoa.dhhs.gov

Agency for Healthcare Research and Quality
2101 E. Jefferson St., Suite 501
Rockville, MD 20852
Phone: (301) 594-1364
E-mail: info@ahrq.gov
Website: http://www.ahrq.gov

Associated Services for the Blind
919 Walnut Street
Philadelphia, PA 19107
Phone: (215) 627-0600
Fax: (215) 922-0692
E-mail: asbinfo@asb.org
Website: http://www.asb.org

Federal Trade Commission (FTC)
CRC-240
Washington, DC 20580
Toll-Free: (877) 382-4357
Phone: (202) 326-2222
Website: http://www.ftc.gov

Resources in this chapter were compiled from many sources deemed accurate; all contact information was verified and updated in August 2002.

National Eye Institute (NEI)
2020 Vision Place
Bethesda, MD 20892-3655
Phone: (301) 496-5248
E-mail: 2020@nei.nih.gov
Website: http://www.nei.nih.gov

National Cancer Institute (NCI)
NCI Public Inquiries Office
Suite 3036A
6116 Executive Boulevard,
MSC8322
Bethesda, MD 20892-8322
Toll-Free: (800) 422-6237
TTY: (800) 332-8615
Website: http://www.cancer.gov

National Institute on Aging
Building 31, Room 5C27
31 Center Drive, MSC 2292
Bethesda, MD 20892
Phone: (301) 496-1752
E-mail: webmaster@nia.nih.gov
Website: http://www.nih.gov/nia

National Institutes of Health (NIH)
9000 Rockville Pike
Bethesda, MD 20892
Phone: (301) 496-4000
E-mail: NIHInfo@OD.NIH.GOV
Website: http://www.nih.gov

U.S. Food and Drug Administration (FDA)
5600 Fishers Lane
Rockville, MD 20857-0001
Toll-Free: (888) 463-6332
Website: http://www.fda.gov

Veterans Health Administration
810 Vermont Avenue NW
Washington, DC 20420
Toll-Free TDD: (800) 829-4833
Phone: (202) 273-5400
Website: http://www.va.gov

Nonprofit and Not-for-Profit Organizations

American Academy of Ophthalmology (AAO)
P.O. Box 7424
San Francisco, CA 94120-7424
Phone: (415) 561-8500
Fax: (415) 561-8533
E-mail:
customer_service@aao.org
Website: http://www.aao.org

American Academy of Optometry
6110 Executive Blvd.
Suite 506
Rockville, MD,20852
Phone: (301) 984-1441
Fax: (301) 984-4737
Website: http://www.aaopt.org

American Association for Pediatric Ophthalmology and Strabismus
P.O. Box 193832
San Francisco, CA 94119-3832
Phone: (415) 561-8505
Fax: (415) 561-8531
E-mail: aapos@aao.org
Website: http://www.aapos.org

American Association of People with Disabilities
1819 H St. NW #330
Washington DC 20006
Toll-Free: (800) 840-8844 (V/TTY)
Phone: (202) 457-0046 (V/TTY)
Fax: (202) 457-0473
E-mail: aapd@aol.com
Website: http://www.aapd-dc.org

American Cancer Society
1599 Clifton Road
Atlanta, GA 30329
Toll-Free: (800) ACS-2345
Website: http://www.cancer.org

American Council of the Blind
1155 15th Street, NW
Suite 1004
Washington, DC 20005
Toll-Free: (800) 424-8666
Phone: (202) 467-5081
Fax: (202) 467-5085
E-mail: info@acb.org
Website: http://www.acb.org

American Foundation for the Blind (AFB)
11 Penn Plaza
Suite 300
New York, NY 10001
Toll-Free: (800) 232-5463
Phone: (212) 502-7600
Fax: (212) 502-7777
E-mail: afbinfo@afb.net
Website: http://www.afb.org

American Optometric Association (AOA)
243 North Lindbergh Blvd.
St. Louis, MO 63141
Phone: (314) 991-4100
Fax: (314) 991-4101
Website: http://www.aoa.org

American Society of Cataract and Refractive Surgery (ASCRS)/LASIK Institute
4000 Legato Road
Suite 850
Fairfax, VA 22033
Phone: (703) 591-2220
Fax: (703) 591-0614
E-mail: info@lasikinstitute.org
Website: http://www.lasikinstitute.org

American Society of Ophthalmic Plastic and Reconstructive Surgery
1133 West Morse Blvd., #201
Winter Park, FL 32789
Phone: (407) 647-8839
Fax: (407) 629-2502
Website: http://www.asoprs.org

American Society of Plastic Surgeons
444 East Algonquin Road
Arlington Heights, IL 60005
Toll-Free: 888-475-2784
Phone: (847) 228-9900
Fax: (847) 228-9131
Toll-Free: (888) 475-2784
Website: http://www.plasticsurgery.org

Eye Bank Association of America
1015 Eighteenth Street NW,
Suite 1010
Washington, DC 20036
Phone: (202) 775-4999
Fax: (202) 429-6036
E-mail: info@restoresight.org
Website: http://www.restoresight.org

Foundation Fighting Blindness
11435 Cronhill Drive
Owings Mills, MD 2117-2220
Toll-Free TDD: (800) 683-5551
Toll-Free: (888) 394-3937
Phone: (410) 568-0150
TDD: (410) 363-7139
E-mail: info@blindness.org
Website: http://www.blindness.org

International Society of Refractive Surgery (ISRS)
1180 Springs Centre South Blvd.,
Suite 116
Altamonte Springs, FL 32714
Phone: (407) 786-7446
Fax: (407) 786-7447
E-mail: ISRShq@ISRS.org
Website: http://www.isrs.org

Knights Templar Eye Foundation
5097 North Elston Avenue,
Suite 100
Chicago, IL 60630-2460
Phone: (773) 205-3838
Fax: (773) 205-1689
E-mail: ktef@knightstemplar.org
Website: http://www.knightstemplar.org/ktef

Lighthouse International
111 East 59th Street
New York, NY 10022-1202
Toll-Free: (800) 829-0500
Phone: (212) 821-9200
TTY: (212) 821-9713
Fax: (212) 821-9707
E-mail: info@lighthouse.org
Website: http://www.lighthouse.org

Lions Clubs International Focus on Sight Program
Lions Clubs International Headquarters
300 West 22nd Street
Oak Brook, IL 60523-8842
Phone: (630) 571-5466
Website: http://www.lionsclubs.org

National Federation of the Blind
1800 Johnson Street
Baltimore, MD 21230
Phone: (410) 659-9314
E-mail: nfb@nfb.org
Website: http://www.nfb.org

National Keratoconus Foundation
Cedars-Sinai Medical Center
8733 Beverly Blvd. Suite 201
Los Angeles, CA 90048
Toll-Free: (800) 521-2524
E-mail: nkcf@csmc.edu
Website: http://www.nkcf.org

New Eyes for the Needy
549 Millburn Avenue
P.O. Box 332
Short Hills, NJ 07078-0332
Phone: (973) 376-4903
Fax: (973) 376-3807

Opticians Association of America
7023 Little River Turnpike, Suite 207
Annandale, VA 22003
Phone: (703) 916-8856
Fax: (703) 916-7966
E-mail: oaa@oaa.org
Website: http://www.opticians.org

Prevent Blindness America
500 E. Remington Rd.
Schaumburg, IL 60173
Toll-Free: (800) 331-2020
Phone: (847) 843-2020
E-mail: info@preventblindness.org
Website: http://www.preventblindness.org

Prevention of Blindness Society of the Metropolitan Area
1775 Church Street, N.W.
Washington, DC 20036
Phone: (202) 234-1010
E-mail: mail@youreyes.org
Website: http://www.youreyes.org

Resources for Rehabilitation
22 Bonad Road
Winchester, MA 01890
Phone: (781) 368-9094
Fax: (781) 368-9096
E-mail: info@rfr.org
Website: http://www.rfr.org

Sjögren's Syndrome Foundation, Inc.
8120 Woodmont Ave.
Suite 530
Bethesda, MD 20814
Toll-Free: (800) 475-6473
Phone: (301) 718-0300
Fax: (301) 718-0322
Website: http://www.sjogrens.com

Vision Council of America
1700 Diagonal Road
Suite 500
Alexandria, VA 22314
Toll-Free: (800) 424-8422
Phone: (703) 548-4560
Fax: (703) 548-4580
E-mail: vca@visionsite.org
Website: http://
www.community.visionsite.org

Diabetic Retinopathy

American Diabetes Association
1701 North Beauregard Street
Alexandria, VA 22311
Toll-Free: (800) DIABETES
E-mail:
customerservice@diabetes.org
Website: http://www.diabetes.org

Diabetic Retinopathy Foundation
350 North LaSalle, Suite 800
Chicago, IL 60610
Website: http://
www.retinopathy.org

National Institute of Diabetic & Digestive & Kidney Diseases (NIDDK)
National Institutes of Health
Building 31, Room 9A04
31 Center Drive, MSC 2560
Bethesda, MD 20892-2560
Phone: (301) 496-3583
Website: http://
www.niddk.nih.gov

Glaucoma

Glaucoma Research Foundation
200 Pine Street, Suite 200
San Francisco, CA 94104
Toll-Free: (800) 826-6693
Fax: (415) 986-3763
E-mail: info@glaucoma.org
Website: http://
www.glaucoma.org

The Glaucoma Foundation
116 John Street
Suite 1605
New York, NY 10038
Phone: (212) 285-0080
Fax: (212) 651-1888
E-mail: info@glaucoma-
foundation.org
Website: http://www.glaucoma-
foundation.org

Macular Degeneration

American Macular Degeneration Foundation
P.O. Box 515
Northampton, MA 01061-0515
Toll-Free: (888) 622-8527
Phone: (413) 268-7660
E-mail: amdf@macular.org
Website: http://www.macular.org

Association for Macular Diseases
210 East 64th Street
8th Floor
New York, NY 10021
Phone: (212) 605-3719
Fax: (212) 605-3795
E-mail: association@retinalresearch.org
Website: http://www.macula.org

Macular Degeneration Foundation, Inc.
P.O. Box 531313
Henderson, NV 89053
E-mail: eyesight@eyesight.org
Website: http://www.eyesight.org

Macular Degeneration International
6700 N. Oracle Rd.
Suite 505
Tucson, AZ 85704
Toll-Free: (800) 393-7634
Phone: (520) 797-2525
E-mail: info@maculardegeneration.org
Website: www.maculardegeneration.org

Chapter 63

Resources for People with Low Vision or Blindness

Organizations

Associated Services for the Blind
919 Walnut Street
Philadelphia, PA 19107
Phone: (215) 627-0600
Fax: (215) 922-0692
E-mail: asbinfo@asb.org
Website: http://www.asb.org

Blinded Veterans Association
477 H Street, NW
Washington, DC 20001-2694
Toll-Free: (800) 669-7079
Phone: (202) 371-8880
Fax: (202) 371-8258
E-mail: bva@bva.org
Website: http://www.bva.org

Council of Citizens with Low Vision International
1155 15th Street NW, Suite 1004
Washington, DC 20005
Toll-Free: (800) 733-2258
Phone: (202) 467-5081
Fax: (202) 467-5085
E-mail: info@acb.org
Website: http://www.cclvi.org

Foundation for Blind Children
1235 E. Harmont Drive
Phoenix, AZ 85020
Phone: (602) 678-5810
Fax: (602) 678-5803
E-mail: info@the-fbc.org
Website: http://www.the-fbc.org

Resources in this chapter were compiled from many sources deemed accurate; all contact information was verified and updated in August 2002.

493

Low Vision Research Group Network (LVRGNet)
Website: http://
www.varrd.emory.edu/
LVRGNET/index.html

National Association for Parents of Children with Visual Impairments (NAPVI)
P.O. Box 317
Watertown, MA 02471
Toll-Free: (800) 562-6265
Phone: (617) 972-7441
Fax: (617) 972-7444
Website: http://www.spedex.com/
NAPVI

National Association for the Visually Handicapped (NAVH)
NAVH—New York City
22 West 21st Street
New York, NY 10010
Phone: (212) 255-2804
Fax: (212) 727-2931
E-mail: staff@navh.org
Website: http://www.navh.org

National Library Service for the Blind and Visually Handicapped
The Library of Congress
1291 Taylor Street NW
Washington, DC 20011
Phone: (202) 707-5100
TDD: (202) 707-0744
Fax: (202) 707-0712
E-mail: nls@loc.gov
Website: http://www.loc.gov/nls

The Center for the Partially Sighted
12301 Wilshire Boulevard
Suite 600
Los Angeles, CA 90025
Phone: (310) 458-3501
Fax: (310) 458-8179
E-mail: info@low-vision.org
Website: http://www.low-
vision.org

VISIONS/Services for the Blind and Visually Impaired
500 Greenwich Street, 3rd Floor
New York, NY 10013-1354
Phone: (212) 625-1616, ext. 117
Fax: (212) 219-4078
E-mail: info@visionsvcb.org
Website: http://
www.visionsvcb.org

Assistive Technology Distributors

Beyond Sight
5650 South Windermere Street
Littleton, CO 80120
Phone: (303) 795-6455
Fax: (303) 795-6425
E-mail:
bsistore@beyondsight.com
Website: http://
www.beyondsight.com/

Closing the Gap
526 Main Street
P.O. Box 68
Henderson, MN 56044
Phone: (507) 248-3294
Fax: (507) 248-3810
E-mail: info@closingthegap.com
Website: http://
www.closingthegap.com

En-Vision America
1013 Porter Lane
Normal, IL 61761
Toll-Free: (800) 890-1180
Phone: (309) 452-3088
Fax: (309) 452-3643
E-mail:
envision@envisionamerica.com
Website: http://
www.envisionamerica.com

Independent Living Aids, Inc.
200 Robbins Lane
Jericho, NY 11753
Toll-Free: (800) 537-2118
Phone: (516) 937-1848
Fax: (516) 937-3906
E-mail: can-
do@independentliving.com
Website: http://
www.independentliving.com

Mons International, Inc.
6595 Roswell Road NE #224
Atlanta, GA 30328
Toll-Free: (800) 541-7903
Phone: (770) 551-8455
E-mail: support@magnifiers.com
Website: http://
www.magnifiers.com

Recording for the Blind and Dyslexic
20 Roszel Road
Princeton, NJ 08540
Toll-Free: (800) 221-4792
Phone: (609) 452-0606
E-mail: custserv@rfbd.org
Website: http://www.rfbd.org

Speak to Me
330 SW 43rd Street
Suite #154
Renton, WA 98055
Toll-Free: (800) 248-9965
Phone: (425) 235-6119
E-mail:
info@speaktomecatalog.com
Website: http://
www.speaktomecatalog.com

Talking Tapes/Textbooks on Tape
16 Sunnen Drive
St. Louis, MO 63143
Toll-Free: (877) 926-0500
Phone: (314) 646-0500
Email: info@talkintapes.org
Website: http://
www.talkingtapes.org

Braille Organizations and Publishers

Braille Authority of North America
919 Walnut Street
Philadelphia, PA 19107
Phone: (215) 627-0600
Fax: (215) 922-0692
Website: http://
www.brailleauthority.org

Braille Institute
741 North Vermont Avenue
Los Angeles, CA 90029-3594
Toll-Free: (800) BRAILLE (272-4553)
Phone: (323) 663-1111
Fax: (323) 663-0867
E-mail: info@BrailleInstitute.org
Website:
www.brailleinstitute.org

Duxbury Systems, Inc.
270 Littleton Road, Unit 6
Westford, MA 01886-3523
Phone: (978) 692-3000
Fax: (978) 692-7912
E-mail: info@duxsys.com
Website: http://
www.duxburysystems.com

National Braille Press
88 St. Stephen Street
Boston, MA 02115
Toll-Free: (888) 965-8965
Phone: (617) 266-6160
Fax: (617) 437-0456
E-mail: orders@nbp.org
Website: http://www.nbp.org

Guide Dog Organizations

Canine Companions for Independence, Inc.
2965 Dutton Avenue
P.O. Box 446
Santa Rosa, CA 95402-0446
Toll-Free: (800) 572-2275 or (866) 224-3647
Phone: (707) 577-1700
TDD: (707) 577-1756
E-mail: info@caninecompanions.org
Website: http://www.caninecompanions.org

Guide Dog Foundation for the Blind, Inc.
371 East Jericho Tpke.
Smithtown, NY 11787-2976
Toll-Free: (800) 548-4337
Phone: (631) 265-2121
Fax: (631) 361-5192
E-mail: info@guidedog.org
Website: http://www.guidedog.org

Index

Index

Page numbers followed by 'n' indicate a footnote. Page numbers in *italics* indicate a table or illustration.

Health Reference Series
COMPLETE CATALOG

Adolescent Health Sourcebook

Basic Consumer Health Information about Common Medical, Mental, and Emotional Concerns in Adolescents, Including Facts about Acne, Body Piercing, Mononucleosis, Nutrition, Eating Disorders, Stress, Depression, Behavior Problems, Peer Pressure, Violence, Gangs, Drug Use, Puberty, Sexuality, Pregnancy, Learning Disabilities, and More

Along with a Glossary of Terms and Other Resources for Further Help and Information

Edited by Chad T. Kimball. 658 pages. 2002. 0-7808-0248-9. $78.

"A good starting point for information related to common medical, mental, and emotional concerns of adolescents."
— School Library Journal, Nov '02

"This book provides accurate information in an easy to access format. It addresses topics that parents and caregivers might not be aware of and provides practical, useable information." — Doody's Health Sciences Book Review Journal, Sep-Oct '02

"Recommended reference source."
— Booklist, American Library Association, Sep '02

■

AIDS Sourcebook, 1st Edition

Basic Information about AIDS and HIV Infection, Featuring Historical and Statistical Data, Current Research, Prevention, and Other Special Topics of Interest for Persons Living with AIDS

Along with Source Listings for Further Assistance

Edited by Karen Bellenir and Peter D. Dresser. 831 pages. 1995. 0-7808-0031-1. $78.

"One strength of this book is its practical emphasis. The intended audience is the lay reader . . . useful as an educational tool for health care providers who work with AIDS patients. Recommended for public libraries as well as hospital or academic libraries that collect consumer materials."
— Bulletin of the Medical Library Association, Jan '96

"This is the most comprehensive volume of its kind on an important medical topic. Highly recommended for all libraries." — Reference Book Review, '96

"Very useful reference for all libraries."
— Choice, Association of College and Research Libraries, Oct '95

"There is a wealth of information here that can provide much educational assistance. It is a must book for all libraries and should be on the desk of each and every congressional leader. Highly recommended."
— AIDS Book Review Journal, Aug '95

"Recommended for most collections."
— Library Journal, Jul '95

AIDS Sourcebook, 2nd Edition

Basic Consumer Health Information about Acquired Immune Deficiency Syndrome (AIDS) and Human Immunodeficiency Virus (HIV) Infection, Featuring Updated Statistical Data, Reports on Recent Research and Prevention Initiatives, and Other Special Topics of Interest for Persons Living with AIDS, Including New Antiretroviral Treatment Options, Strategies for Combating Opportunistic Infections, Information about Clinical Trials, and More

Along with a Glossary of Important Terms and Resource Listings for Further Help and Information

Edited by Karen Bellenir. 751 pages. 1999. 0-7808-0225-X. $78.

"Highly recommended."
—American Reference Books Annual, 2000

"Excellent sourcebook. This continues to be a highly recommended book. There is no other book that provides as much information as this book provides."
— AIDS Book Review Journal, Dec-Jan 2000

"Recommended reference source."
—Booklist, American Library Association, Dec '99

"A solid text for college-level health libraries."
—The Bookwatch, Aug '99

Cited in Reference Sources for Small and Medium-Sized Libraries, American Library Association, 1999

■

AIDS Sourcebook, 3rd Edition

Basic Consumer Health Information about Acquired Immune Deficiency Syndrome (AIDS) and Human Immunodeficiency Virus (HIV) Infection, Including Facts about Transmission, Prevention, Diagnosis, Treatment, Opportunistic Infections, and Other Complications, with a Section for Women and Children, Including Details about Associated Gynecological Concerns, Pregnancy, and Pediatric Care

Along with Updated Statistical Information, Reports on Current Research Initiatives, a Glossary, and Directories of Internet, Hotline, and Other Resources

Edited by Dawn D. Matthews. 675 pages. 2003. 0-7808-0631-X. $78.

■

Alcoholism Sourcebook

Basic Consumer Health Information about the Physical and Mental Consequences of Alcohol Abuse, Including Liver Disease, Pancreatitis, Wernicke-Korsakoff Syndrome (Alcoholic Dementia), Fetal Alcohol Syndrome, Heart Disease, Kidney Disorders, Gastrointestinal Problems, and Immune System Compromise and Featuring Facts about Addiction, Detoxification, Alcohol Withdrawal, Recovery, and the Maintenance of Sobriety

Along with a Glossary and Directories of Resources for Further Help and Information

Edited by Karen Bellenir. 613 pages. 2000. 0-7808-0325-6. $78.

"This title is one of the few reference works on alcoholism for general readers. For some readers this will be a welcome complement to the many self-help books on the market. Recommended for collections serving general readers and consumer health collections."
— *E-Streams, Mar '01*

"This book is an excellent choice for public and academic libraries."
— *American Reference Books Annual, 2001*

"Recommended reference source."
— *Booklist, American Library Association, Dec '00*

"Presents a wealth of information on alcohol use and abuse and its effects on the body and mind, treatment, and prevention." — *SciTech Book News, Dec '00*

"Important new health guide which packs in the latest consumer information about the problems of alcoholism." — *Reviewer's Bookwatch, Nov '00*

SEE ALSO *Drug Abuse Sourcebook, Substance Abuse Sourcebook*

Allergies Sourcebook, 1st Edition

Basic Information about Major Forms and Mechanisms of Common Allergic Reactions, Sensitivities, and Intolerances, Including Anaphylaxis, Asthma, Hives and Other Dermatologic Symptoms, Rhinitis, and Sinusitis

Along with Their Usual Triggers Like Animal Fur, Chemicals, Drugs, Dust, Foods, Insects, Latex, Pollen, and Poison Ivy, Oak, and Sumac; Plus Information on Prevention, Identification, and Treatment

Edited by Allan R. Cook. 611 pages. 1997. 0-7808-0036-2. $78.

Allergies Sourcebook, 2nd Edition

Basic Consumer Health Information about Allergic Disorders, Triggers, Reactions, and Related Symptoms, Including Anaphylaxis, Rhinitis, Sinusitis, Asthma, Dermatitis, Conjunctivitis, and Multiple Chemical Sensitivity

Along with Tips on Diagnosis, Prevention, and Treatment, Statistical Data, a Glossary, and a Directory of Sources for Further Help and Information

Edited by Annemarie S. Muth. 598 pages. 2002. 0-7808-0376-0. $78.

"This second edition would be useful to laypersons with little or advanced knowledge of the subject matter. This book would also serve as a resource for nursing and other health care professions students. It would be useful in public, academic, and hospital libraries with consumer health collections." — *E-Streams, Jul '02*

Alternative Medicine Sourcebook, 1st Edition

Basic Consumer Health Information about Alternatives to Conventional Medicine, Including Acupressure, Acupuncture, Aromatherapy, Ayurveda, Bioelectromagnetics, Environmental Medicine, Essence Therapy, Food and Nutrition Therapy, Herbal Therapy, Homeopathy, Imaging, Massage, Naturopathy, Reflexology, Relaxation and Meditation, Sound Therapy, Vitamin and Mineral Therapy, and Yoga, and More

Edited by Allan R. Cook. 737 pages. 1999. 0-7808-0200-4. $78.

"Recommended reference source."
— *Booklist, American Library Association, Feb '00*

"A great addition to the reference collection of every type of library." — *American Reference Books Annual, 2000*

Alternative Medicine Sourcebook, 2nd Edition

Basic Consumer Health Information about Alternative and Complementary Medical Practices, Including Acupuncture, Chiropractic, Herbal Medicine, Homeopathy, Naturopathic Medicine, Mind-Body Interventions, Ayurveda, and Other Non-Western Medical Traditions

Along with Facts about such Specific Therapies as Massage Therapy, Aromatherapy, Qigong, Hypnosis, Prayer, Dance, and Art Therapies, a Glossary, and Resources for Further Information

Edited by Dawn D. Matthews. 618 pages. 2002. 0-7808-0605-0. $78.

"An important alternate health reference."
— *MBR Bookwatch, Oct '02*

Alzheimer's, Stroke & 29 Other Neurological Disorders Sourcebook, 1st Edition

Basic Information for the Layperson on 31 Diseases or Disorders Affecting the Brain and Nervous System, First Describing the Illness, Then Listing Symptoms, Diagnostic Methods, and Treatment Options, and Including Statistics on Incidences and Causes

Edited by Frank E. Bair. 579 pages. 1993. 1-55888-748-2. $78.

"Nontechnical reference book that provides reader-friendly information."
— *Family Caregiver Alliance Update, Winter '96*

"Should be included in any library's patient education section." — *American Reference Books Annual, 1994*

"Written in an approachable and accessible style. Recommended for patient education and consumer health collections in health science center and public libraries." — *Academic Library Book Review, Dec '93*

"It is very handy to have information on more than thirty neurological disorders under one cover, and there is no recent source like it." — *Reference Quarterly, American Library Association, Fall '93*

SEE ALSO *Brain Disorders Sourcebook*

■

Alzheimer's Disease Sourcebook, 2nd Edition

Basic Consumer Health Information about Alzheimer's Disease, Related Disorders, and Other Dementias, Including Multi-Infarct Dementia, AIDS-Related Dementia, Alcoholic Dementia, Huntington's Disease, Delirium, and Confusional States

Along with Reports Detailing Current Research Efforts in Prevention and Treatment, Long-Term Care Issues, and Listings of Sources for Additional Help and Information

Edited by Karen Bellenir. 524 pages. 1999. 0-7808-0223-3. $78.

"Provides a wealth of useful information not otherwise available in one place. This resource is recommended for all types of libraries." — *American Reference Books Annual, 2000*

"Recommended reference source." — *Booklist, American Library Association, Oct '99*

■

Arthritis Sourcebook

Basic Consumer Health Information about Specific Forms of Arthritis and Related Disorders, Including Rheumatoid Arthritis, Osteoarthritis, Gout, Polymyalgia Rheumatica, Psoriatic Arthritis, Spondyloarthropathies, Juvenile Rheumatoid Arthritis, and Juvenile Ankylosing Spondylitis

Along with Information about Medical, Surgical, and Alternative Treatment Options, and Including Strategies for Coping with Pain, Fatigue, and Stress

Edited by Allan R. Cook. 550 pages. 1998. 0-7808-0201-2. $78.

". . . accessible to the layperson." — *Reference and Research Book News, Feb '99*

■

Asthma Sourcebook

Basic Consumer Health Information about Asthma, Including Symptoms, Traditional and Nontraditional Remedies, Treatment Advances, Quality-of-Life Aids, Medical Research Updates, and the Role of Allergies, Exercise, Age, the Environment, and Genetics in the Development of Asthma

Along with Statistical Data, a Glossary, and Directories of Support Groups, and Other Resources for Further Information

Edited by Annemarie S. Muth. 628 pages. 2000. 0-7808-0381-7. $78.

"A worthwhile reference acquisition for public libraries and academic medical libraries whose readers desire a quick introduction to the wide range of asthma information." — *Choice, Association of College & Research Libraries, Jun '01*

"Recommended reference source." — *Booklist, American Library Association, Feb '01*

"Highly recommended." — *The Bookwatch, Jan '01*

"There is much good information for patients and their families who deal with asthma daily." — *American Medical Writers Association Journal, Winter '01*

"This informative text is recommended for consumer health collections in public, secondary school, and community college libraries and the libraries of universities with a large undergraduate population." — *American Reference Books Annual, 2001*

■

Attention Deficit Disorder Sourcebook

Basic Consumer Health Information about Attention Deficit/Hyperactivity Disorder in Children and Adults, Including Facts about Causes, Symptoms, Diagnostic Criteria, and Treatment Options Such as Medications, Behavior Therapy, Coaching, and Homeopathy

Along with Reports on Current Research Initiatives, Legal Issues, and Government Regulations, and Featuring a Glossary of Related Terms, Internet Resources, and a List of Additional Reading Material

Edited by Dawn D. Matthews. 470 pages. 2002. 0-7808-0624-7. $78.

■

Back & Neck Disorders Sourcebook

Basic Information about Disorders and Injuries of the Spinal Cord and Vertebrae, Including Facts on Chiropractic Treatment, Surgical Interventions, Paralysis, and Rehabilitation

Along with Advice for Preventing Back Trouble

Edited by Karen Bellenir. 548 pages. 1997. 0-7808-0202-0. $78.

"The strength of this work is its basic, easy-to-read format. Recommended." — *Reference and User Services Quarterly, American Library Association, Winter '97*

■

Blood & Circulatory Disorders Sourcebook

Basic Information about Blood and Its Components, Anemias, Leukemias, Bleeding Disorders, and Circulatory Disorders, Including Aplastic Anemia, Thalassemia, Sickle-Cell Disease, Hemochromatosis, Hemophilia, Von Willebrand Disease, and Vascular Diseases

Along with a Special Section on Blood Transfusions and Blood Supply Safety, a Glossary, and Source Listings for Further Help and Information

Edited by Karen Bellenir and Linda M. Shin. 554 pages. 1998. 0-7808-0203-9. $78.

"Recommended reference source."
—Booklist, American Library Association, Feb '99

"An important reference sourcebook written in simple language for everyday, non-technical users. "
— Reviewer's Bookwatch, Jan '99

■

Brain Disorders Sourcebook

Basic Consumer Health Information about Strokes, Epilepsy, Amyotrophic Lateral Sclerosis (ALS/Lou Gehrig's Disease), Parkinson's Disease, Brain Tumors, Cerebral Palsy, Headache, Tourette Syndrome, and More

Along with Statistical Data, Treatment and Rehabilitation Options, Coping Strategies, Reports on Current Research Initiatives, a Glossary, and Resource Listings for Additional Help and Information

Edited by Karen Bellenir. 481 pages. 1999. 0-7808-0229-2. $78.

"Belongs on the shelves of any library with a consumer health collection."   *— E-Streams, Mar '00*

"Recommended reference source."
— Booklist, American Library Association, Oct '99

SEE ALSO *Alzheimer's Disease Sourcebook, 2nd Edition*

■

Breast Cancer Sourcebook

Basic Consumer Health Information about Breast Cancer, Including Diagnostic Methods, Treatment Options, Alternative Therapies, Self-Help Information, Related Health Concerns, Statistical and Demographic Data, and Facts for Men with Breast Cancer

Along with Reports on Current Research Initiatives, a Glossary of Related Medical Terms, and a Directory of Sources for Further Help and Information

Edited by Edward J. Prucha and Karen Bellenir. 580 pages. 2001. 0-7808-0244-6. $78.

"Recommended reference source."
— Booklist, American Library Association, Jan '02

"This reference source is highly recommended. It is quite informative, comprehensive and detailed in nature, and yet it offers practical advice in easy-to-read language. It could be thought of as the 'bible' of breast cancer for the consumer."   *— E-Streams, Jan '02*

"The broad range of topics covered in lay language make the *Breast Cancer Sourcebook* an excellent addition to public and consumer health library collections."
— American Reference Books Annual 2002

"From the pros and cons of different screening methods and results to treatment options, *Breast Cancer Sourcebook* provides the latest information on the subject."
— Library Bookwatch, Dec '01

"This thoroughgoing, very readable reference covers all aspects of breast health and cancer. . . . Readers will find much to consider here. Recommended for all public and patient health collections."
—Library Journal, Sep '01

SEE ALSO *Cancer Sourcebook for Women, 1st and 2nd Editions, Women's Health Concerns Sourcebook*

■

Breastfeeding Sourcebook

Basic Consumer Health Information about the Benefits of Breastmilk, Preparing to Breastfeed, Breastfeeding as a Baby Grows, Nutrition, and More, Including Information on Special Situations and Concerns Such as Mastitis, Illness, Medications, Allergies, Multiple Births, Prematurity, Special Needs, and Adoption

Along with a Glossary and Resources for Additional Help and Information

Edited by Jenni Lynn Colson. 388 pages. 2002. 0-7808-0332-9. $78.

SEE ALSO *Pregnancy & Birth Sourcebook*

■

Burns Sourcebook

Basic Consumer Health Information about Various Types of Burns and Scalds, Including Flame, Heat, Cold, Electrical, Chemical, and Sun Burns

Along with Information on Short-Term and Long-Term Treatments, Tissue Reconstruction, Plastic Surgery, Prevention Suggestions, and First Aid

Edited by Allan R. Cook. 604 pages. 1999. 0-7808-0204-7. $78.

"This is an exceptional addition to the series and is highly recommended for all consumer health collections, hospital libraries, and academic medical centers."
— E-Streams, Mar '00

"This key reference guide is an invaluable addition to all health care and public libraries in confronting this ongoing health issue."
—American Reference Books Annual, 2000

"Recommended reference source."
—Booklist, American Library Association, Dec '99

SEE ALSO *Skin Disorders Sourcebook*

■

Cancer Sourcebook, 1st Edition

Basic Information on Cancer Types, Symptoms, Diagnostic Methods, and Treatments, Including Statistics on Cancer Occurrences Worldwide and the Risks Associated with Known Carcinogens and Activities

Edited by Frank E. Bair. 932 pages. 1990. 1-55888-888-8. $78.

Cited in *Reference Sources for Small and Medium-Sized Libraries, American Library Association, 1999*

"Written in nontechnical language. Useful for patients, their families, medical professionals, and librarians."
—Guide to Reference Books, 1996

"Designed with the non-medical professional in mind. Libraries and medical facilities interested in patient education should certainly consider adding the *Cancer Sourcebook* to their holdings. This compact collection of reliable information . . . is an invaluable tool for helping patients and patients' families and friends to take the first steps in coping with the many difficulties of cancer."
— *Medical Reference Services Quarterly, Winter '91*

"Specifically created for the nontechnical reader . . . an important resource for the general reader trying to understand the complexities of cancer."
— *American Reference Books Annual, 1991*

"This publication's nontechnical nature and very comprehensive format make it useful for both the general public and undergraduate students."
— *Choice, Association of College and Research Libraries, Oct '90*

∎

New Cancer Sourcebook, 2nd Edition

Basic Information about Major Forms and Stages of Cancer, Featuring Facts about Primary and Secondary Tumors of the Respiratory, Nervous, Lymphatic, Circulatory, Skeletal, and Gastrointestinal Systems, and Specific Organs; Statistical and Demographic Data; Treatment Options; and Strategies for Coping

Edited by Allan R. Cook. 1,313 pages. 1996. 0-7808-0041-9. $78.

"An excellent resource for patients with newly diagnosed cancer and their families. The dialogue is simple, direct, and comprehensive. Highly recommended for patients and families to aid in their understanding of cancer and its treatment."
— *Booklist Health Sciences Supplement, American Library Association, Oct '97*

"The amount of factual and useful information is extensive. The writing is very clear, geared to general readers. Recommended for all levels." — *Choice, Association of College & Research Libraries, Jan '97*

∎

Cancer Sourcebook, 3rd Edition

Basic Consumer Health Information about Major Forms and Stages of Cancer, Featuring Facts about Primary and Secondary Tumors of the Respiratory, Nervous, Lymphatic, Circulatory, Skeletal, and Gastrointestinal Systems, and Specific Organs

Along with Statistical and Demographic Data, Treatment Options, Strategies for Coping, a Glossary, and a Directory of Sources for Additional Help and Information

Edited by Edward J. Prucha. 1,069 pages. 2000. 0-7808-0227-6. $78.

"This title is recommended for health sciences and public libraries with consumer health collections."
— *E-Streams, Feb '01*

"... can be effectively used by cancer patients and their families who are looking for answers in a language they can understand. Public and hospital libraries should have it on their shelves."
— *American Reference Books Annual, 2001*

"Recommended reference source."
— *Booklist, American Library Association, Dec '00*

∎

Cancer Sourcebook for Women, 1st Edition

Basic Information about Specific Forms of Cancer That Affect Women, Featuring Facts about Breast Cancer, Cervical Cancer, Ovarian Cancer, Cancer of the Uterus and Uterine Sarcoma, Cancer of the Vagina, and Cancer of the Vulva; Statistical and Demographic Data; Treatments, Self-Help Management Suggestions, and Current Research Initiatives

Edited by Allan R. Cook and Peter D. Dresser. 524 pages. 1996. 0-7808-0076-1. $78.

". . . written in easily understandable, non-technical language. Recommended for public libraries or hospital and academic libraries that collect patient education or consumer health materials."
— *Medical Reference Services Quarterly, Spring '97*

"Would be of value in a consumer health library. . . . written with the health care consumer in mind. Medical jargon is at a minimum, and medical terms are explained in clear, understandable sentences."
— *Bulletin of the Medical Library Association, Oct '96*

"The availability under one cover of all these pertinent publications, grouped under cohesive headings, makes this certainly a most useful sourcebook." — *Choice, Association of College & Research Libraries, Jun '96*

"Presents a comprehensive knowledge base for general readers. Men and women both benefit from the gold mine of information nestled between the two covers of this book. Recommended."
— *Academic Library Book Review, Summer '96*

"This timely book is highly recommended for consumer health and patient education collections in all libraries." — *Library Journal, Apr '96*

∎

Cancer Sourcebook for Women, 2nd Edition

Basic Consumer Health Information about Gynecologic Cancers and Related Concerns, Including Cervical Cancer, Endometrial Cancer, Gestational Trophoblastic Tumor, Ovarian Cancer, Uterine Cancer, Vaginal Cancer, Vulvar Cancer, Breast Cancer, and Common Non-Cancerous Uterine Conditions, with Facts about Cancer Risk Factors, Screening and Prevention, Treatment Options, and Reports on Current Research Initiatives

Along with a Glossary of Cancer Terms and a Directory of Resources for Additional Help and Information

Edited by Karen Bellenir. 604 pages. 2002. 0-7808-0226-8. $78.

525

SEE ALSO Breast Cancer Sourcebook, Women's Health Concerns Sourcebook

■

Cardiovascular Diseases & Disorders Sourcebook, 1st Edition

Basic Information about Cardiovascular Diseases and Disorders, Featuring Facts about the Cardiovascular System, Demographic and Statistical Data, Descriptions of Pharmacological and Surgical Interventions, Lifestyle Modifications, and a Special Section Focusing on Heart Disorders in Children

Edited by Karen Bellenir and Peter D. Dresser. 683 pages. 1995. 0-7808-0032-X. $78.

SEE ALSO Healthy Heart Sourcebook for Women, Heart Diseases & Disorders Sourcebook, 2nd Edition

■

Caregiving Sourcebook

Basic Consumer Health Information for Caregivers, Including a Profile of Caregivers, Caregiving Responsibilities and Concerns, Tips for Specific Conditions, Care Environments, and the Effects of Caregiving

Along with Facts about Legal Issues, Financial Information, and Future Planning, a Glossary, and a Listing of Additional Resources

Edited by Joyce Brennfleck Shannon. 600 pages. 2001. 0-7808-0331-0. $78.

Colds, Flu & Other Common Ailments Sourcebook

Basic Consumer Health Information about Common Ailments and Injuries, Including Colds, Coughs, the Flu, Sinus Problems, Headaches, Fever, Nausea and Vomiting, Menstrual Cramps, Diarrhea, Constipation, Hemorrhoids, Back Pain, Dandruff, Dry and Itchy Skin, Cuts, Scrapes, Sprains, Bruises, and More

Along with Information about Prevention, Self-Care, Choosing a Doctor, Over-the-Counter Medications, Folk Remedies, and Alternative Therapies, and Including a Glossary of Important Terms and a Directory of Resources for Further Help and Information

Edited by Chad T. Kimball. 638 pages. 2001. 0-7808-0435-X. $78.

■

Communication Disorders Sourcebook

Basic Information about Deafness and Hearing Loss, Speech and Language Disorders, Voice Disorders, Balance and Vestibular Disorders, and Disorders of Smell, Taste, and Touch

Edited by Linda M. Ross. 533 pages. 1996. 0-7808-0077-X. $78.

■

Congenital Disorders Sourcebook

Basic Information about Disorders Acquired during Gestation, Including Spina Bifida, Hydrocephalus, Cerebral Palsy, Heart Defects, Craniofacial Abnormalities, Fetal Alcohol Syndrome, and More

Along with Current Treatment Options and Statistical Data

Edited by Karen Bellenir. 607 pages. 1997. 0-7808-0205-5. $78.

SEE ALSO Pregnancy & Birth Sourcebook

Consumer Issues in Health Care Sourcebook

Basic Information about Health Care Fundamentals and Related Consumer Issues, Including Exams and Screening Tests, Physician Specialties, Choosing a Doctor, Using Prescription and Over-the-Counter Medications Safely, Avoiding Health Scams, Managing Common Health Risks in the Home, Care Options for Chronically or Terminally Ill Patients, and a List of Resources for Obtaining Help and Further Information

Edited by Karen Bellenir. 618 pages. 1998. 0-7808-0221-7. $78.

"Both public and academic libraries will want to have a copy in their collection for readers who are interested in self-education on health issues."
— *American Reference Books Annual, 2000*

"The editor has researched the literature from government agencies and others, saving readers the time and effort of having to do the research themselves. Recommended for public libraries."
— *Reference and User Services Quarterly, American Library Association, Spring '99*

"Recommended reference source."
— *Booklist, American Library Association, Dec '98*

■

Contagious & Non-Contagious Infectious Diseases Sourcebook

Basic Information about Contagious Diseases like Measles, Polio, Hepatitis B, and Infectious Mononucleosis, and Non-Contagious Infectious Diseases like Tetanus and Toxic Shock Syndrome, and Diseases Occurring as Secondary Infections Such as Shingles and Reye Syndrome

Along with Vaccination, Prevention, and Treatment Information, and a Section Describing Emerging Infectious Disease Threats

Edited by Karen Bellenir and Peter D. Dresser. 566 pages. 1996. 0-7808-0075-3. $78.

■

Death & Dying Sourcebook

Basic Consumer Health Information for the Layperson about End-of-Life Care and Related Ethical and Legal Issues, Including Chief Causes of Death, Autopsies, Pain Management for the Terminally Ill, Life Support Systems, Insurance, Euthanasia, Assisted Suicide, Hospice Programs, Living Wills, Funeral Planning, Counseling, Mourning, Organ Donation, and Physician Training

Along with Statistical Data, a Glossary, and Listings of Sources for Further Help and Information

Edited by Annemarie S. Muth. 641 pages. 1999. 0-7808-0230-6. $78.

"Public libraries, medical libraries, and academic libraries will all find this sourcebook a useful addition to their collections."
— *American Reference Books Annual, 2001*

"An extremely useful resource for those concerned with death and dying in the United States."
— *Respiratory Care, Nov '00*

"Recommended reference source."
— *Booklist, American Library Association, Aug '00*

"This book is a definite must for all those involved in end-of-life care." — *Doody's Review Service, 2000*

■

Depression Sourcebook

Basic Consumer Health Information about Unipolar Depression, Bipolar Disorder, Postpartum Depression, Seasonal Affective Disorder, and Other Types of Depression in Children, Adolescents, Women, Men, the Elderly, and Other Selected Populations

Along with Facts about Causes, Risk Factors, Diagnostic Criteria, Treatment Options, Coping Strategies, Suicide Prevention, a Glossary, and a Directory of Sources for Additional Help and Information

Edited by Karen Belleni. 602 pages. 2002. 0-7808-0611-5. $78.

■

Diabetes Sourcebook, 1st Edition

Basic Information about Insulin-Dependent and Non-insulin-Dependent Diabetes Mellitus, Gestational Diabetes, and Diabetic Complications, Symptoms, Treatment, and Research Results, Including Statistics on Prevalence, Morbidity, and Mortality

Along with Source Listings for Further Help and Information

Edited by Karen Bellenir and Peter D. Dresser. 827 pages. 1994. 1-55888-751-2. $78.

". . . very informative and understandable for the layperson without being simplistic. It provides a comprehensive overview for laypersons who want a general understanding of the disease or who want to focus on various aspects of the disease."
— *Bulletin of the Medical Library Association, Jan '96*

■

Diabetes Sourcebook, 2nd Edition

Basic Consumer Health Information about Type 1 Diabetes (Insulin-Dependent or Juvenile-Onset Diabetes), Type 2 (Noninsulin-Dependent or Adult-Onset Diabetes), Gestational Diabetes, and Related Disorders, Including Diabetes Prevalence Data, Management Issues, the Role of Diet and Exercise in Controlling Diabetes, Insulin and Other Diabetes Medicines, and Complications of Diabetes Such as Eye Diseases, Periodontal Disease, Amputation, and End-Stage Renal Disease

Along with Reports on Current Research Initiatives, a Glossary, and Resource Listings for Further Help and Information

Edited by Karen Bellenir. 688 pages. 1998. 0-7808-0224-1. $78.

"An invaluable reference." — *Library Journal, May '00*

Selected as one of the 250 "Best Health Sciences Books of 1999." — *Doody's Rating Service, Mar-Apr 2000*

"This comprehensive book is an excellent addition for high school, academic, medical, and public libraries. This volume is highly recommended."
— *American Reference Books Annual, 2000*

"Provides useful information for the general public."
— *Healthlines, University of Michigan Health Management Research Center, Sep/Oct '99*

". . . provides reliable mainstream medical information . . . belongs on the shelves of any library with a consumer health collection." — *E-Streams, Sep '99*

"Recommended reference source."
— *Booklist, American Library Association, Feb '99*

■

Diabetes Sourcebook, 3rd Edition

Basic Consumer Health Information about Type 1 Diabetes (Insulin-Dependent or Juvenile-Onset Diabetes), Type 2 Diabetes (Noninsulin-Dependent or Adult-Onset Diabetes), Gestational Diabetes, Impaired Glucose Tolerance (IGT), and Related Complications, Such as Amputation, Eye Disease, Gum Disease, Nerve Damage, and End-Stage Renal Disease, Including Facts about Insulin, Oral Diabetes Medications, Blood Sugar Testing, and the Role of Exercise and Nutrition in the Control of Diabetes

Along with a Glossary and Resources for Further Help and Information

Edited by Dawn D. Matthews. 622 pages. 2003. 0-7808-0629-8. $78.

■

Diet & Nutrition Sourcebook, 1st Edition

Basic Information about Nutrition, Including the Dietary Guidelines for Americans, the Food Guide Pyramid, and Their Applications in Daily Diet, Nutritional Advice for Specific Age Groups, Current Nutritional Issues and Controversies, the New Food Label and How to Use It to Promote Healthy Eating, and Recent Developments in Nutritional Research

Edited by Dan R. Harris. 662 pages. 1996. 0-7808-0084-2. $78.

"Useful reference as a food and nutrition sourcebook for the general consumer." — *Booklist Health Sciences Supplement, American Library Association, Oct '97*

"Recommended for public libraries and medical libraries that receive general information requests on nutrition. It is readable and will appeal to those interested in learning more about healthy dietary practices."
— *Medical Reference Services Quarterly, Fall '97*

"An abundance of medical and social statistics is translated into readable information geared toward the general reader." — *Bookwatch, Mar '97*

"With dozens of questionable diet books on the market, it is so refreshing to find a reliable and factual reference book. Recommended to aspiring professionals, librarians, and others seeking and giving reliable dietary advice. An excellent compilation." — *Choice, Association of College and Research Libraries, Feb '97*

SEE ALSO Digestive Diseases & Disorders Sourcebook, Gastrointestinal Diseases & Disorders Sourcebook

■

Diet & Nutrition Sourcebook, 2nd Edition

Basic Consumer Health Information about Dietary Guidelines, Recommended Daily Intake Values, Vitamins, Minerals, Fiber, Fat, Weight Control, Dietary Supplements, and Food Additives

Along with Special Sections on Nutrition Needs throughout Life and Nutrition for People with Such Specific Medical Concerns as Allergies, High Blood Cholesterol, Hypertension, Diabetes, Celiac Disease, Seizure Disorders, Phenylketonuria (PKU), Cancer, and Eating Disorders, and Including Reports on Current Nutrition Research and Source Listings for Additional Help and Information

Edited by Karen Bellenir. 650 pages. 1999. 0-7808-0228-4. $78.

"This book is an excellent source of basic diet and nutrition information." — *Booklist Health Sciences Supplement, American Library Association, Dec '00*

"This reference document should be in any public library, but it would be a very good guide for beginning students in the health sciences. If the other books in this publisher's series are as good as this, they should all be in the health sciences collections."
— *American Reference Books Annual, 2000*

"This book is an excellent general nutrition reference for consumers who desire to take an active role in their health care for prevention. Consumers of all ages who select this book can feel confident they are receiving current and accurate information." — *Journal of Nutrition for the Elderly, Vol. 19, No. 4, '00*

"Recommended reference source."
— *Booklist, American Library Association, Dec '99*

SEE ALSO Digestive Diseases & Disorders Sourcebook, Gastrointestinal Diseases & Disorders Sourcebook

■

Digestive Diseases & Disorders Sourcebook

Basic Consumer Health Information about Diseases and Disorders that Impact the Upper and Lower Digestive System, Including Celiac Disease, Constipation, Crohn's Disease, Cyclic Vomiting Syndrome, Diarrhea, Diverticulosis and Diverticulitis, Gallstones, Heartburn, Hemorrhoids, Hernias, Indigestion (Dyspepsia), Irritable Bowel Syndrome, Lactose Intolerance, Ulcers, and More

Along with Information about Medications and Other Treatments, Tips for Maintaining a Healthy Digestive Tract, a Glossary, and Directory of Digestive Diseases Organizations

Edited by Karen Bellenir. 335 pages. 2000. 0-7808-0327-2. $78.

"This title would be an excellent addition to all public or patient-research libraries."
—*American Reference Books Annual, 2001*

"This title is recommended for public, hospital, and health sciences libraries with consumer health collections." —*E-Streams, Jul-Aug '00*

"Recommended reference source."
—*Booklist, American Library Association, May '00*

SEE ALSO *Diet & Nutrition Sourcebook, 1st and 2nd Editions, Gastrointestinal Diseases & Disorders Sourcebook*

Disabilities Sourcebook

Basic Consumer Health Information about Physical and Psychiatric Disabilities, Including Descriptions of Major Causes of Disability, Assistive and Adaptive Aids, Workplace Issues, and Accessibility Concerns

Along with Information about the Americans with Disabilities Act, a Glossary, and Resources for Additional Help and Information

Edited by Dawn D. Matthews. 616 pages. 2000. 0-7808-0389-2. $78.

"It is a must for libraries with a consumer health section." —*American Reference Books Annual 2002*

"A much needed addition to the Omnigraphics *Health Reference Series*. A current reference work to provide people with disabilities, their families, caregivers or those who work with them, a broad range of information in one volume, has not been available until now. . . . It is recommended for all public and academic library reference collections." —*E-Streams, May '01*

"An excellent source book in easy-to-read format covering many current topics; highly recommended for all libraries." —*Choice, Association of College and Research Libraries, Jan '01*

"Recommended reference source."
—*Booklist, American Library Association, Jul '00*

Domestic Violence & Child Abuse Sourcebook

Basic Consumer Health Information about Spousal/ Partner, Child, Sibling, Parent, and Elder Abuse, Covering Physical, Emotional, and Sexual Abuse, Teen Dating Violence, and Stalking; Includes Information about Hotlines, Safe Houses, Safety Plans, and Other Resources for Support and Assistance, Community Initiatives, and Reports on Current Directions in Research and Treatment

Along with a Glossary, Sources for Further Reading, and Governmental and Non-Governmental Organizations Contact Information

Edited by Helene Henderson. 1,064 pages. 2001. 0-7808-0235-7. $78.

"This is important information. The Web has many resources but this sourcebook fills an important societal need. I am not aware of any other resources of this type." —*Doody's Review Service, Sep '01*

"Recommended for all libraries, scholars, and practitioners." —*Choice, Association of College & Research Libraries, Jul '01*

"Recommended reference source."
—*Booklist, American Library Association, Apr '01*

"Important pick for college-level health reference libraries." —*The Bookwatch, Mar '01*

"Because this problem is so widespread and because this book includes a lot of issues within one volume, this work is recommended for all public libraries." —*American Reference Books Annual, 2001*

Drug Abuse Sourcebook

Basic Consumer Health Information about Illicit Substances of Abuse and the Diversion of Prescription Medications, Including Depressants, Hallucinogens, Inhalants, Marijuana, Narcotics, Stimulants, and Anabolic Steroids

Along with Facts about Related Health Risks, Treatment Issues, and Substance Abuse Prevention Programs, a Glossary of Terms, Statistical Data, and Directories of Hotline Services, Self-Help Groups, and Organizations Able to Provide Further Information

Edited by Karen Bellenir. 629 pages. 2000. 0-7808-0242-X. $78.

"Containing a wealth of information, this book will be useful to the college student just beginning to explore the topic of substance abuse. This resource belongs in libraries that serve a lower-division undergraduate or community college clientele as well as the general public." —*Choice, Association of College and Research Libraries, Jun '01*

"Recommended reference source."
—*Booklist, American Library Association, Feb '01*

"Highly recommended." —*The Bookwatch, Jan '01*

"Even though there is a plethora of books on drug abuse, this volume is recommended for school, public, and college libraries." —*American Reference Books Annual, 2001*

SEE ALSO *Alcoholism Sourcebook, Substance Abuse Sourcebook*

Ear, Nose & Throat Disorders Sourcebook

Basic Information about Disorders of the Ears, Nose, Sinus Cavities, Pharynx, and Larynx, Including Ear Infections, Tinnitus, Vestibular Disorders, Allergic and Non-Allergic Rhinitis, Sore Throats, Tonsillitis, and Cancers That Affect the Ears, Nose, Sinuses, and Throat

Along with Reports on Current Research Initiatives, a Glossary of Related Medical Terms, and a Directory of Sources for Further Help and Information

Edited by Karen Bellenir and Linda M. Shin. 576 pages. 1998. 0-7808-0206-3. $78.

529

■

Eating Disorders Sourcebook

Basic Consumer Health Information about Eating Disorders, Including Information about Anorexia Nervosa, Bulimia Nervosa, Binge Eating, Body Dysmorphic Disorder, Pica, Laxative Abuse, and Night Eating Syndrome

Along with Information about Causes, Adverse Effects, and Treatment and Prevention Issues, and Featuring a Section on Concerns Specific to Children and Adolescents, a Glossary, and Resources for Further Help and Information

Edited by Dawn D. Matthews. 322 pages. 2001. 0-7808-0335-3. $78.

■

Emergency Medical Services Sourcebook

Basic Consumer Health Information about Preventing, Preparing for, and Managing Emergency Situations, When and Who to Call for Help, What to Expect in the Emergency Room, the Emergency Medical Team, Patient Issues, and Current Topics in Emergency Medicine

Along with Statistical Data, a Glossary, and Sources of Additional Help and Information

Edited by Jenni Lynn Colson. 494 pages. 2002. 0-7808-0420-1. $78.

■

Endocrine & Metabolic Disorders Sourcebook

Basic Information for the Layperson about Pancreatic and Insulin-Related Disorders Such as Pancreatitis, Diabetes, and Hypoglycemia; Adrenal Gland Disorders Such as Cushing's Syndrome, Addison's Disease, and Congenital Adrenal Hyperplasia; Pituitary Gland Disorders Such as Growth Hormone Deficiency, Acromegaly, and Pituitary Tumors; Thyroid Disorders Such as Hypothyroidism, Graves' Disease, Hashimoto's Disease, and Goiter; Hyperparathyroidism; and Other Diseases and Syndromes of Hormone Imbalance or Metabolic Dysfunction

Along with Reports on Current Research Initiatives

Edited by Linda M. Shin. 574 pages. 1998. 0-7808-0207-1. $78.

■

Environmentally Induced Disorders Sourcebook

Basic Information about Diseases and Syndromes Linked to Exposure to Pollutants and Other Substances in Outdoor and Indoor Environments Such as Lead, Asbestos, Formaldehyde, Mercury, Emissions, Noise, and More

Edited by Allan R. Cook. 620 pages. 1997. 0-7808-0083-4. $78.

■

Ethnic Diseases Sourcebook

Basic Consumer Health Information for Ethnic and Racial Minority Groups in the United States, Including General Health. Indicators and Behaviors, Ethnic Diseases, Genetic Testing, the Impact of Chronic Diseases, Women's Health, Mental Health Issues, and Preventive Health Care Services

Along with a Glossary and a Listing of Additional Resources

Edited by Joyce Brennfleck Shannon. 664 pages. 2001. 0-7808-0336-1. $78.

"Will prove valuable to any library seeking to maintain a current, comprehensive reference collection of health resources.... An excellent source of health information about genetic disorders which affect particular ethnic and racial minorities in the U.S."
— *The Bookwatch, Aug '01*

■

Eye Care Sourcebook, 2nd Edition

Basic Consumer Health Information about Eye Care and Eye Disorders, Including Facts about the Diagnosis, Prevention, and Treatment of Common Refractive Problems Such as Myopia, Hyperopia, Astigmatism, and Presbyopia, and Eye Diseases, Including Glaucoma, Cataract, Age-Related Macular Degeneration, and Diabetic Retinopathy

Along with a Section on Vision Correction and Refractive Surgeries, Including LASIK and LASEK, a Glossary, and Directories of Resources for Additional Help and Information

Edited by Amy L. Sutton. 543 pages. 2003. 0-7808-0635-2. $78.

■

Family Planning Sourcebook

Basic Consumer Health Information about Planning for Pregnancy and Contraception, Including Traditional Methods, Barrier Methods, Hormonal Methods, Permanent Methods, Future Methods, Emergency Contraception, and Birth Control Choices for Women at Each Stage of Life

Along with Statistics, a Glossary, and Sources of Additional Information

Edited by Amy Marcaccio Keyzer. 520 pages. 2001. 0-7808-0379-5. $78.

"Recommended for public, health, and undergraduate libraries as part of the circulating collection."
— *E-Streams, Mar '02*

"Information is presented in an unbiased, readable manner, and the sourcebook will certainly be a necessary addition to those public and high school libraries where Internet access is restricted or otherwise problematic." — *American Reference Books Annual 2002*

"Recommended reference source."
— *Booklist, American Library Association, Oct '01*

"Will prove valuable to any library seeking to maintain a current, comprehensive reference collection of health resources.... Excellent reference."
— *The Bookwatch, Aug '01*

SEE ALSO *Pregnancy & Birth Sourcebook*

■

Fitness & Exercise Sourcebook, 1st Edition

Basic Information on Fitness and Exercise, Including Fitness Activities for Specific Age Groups, Exercise for People with Specific Medical Conditions, How to Begin a Fitness Program in Running, Walking, Swimming, Cycling, and Other Athletic Activities, and Recent Research in Fitness and Exercise

Edited by Dan R. Harris. 663 pages. 1996. 0-7808-0186-5. $78.

"A good resource for general readers." — *Choice, Association of College and Research Libraries, Nov '97*

"The perennial popularity of the topic . . . make this an appealing selection for public libraries."
— *Rettig on Reference, Jun/Jul '97*

■

Fitness & Exercise Sourcebook, 2nd Edition

Basic Consumer Health Information about the Fundamentals of Fitness and Exercise, Including How to Begin and Maintain a Fitness Program, Fitness as a Lifestyle, the Link between Fitness and Diet, Advice for Specific Groups of People, Exercise as It Relates to Specific Medical Conditions, and Recent Research in Fitness and Exercise

Along with a Glossary of Important Terms and Resources for Additional Help and Information

Edited by Kristen M. Gledhill. 646 pages. 2001. 0-7808-0334-5. $78.

"This work is recommended for all general reference collections."
— *American Reference Books Annual 2002*

"Highly recommended for public, consumer, and school grades fourth through college."
— *E-Streams, Nov '01*

"Recommended reference source." — *Booklist, American Library Association, Oct '01*

"The information appears quite comprehensive and is considered reliable. . . . This second edition is a welcomed addition to the series."
— *Doody's Review Service, Sep '01*

"This reference is a valuable choice for those who desire a broad source of information on exercise, fitness, and chronic-disease prevention through a healthy lifestyle." — *American Medical Writers Association Journal, Fall '01*

"Will prove valuable to any library seeking to maintain a current, comprehensive reference collection of health resources. . . . Excellent reference."
— *The Bookwatch, Aug '01*

■

Food & Animal Borne Diseases Sourcebook

Basic Information about Diseases That Can Be Spread to Humans through the Ingestion of Contaminated Food or Water or by Contact with Infected Animals and Insects, Such as Botulism, E. Coli, Hepatitis A, Trichinosis, Lyme Disease, and Rabies

Along with Information Regarding Prevention and Treatment Methods, and Including a Special Section for International Travelers Describing Diseases Such as Cholera, Malaria, Travelers' Diarrhea, and Yellow Fever, and Offering Recommendations for Avoiding Illness

Edited by Karen Bellenir and Peter D. Dresser. 535 pages. 1995. 0-7808-0033-8. $78.

"Targeting general readers and providing them with a single, comprehensive source of information on selected topics, this book continues, with the excellent caliber of its predecessors, to catalog topical information on health matters of general interest. Readable and thorough, this valuable resource is highly recommended for all libraries."
— *Academic Library Book Review, Summer '96*

"A comprehensive collection of authoritative information."   — *Emergency Medical Services, Oct '95*

■

Food Safety Sourcebook

Basic Consumer Health Information about the Safe Handling of Meat, Poultry, Seafood, Eggs, Fruit Juices, and Other Food Items, and Facts about Pesticides, Drinking Water, Food Safety Overseas, and the Onset, Duration, and Symptoms of Foodborne Illnesses, Including Types of Pathogenic Bacteria, Parasitic Protozoa, Worms, Viruses, and Natural Toxins

Along with the Role of the Consumer, the Food Handler, and the Government in Food Safety; a Glossary, and Resources for Additional Help and Information

Edited by Dawn D. Matthews. 339 pages. 1999. 0-7808-0326-4. $78.

"This book is recommended for public libraries and universities with home economic and food science programs."   — *E-Streams, Nov '00*

"Recommended reference source."
— *Booklist, American Library Association, May '00*

"This book takes the complex issues of food safety and foodborne pathogens and presents them in an easily understood manner. [It does] an excellent job of covering a large and often confusing topic."
— *American Reference Books Annual, 2000*

■

Forensic Medicine Sourcebook

Basic Consumer Information for the Layperson about Forensic Medicine, Including Crime Scene Investigation, Evidence Collection and Analysis, Expert Testimony, Computer-Aided Criminal Identification, Digital Imaging in the Courtroom, DNA Profiling, Accident Reconstruction, Autopsies, Ballistics, Drugs and Explosives Detection, Latent Fingerprints, Product Tampering, and Questioned Document Examination

Along with Statistical Data, a Glossary of Forensics Terminology, and Listings of Sources for Further Help and Information

Edited by Annemarie S. Muth. 574 pages. 1999. 0-7808-0232-2. $78.

"Given the expected widespread interest in its content and its easy to read style, this book is recommended for most public and all college and university libraries."
— *E-Streams, Feb '01*

"Recommended for public libraries."
— *Reference & User Services Quarterly, American Library Association, Spring 2000*

"Recommended reference source."
— *Booklist, American Library Association, Feb '00*

"A wealth of information, useful statistics, references are up-to-date and extremely complete. This wonderful collection of data will help students who are interested in a career in any type of forensic field. It is a great resource for attorneys who need information about types of expert witnesses needed in a particular case. It also offers useful information for fiction and nonfiction writers whose work involves a crime. A fascinating compilation. All levels."   — *Choice, Association of College and Research Libraries, Jan 2000*

"There are several items that make this book attractive to consumers who are seeking certain forensic data. . . . This is a useful current source for those seeking general forensic medical answers."
— *American Reference Books Annual, 2000*

■

Gastrointestinal Diseases & Disorders Sourcebook

Basic Information about Gastroesophageal Reflux Disease (Heartburn), Ulcers, Diverticulosis, Irritable Bowel Syndrome, Crohn's Disease, Ulcerative Colitis, Diarrhea, Constipation, Lactose Intolerance, Hemorrhoids, Hepatitis, Cirrhosis, and Other Digestive Problems, Featuring Statistics, Descriptions of Symptoms, and Current Treatment Methods of Interest for Persons Living with Upper and Lower Gastrointestinal Maladies

Edited by Linda M. Ross. 413 pages. 1996. 0-7808-0078-8. $78.

". . . very readable form. The successful editorial work that brought this material together into a useful and understandable reference makes accessible to all readers information that can help them more effectively understand and obtain help for digestive tract problems."
— *Choice, Association of College & Research Libraries, Feb '97*

SEE ALSO Diet & Nutrition Sourcebook, 1st and 2nd Editions, Digestive Diseases & Disorders

■

Genetic Disorders Sourcebook, 1st Edition

Basic Information about Heritable Diseases and Disorders Such as Down Syndrome, PKU, Hemophilia, Von Willebrand Disease, Gaucher Disease, Tay-Sachs Disease, and Sickle-Cell Disease, Along with Information about Genetic Screening, Gene Therapy, Home Care, and Including Source Listings for Further Help and Information on More Than 300 Disorders

Edited by Karen Bellenir. 642 pages. 1996. 0-7808-0034-6. $78.

"Recommended for undergraduate libraries or libraries that serve the public."
— *Science & Technology Libraries, Vol. 18, No. 1, '99*

"Provides essential medical information to both the general public and those diagnosed with a serious or fatal genetic disease or disorder." —*Choice, Association of College and Research Libraries, Jan '97*

"Geared toward the lay public. It would be well placed in all public libraries and in those hospital and medical libraries in which access to genetic references is limited." — *Doody's Health Sciences Book Review, Oct '96*

Genetic Disorders Sourcebook, 2nd Edition

Basic Consumer Health Information about Hereditary Diseases and Disorders, Including Cystic Fibrosis, Down Syndrome, Hemophilia, Huntington's Disease, Sickle Cell Anemia, and More; Facts about Genes, Gene Research and Therapy, Genetic Screening, Ethics of Gene Testing, Genetic Counseling, and Advice on Coping and Caring

Along with a Glossary of Genetic Terminology and a Resource List for Help, Support, and Further Information

Edited by Kathy Massimini. 768 pages. 2001. 0-7808-0241-1. $78.

"Recommended for public libraries and medical and hospital libraries with consumer health collections." —*E-Streams, May '01*

"Recommended reference source." —*Booklist, American Library Association, Apr '01*

"Important pick for college-level health reference libraries." —*The Bookwatch, Mar '01*

Head Trauma Sourcebook

Basic Information for the Layperson about Open-Head and Closed-Head Injuries, Treatment Advances, Recovery, and Rehabilitation

Along with Reports on Current Research Initiatives

Edited by Karen Bellenir. 414 pages. 1997. 0-7808-0208-X. $78.

Headache Sourcebook

Basic Consumer Health Information about Migraine, Tension, Cluster, Rebound and Other Types of Headaches, with Facts about the Cause and Prevention of Headaches, the Effects of Stress and the Environment, Headaches during Pregnancy and Menopause, and Childhood Headaches

Along with a Glossary and Other Resources for Additional Help and Information

Edited by Dawn D. Matthews. 362 pages. 2002. 0-7808-0337-X. $78.

"Highly recommended for academic and medical reference collections." —*Library Bookwatch, Sep '02*

Health Insurance Sourcebook

Basic Information about Managed Care Organizations, Traditional Fee-for-Service Insurance, Insurance Portability and Pre-Existing Conditions Clauses, Medicare, Medicaid, Social Security, and Military Health Care

Along with Information about Insurance Fraud

Edited by Wendy Wilcox. 530 pages. 1997. 0-7808-0222-5. $78.

"Particularly useful because it brings much of this information together in one volume. This book will be a handy reference source in the health sciences library, hospital library, college and university library, and medium to large public library." —*Medical Reference Services Quarterly, Fall '98*

Awarded "Books of the Year Award" —*American Journal of Nursing, 1997*

"The layout of the book is particularly helpful as it provides easy access to reference material. A most useful addition to the vast amount of information about health insurance. The use of data from U.S. government agencies is most commendable. Useful in a library or learning center for healthcare professional students." —*Doody's Health Sciences Book Reviews, Nov '97*

Health Reference Series Cumulative Index 1999

A Comprehensive Index to the Individual Volumes of the Health Reference Series, Including a Subject Index, Name Index, Organization Index, and Publication Index

Along with a Master List of Acronyms and Abbreviations

Edited by Edward J. Prucha, Anne Holmes, and Robert Rudnick. 990 pages. 2000. 0-7808-0382-5. $78.

"This volume will be most helpful in libraries that have a relatively complete collection of the Health Reference Series." —*American Reference Books Annual, 2001*

"Essential for collections that hold any of the numerous *Health Reference Series* titles." —*Choice, Association of College and Research Libraries, Nov '00*

Healthy Aging Sourcebook

Basic Consumer Health Information about Maintaining Health through the Aging Process, Including Advice on Nutrition, Exercise, and Sleep, Help in Making Decisions about Midlife Issues and Retirement, and Guidance Concerning Practical and Informed Choices in Health Consumerism

Along with Data Concerning the Theories of Aging, Different Experiences in Aging by Minority Groups, and Facts about Aging Now and Aging in the Future; and Featuring a Glossary, a Guide to Consumer Help, Additional Suggested Reading, and Practical Resource Directory

Edited by Jenifer Swanson. 536 pages. 1999. 0-7808-0390-6. $78.

"Recommended reference source."
—*Booklist, American Library Association, Feb '00*

SEE ALSO Physical & Mental Issues in Aging Sourcebook

Healthy Heart Sourcebook for Women

Basic Consumer Health Information about Cardiac Issues Specific to Women, Including Facts about Major Risk Factors and Prevention, Treatment and Control Strategies, and Important Dietary Issues

Along with a Special Section Regarding the Pros and Cons of Hormone Replacement Therapy and Its Impact on Heart Health, and Additional Help, Including Recipes, a Glossary, and a Directory of Resources

Edited by Dawn D. Matthews. 336 pages. 2000. 0-7808-0329-9. $78.

"A good reference source and recommended for all public, academic, medical, and hospital libraries."
—*Medical Reference Services Quarterly, Summer '01*

"Because of the lack of information specific to women on this topic, this book is recommended for public libraries and consumer libraries."
—*American Reference Books Annual, 2001*

"Contains very important information about coronary artery disease that all women should know. The information is current and presented in an easy-to-read format. The book will make a good addition to any library." —*American Medical Writers Association Journal, Summer '00*

"Important, basic reference."
—*Reviewer's Bookwatch, Jul '00*

SEE ALSO Cardiovascular Diseases & Disorders Sourcebook, 1st Edition, Heart Diseases & Disorders Sourcebook, 2nd Edition, Women's Health Concerns Sourcebook

---

Heart Diseases & Disorders Sourcebook, 2nd Edition

Basic Consumer Health Information about Heart Attacks, Angina, Rhythm Disorders, Heart Failure, Valve Disease, Congenital Heart Disorders, and More, Including Descriptions of Surgical Procedures and Other Interventions, Medications, Cardiac Rehabilitation, Risk Identification, and Prevention Tips

Along with Statistical Data, Reports on Current Research Initiatives, a Glossary of Cardiovascular Terms, and Resource Directory

Edited by Karen Bellenir. 612 pages. 2000. 0-7808-0238-1. $78.

"This work stands out as an imminently accessible resource for the general public. It is recommended for the reference and circulating shelves of school, public, and academic libraries."
—*American Reference Books Annual, 2001*

"Recommended reference source."
—*Booklist, American Library Association, Dec '00*

"Provides comprehensive coverage of matters related to the heart. This title is recommended for health sciences and public libraries with consumer health collections."
—*E-Streams, Oct '00*

SEE ALSO Cardiovascular Diseases & Disorders Sourcebook, 1st Edition; Healthy Heart Sourcebook for Women

---

Household Safety Sourcebook

Basic Consumer Health Information about Household Safety, Including Information about Poisons, Chemicals, Fire, and Water Hazards in the Home

Along with Advice about the Safe Use of Home Maintenance Equipment, Choosing Toys and Nursery Furniture, Holiday and Recreation Safety, a Glossary, and Resources for Further Help and Information

Edited by Dawn D. Matthews. 606 pages. 2002. 0-7808-0338-8. $78.

"As a sourcebook on household safety this book meets its mark. It is encyclopedic in scope and covers a wide range of safety issues that are commonly seen in the home." —*E-Streams, Jul '02*

Immune System Disorders Sourcebook

Basic Information about Lupus, Multiple Sclerosis, Guillain-Barré Syndrome, Chronic Granulomatous Disease, and More

Along with Statistical and Demographic Data and Reports on Current Research Initiatives

Edited by Allan R. Cook. 608 pages. 1997. 0-7808-0209-8. $78.

Infant & Toddler Health Sourcebook

Basic Consumer Health Information about the Physical and Mental Development of Newborns, Infants, and Toddlers, Including Neonatal Concerns, Nutrition Recommendations, Immunization Schedules, Common Pediatric Disorders, Assessments and Milestones, Safety Tips, and Advice for Parents and Other Caregivers

Along with a Glossary of Terms and Resource Listings for Additional Help

Edited by Jenifer Swanson. 585 pages. 2000. 0-7808-0246-2. $78.

"As a reference for the general public, this would be useful in any library." —*E-Streams, May '01*

"Recommended reference source."
—*Booklist, American Library Association, Feb '01*

"This is a good source for general use."
—*American Reference Books Annual, 2001*

Injury & Trauma Sourcebook

Basic Consumer Health Information about the Impact of Injury, the Diagnosis and Treatment of Common and Traumatic Injuries, Emergency Care, and Specific Injuries Related to Home, Community, Workplace, Transportation, and Recreation

Along with Guidelines for Injury Prevention, a Glossary, and a Directory of Additional Resources

Edited by Joyce Brennfleck Shannon. 696 pages. 2002. 0-7808-0421-X. $78.

"Practitioners should be aware of guides such as this in order to facilitate their use by patients and their families." — *Doody's Health Sciences Book Review Journal, Sep-Oct '02*

"Recommended reference source." — *Booklist, American Library Association, Sep '02*

"Highly recommended for academic and medical reference collections." — *Library Bookwatch, Sep '02*

■

Kidney & Urinary Tract Diseases & Disorders Sourcebook

Basic Information about Kidney Stones, Urinary Incontinence, Bladder Disease, End Stage Renal Disease, Dialysis, and More

Along with Statistical and Demographic Data and Reports on Current Research Initiatives

Edited by Linda M. Ross. 602 pages. 1997. 0-7808-0079-6. $78.

■

Learning Disabilities Sourcebook, 1st Edition

Basic Information about Disorders Such as Dyslexia, Visual and Auditory Processing Deficits, Attention Deficit/Hyperactivity Disorder, and Autism

Along with Statistical and Demographic Data, Reports on Current Research Initiatives, an Explanation of the Assessment Process, and a Special Section for Adults with Learning Disabilities

Edited by Linda M. Shin. 579 pages. 1998. 0-7808-0210-1. $78.

Named "Outstanding Reference Book of 1999." — *New York Public Library, Feb 2000*

"An excellent candidate for inclusion in a public library reference section. It's a great source of information. Teachers will also find the book useful. Definitely worth reading." — *Journal of Adolescent & Adult Literacy, Feb 2000*

"Readable . . . provides a solid base of information regarding successful techniques used with individuals who have learning disabilities, as well as practical suggestions for educators and family members. Clear language, concise descriptions, and pertinent information for contacting multiple resources add to the strength of this book as a useful tool." — *Choice, Association of College and Research Libraries, Feb '99*

"Recommended reference source." — *Booklist, American Library Association, Sep '98*

"A useful resource for libraries and for those who don't have the time to identify and locate the individual publications." — *Disability Resources Monthly, Sep '98*

■

Learning Disabilities Sourcebook, 2nd Edition

Basic Consumer Health Information about Learning Disabilities, Including Dyslexia, Developmental Speech and Language Disabilities, Non-Verbal Learning Disorders, Developmental Arithmetic Disorder, Developmental Writing Disorder, and Other Conditions That Impede Learning Such as Attention Deficit/ Hyperactivity Disorder, Brain Injury, Hearing Impairment, Klinefelter Syndrome, Dyspraxia, and Tourette Syndrome

Along with Facts about Educational Issues and Assistive Technology, Coping Strategies, a Glossary of Related Terms, and Resources for Further Help and Information

Edited by Dawn D. Matthews. 621 pages. 2003. 0-7808-0626-3. $78.

■

Liver Disorders Sourcebook

Basic Consumer Health Information about the Liver and How It Works; Liver Diseases, Including Cancer, Cirrhosis, Hepatitis, and Toxic and Drug Related Diseases; Tips for Maintaining a Healthy Liver; Laboratory Tests, Radiology Tests, and Facts about Liver Transplantation

Along with a Section on Support Groups, a Glossary, and Resource Listings

Edited by Joyce Brennfleck Shannon. 591 pages. 2000. 0-7808-0383-3. $78.

"A valuable resource." — *American Reference Books Annual, 2001*

"This title is recommended for health sciences and public libraries with consumer health collections." — *E-Streams, Oct '00*

"Recommended reference source." — *Booklist, American Library Association, Jun '00*

■

Lung Disorders Sourcebook

Basic Consumer Health Information about Emphysema, Pneumonia, Tuberculosis, Asthma, Cystic Fibrosis, and Other Lung Disorders, Including Facts about Diagnostic Procedures, Treatment Strategies, Disease Prevention Efforts, and Such Risk Factors as Smoking, Air Pollution, and Exposure to Asbestos, Radon, and Other Agents

Along with a Glossary and Resources for Additional Help and Information

Edited by Dawn D. Matthews. 678 pages. 2002. 0-7808-0339-6. $78.

■

Medical Tests Sourcebook

Basic Consumer Health Information about Medical Tests, Including Periodic Health Exams, General Screening Tests, Tests You Can Do at Home, Findings of the U.S. Preventive Services Task Force, X-ray and Radiology Tests, Electrical Tests, Tests of Blood and Other Body Fluids and Tissues, Scope Tests, Lung Tests, Genetic Tests, Pregnancy Tests, Newborn Screening Tests, Sexually Transmitted Disease Tests, and Computer Aided Diagnoses

Along with a Section on Paying for Medical Tests, a Glossary, and Resource Listings

Edited by Joyce Brennfleck Shannon. 691 pages. 1999. 0-7808-0243-8. $78.

■

Men's Health Concerns Sourcebook

Basic Information about Health Issues That Affect Men, Featuring Facts about the Top Causes of Death in Men, Including Heart Disease, Stroke, Cancers, Prostate Disorders, Chronic Obstructive Pulmonary Disease, Pneumonia and Influenza, Human Immunodeficiency Virus and Acquired Immune Deficiency Syndrome, Diabetes Mellitus, Stress, Suicide, Accidents and Homicides; and Facts about Common Concerns for Men, Including Impotence, Contraception, Circumcision, Sleep Disorders, Snoring, Hair Loss, Diet, Nutrition, Exercise, Kidney and Urological Disorders, and Backaches

Edited by Allan R. Cook. 738 pages. 1998. 0-7808-0212-8. $78.

Mental Health Disorders Sourcebook, 1st Edition

Basic Information about Schizophrenia, Depression, Bipolar Disorder, Panic Disorder, Obsessive-Compulsive Disorder, Phobias and Other Anxiety Disorders, Paranoia and Other Personality Disorders, Eating Disorders, and Sleep Disorders

Along with Information about Treatment and Therapies

Edited by Karen Bellenir. 548 pages. 1995. 0-7808-0040-0. $78.

■

Mental Health Disorders Sourcebook, 2nd Edition

Basic Consumer Health Information about Anxiety Disorders, Depression and Other Mood Disorders, Eating Disorders, Personality Disorders, Schizophrenia, and More, Including Disease Descriptions, Treatment Options, and Reports on Current Research Initiatives

Along with Statistical Data, Tips for Maintaining Mental Health, a Glossary, and Directory of Sources for Additional Help and Information

Edited by Karen Bellenir. 605 pages. 2000. 0-7808-0240-3. $78.

Mental Retardation Sourcebook

Basic Consumer Health Information about Mental Retardation and Its Causes, Including Down Syndrome, Fetal Alcohol Syndrome, Fragile X Syndrome, Genetic Conditions, Injury, and Environmental Sources

Along with Preventive Strategies, Parenting Issues, Educational Implications, Health Care Needs, Employment and Economic Matters, Legal Issues, a Glossary, and a Resource Listing for Additional Help and Information

Edited by Joyce Brennfleck Shannon. 642 pages. 2000. 0-7808-0377-9. $78.

"Public libraries will find the book useful for reference and as a beginning research point for students, parents, and caregivers."
—*American Reference Books Annual, 2001*

"The strength of this work is that it compiles many basic fact sheets and addresses for further information in one volume. It is intended and suitable for the general public. This sourcebook is relevant to any collection providing health information to the general public."
—*E-Streams, Nov '00*

"From preventing retardation to parenting and family challenges, this covers health, social and legal issues and will prove an invaluable overview."
—*Reviewer's Bookwatch, Jul '00*

■

Movement Disorders Sourcebook

Basic Consumer Health Information about Neurological Movement Disorders, Including Essential Tremor, Parkinson's Disease, Dystonia, Cerebral Palsy, Huntington's Disease, Myasthenia Gravis, Multiple Sclerosis, and Other Early-Onset and Adult-Onset Movement Disorders, Their Symptoms and Causes, Diagnostic Tests, and Treatments

Along with Mobility and Assistive Technology Information, a Glossary, and a Directory of Additional Resources

Edited by Joyce Brennfleck Shannon. 655 pages. 2003. 0-7808-0628-X. $78.

■

Obesity Sourcebook

Basic Consumer Health Information about Diseases and Other Problems Associated with Obesity, and Including Facts about Risk Factors, Prevention Issues, and Management Approaches

Along with Statistical and Demographic Data, Information about Special Populations, Research Updates, a Glossary, and Source Listings for Further Help and Information

Edited by Wilma Caldwell and Chad T. Kimball. 376 pages. 2001. 0-7808-0333-7. $78.

"The book synthesizes the reliable medical literature on obesity into one easy-to-read and useful resource for the general public."
—*American Reference Books Annual 2002*

"This is a very useful resource book for the lay public."
—*Doody's Review Service, Nov '01*

"Well suited for the health reference collection of a public library or an academic health science library that serves the general population." —*E-Streams, Sep '01*

"Recommended reference source."
—*Booklist, American Library Association, Apr '01*

" Recommended pick both for specialty health library collections and any general consumer health reference collection." —*The Bookwatch, Apr '01*

■

Ophthalmic Disorders Sourcebook

Basic Information about Glaucoma, Cataracts, Macular Degeneration, Strabismus, Refractive Disorders, and More

Along with Statistical and Demographic Data and Reports on Current Research Initiatives

Edited by Linda M. Ross. 631 pages. 1996. 0-7808-0081-8. $78.

SEE ALSO *Eye Care Sourcebook, 2nd Edition*

■

Oral Health Sourcebook

Basic Information about Diseases and Conditions Affecting Oral Health, Including Cavities, Gum Disease, Dry Mouth, Oral Cancers, Fever Blisters, Canker Sores, Oral Thrush, Bad Breath, Temporomandibular Disorders, and other Craniofacial Syndromes

Along with Statistical Data on the Oral Health of Americans, Oral Hygiene, Emergency First Aid, Information on Treatment Procedures and Methods of Replacing Lost Teeth

Edited by Allan R. Cook. 558 pages. 1997. 0-7808-0082-6. $78.

"Unique source which will fill a gap in dental sources for patients and the lay public. A valuable reference tool even in a library with thousands of books on dentistry. Comprehensive, clear, inexpensive, and easy to read and use. It fills an enormous gap in the health care literature." —*Reference and User Services Quarterly, American Library Association, Summer '98*

"Recommended reference source."
—*Booklist, American Library Association, Dec '97*

■

Osteoporosis Sourcebook

Basic Consumer Health Information about Primary and Secondary Osteoporosis and Juvenile Osteoporosis and Related Conditions, Including Fibrous Dysplasia, Gaucher Disease, Hyperthyroidism, Hypophosphatasia, Myeloma, Osteopetrosis, Osteogenesis Imperfecta, and Paget's Disease

Along with Information about Risk Factors, Treatments, Traditional and Non-Traditional Pain Management, a Glossary of Related Terms, and a Directory of Resources

Edited by Allan R. Cook. 584 pages. 2001. 0-7808-0239-X. $78.

"This would be a book to be kept in a staff or patient library. The targeted audience is the layperson, but the therapist who needs a quick bit of information on a particular topic will also find the book useful."
— *Physical Therapy, Jan '02*

"This resource is recommended as a great reference source for public, health, and academic libraries, and is another triumph for the editors of Omnigraphics."
— *American Reference Books Annual 2002*

"Recommended for all public libraries and general health collections, especially those supporting patient education or consumer health programs."
—*E-Streams, Nov '01*

"Will prove valuable to any library seeking to maintain a current, comprehensive reference collection of health resources. . . . From prevention to treatment and associated conditions, this provides an excellent survey."
—*The Bookwatch, Aug '01*

"Recommended reference source."
—*Booklist, American Library Association, July '01*

SEE ALSO *Women's Health Concerns Sourcebook*

■

Pain Sourcebook, 1st Edition

Basic Information about Specific Forms of Acute and Chronic Pain, Including Headaches, Back Pain, Muscular Pain, Neuralgia, Surgical Pain, and Cancer Pain

Along with Pain Relief Options Such as Analgesics, Narcotics, Nerve Blocks, Transcutaneous Nerve Stimulation, and Alternative Forms of Pain Control, Including Biofeedback, Imaging, Behavior Modification, and Relaxation Techniques

Edited by Allan R. Cook. 667 pages. 1997. 0-7808-0213-6. $78.

"The text is readable, easily understood, and well indexed. This excellent volume belongs in all patient education libraries, consumer health sections of public libraries, and many personal collections."
— *American Reference Books Annual, 1999*

"A beneficial reference." — *Booklist Health Sciences Supplement, American Library Association, Oct '98*

"The information is basic in terms of scholarship and is appropriate for general readers. Written in journalistic style . . . intended for non-professionals. Quite thorough in its coverage of different pain conditions and summarizes the latest clinical information regarding pain treatment." — *Choice, Association of College and Research Libraries, Jun '98*

"Recommended reference source."
—*Booklist, American Library Association, Mar '98*

■

Pain Sourcebook, 2nd Edition

Basic Consumer Health Information about Specific Forms of Acute and Chronic Pain, Including Muscle and Skeletal Pain, Nerve Pain, Cancer Pain, and Disorders Characterized by Pain, Such as Fibromyalgia, Shingles, Angina, Arthritis, and Headaches

Along with Information about Pain Medications and Management Techniques, Complementary and Alternative Pain Relief Options, Tips for People Living with Chronic Pain, a Glossary, and a Directory of Sources for Further Information

Edited by Karen Bellenir. 670 pages. 2002. 0-7808-0612-3. $78.

■

Pediatric Cancer Sourcebook

Basic Consumer Health Information about Leukemias, Brain Tumors, Sarcomas, Lymphomas, and Other Cancers in Infants, Children, and Adolescents, Including Descriptions of Cancers, Treatments, and Coping Strategies

Along with Suggestions for Parents, Caregivers, and Concerned Relatives, a Glossary of Cancer Terms, and Resource Listings

Edited by Edward J. Prucha. 587 pages. 1999. 0-7808-0245-4. $78.

"An excellent source of information. Recommended for public, hospital, and health science libraries with consumer health collections." — *E-Streams, Jun '00*

"Recommended reference source."
— *Booklist, American Library Association, Feb '00*

"A valuable addition to all libraries specializing in health services and many public libraries."
—*American Reference Books Annual, 2000*

■

Physical & Mental Issues in Aging Sourcebook

Basic Consumer Health Information on Physical and Mental Disorders Associated with the Aging Process, Including Concerns about Cardiovascular Disease, Pulmonary Disease, Oral Health, Digestive Disorders, Musculoskeletal and Skin Disorders, Metabolic Changes, Sexual and Reproductive Issues, and Changes in Vision, Hearing, and Other Senses

Along with Data about Longevity and Causes of Death, Information on Acute and Chronic Pain, Descriptions of Mental Concerns, a Glossary of Terms, and Resource Listings for Additional Help

Edited by Jenifer Swanson. 660 pages. 1999. 0-7808-0233-0. $78.

"This is a treasure of health information for the layperson." — *Choice Health Sciences Supplement, Association of College & Research Libraries, May 2000*

"Recommended for public libraries."
—*American Reference Books Annual, 2000*

"Recommended reference source."
— *Booklist, American Library Association, Oct '99*

SEE ALSO *Healthy Aging Sourcebook*

Podiatry Sourcebook

Basic Consumer Health Information about Foot Conditions, Diseases, and Injuries, Including Bunions, Corns, Calluses, Athlete's Foot, Plantar Warts, Hammertoes and Clawtoes, Clubfoot, Heel Pain, Gout, and More

Along with Facts about Foot Care, Disease Prevention, Foot Safety, Choosing a Foot Care Specialist, a Glossary of Terms, and Resource Listings for Additional Information

Edited by M. Lisa Weatherford. 380 pages. 2001. 0-7808-0215-2. $78.

"Recommended reference source."
— *Booklist, American Library Association, Feb '02*

"There is a lot of information presented here on a topic that is usually only covered sparingly in most larger comprehensive medical encyclopedias."
— *American Reference Books Annual 2002*

■

Pregnancy & Birth Sourcebook

Basic Information about Planning for Pregnancy, Maternal Health, Fetal Growth and Development, Labor and Delivery, Postpartum and Perinatal Care, Pregnancy in Mothers with Special Concerns, and Disorders of Pregnancy, Including Genetic Counseling, Nutrition and Exercise, Obstetrical Tests, Pregnancy Discomfort, Multiple Births, Cesarean Sections, Medical Testing of Newborns, Breastfeeding, Gestational Diabetes, and Ectopic Pregnancy

Edited by Heather E. Aldred. 737 pages. 1997. 0-7808-0216-0. $78.

"A well-organized handbook. Recommended."
— *Choice, Association of College and Research Libraries, Apr '98*

"Recommended reference source."
— *Booklist, American Library Association, Mar '98*

"Recommended for public libraries."
— *American Reference Books Annual, 1998*

SEE ALSO *Congenital Disorders Sourcebook, Family Planning Sourcebook*

■

Prostate Cancer Sourcebook

Basic Consumer Health Information about Prostate Cancer, Including Information about the Associated Risk Factors, Detection, Diagnosis, and Treatment of Prostate Cancer

Along with Information on Non-Malignant Prostate Conditions, and Featuring a Section Listing Support and Treatment Centers and a Glossary of Related Terms

Edited by Dawn D. Matthews. 358 pages. 2001. 0-7808-0324-8. $78.

"Recommended reference source."
— *Booklist, American Library Association, Jan '02*

"A valuable resource for health care consumers seeking information on the subject. . . .All text is written in a clear, easy-to-understand language that avoids technical jargon. Any library that collects consumer health resources would strengthen their collection with the addition of the *Prostate Cancer Sourcebook.*"
— *American Reference Books Annual 2002*

■

Public Health Sourcebook

Basic Information about Government Health Agencies, Including National Health Statistics and Trends, Healthy People 2000 Program Goals and Objectives, the Centers for Disease Control and Prevention, the Food and Drug Administration, and the National Institutes of Health

Along with Full Contact Information for Each Agency

Edited by Wendy Wilcox. 698 pages. 1998. 0-7808-0220-9. $78.

"Recommended reference source."
— *Booklist, American Library Association, Sep '98*

"This consumer guide provides welcome assistance in navigating the maze of federal health agencies and their data on public health concerns."
— *SciTech Book News, Sep '98*

■

Reconstructive & Cosmetic Surgery Sourcebook

Basic Consumer Health Information on Cosmetic and Reconstructive Plastic Surgery, Including Statistical Information about Different Surgical Procedures, Things to Consider Prior to Surgery, Plastic Surgery Techniques and Tools, Emotional and Psychological Considerations, and Procedure-Specific Information

Along with a Glossary of Terms and a Listing of Resources for Additional Help and Information

Edited by M. Lisa Weatherford. 374 pages. 2001. 0-7808-0214-4. $78.

"An excellent reference that addresses cosmetic and medically necessary reconstructive surgeries. . . . The style of the prose is calm and reassuring, discussing the many positive outcomes now available due to advances in surgical techniques."
— *American Reference Books Annual 2002*

"Recommended for health science libraries that are open to the public, as well as hospital libraries that are open to the patients. This book is a good resource for the consumer interested in plastic surgery."
— *E-Streams, Dec '01*

"Recommended reference source."
— *Booklist, American Library Association, July '01*

■

Rehabilitation Sourcebook

Basic Consumer Health Information about Rehabilitation for People Recovering from Heart Surgery, Spinal Cord Injury, Stroke, Orthopedic Impairments, Amputation, Pulmonary Impairments, Traumatic Injury, and More, Including Physical Therapy, Occupational Therapy, Speech/ Language Therapy, Massage Therapy, Dance Therapy, Art Therapy, and Recreational Therapy

Along with Information on Assistive and Adaptive Devices, a Glossary, and Resources for Additional Help and Information

Edited by Dawn D. Matthews. 531 pages. 1999. 0-7808-0236-5. $78.

"This is an excellent resource for public library reference and health collections."
—American Reference Books Annual, 2001

"Recommended reference source."
—Booklist, American Library Association, May '00

■

Respiratory Diseases & Disorders Sourcebook

Basic Information about Respiratory Diseases and Disorders, Including Asthma, Cystic Fibrosis, Pneumonia, the Common Cold, Influenza, and Others, Featuring Facts about the Respiratory System, Statistical and Demographic Data, Treatments, Self-Help Management Suggestions, and Current Research Initiatives

Edited by Allan R. Cook and Peter D. Dresser. 771 pages. 1995. 0-7808-0037-0. $78.

"Designed for the layperson and for patients and their families coping with respiratory illness. . . . an extensive array of information on diagnosis, treatment, management, and prevention of respiratory illnesses for the general reader."
—Choice, Association of College and Research Libraries, Jun '96

"A highly recommended text for all collections. It is a comforting reminder of the power of knowledge that good books carry between their covers."
—Academic Library Book Review, Spring '96

"A comprehensive collection of authoritative information presented in a nontechnical, humanitarian style for patients, families, and caregivers."
—Association of Operating Room Nurses, Sep/Oct '95

■

Sexually Transmitted Diseases Sourcebook, 1st Edition

Basic Information about Herpes, Chlamydia, Gonorrhea, Hepatitis, Nongonoccocal Urethritis, Pelvic Inflammatory Disease, Syphilis, AIDS, and More

Along with Current Data on Treatments and Preventions

Edited by Linda M. Ross. 550 pages. 1997. 0-7808-0217-9. $78.

■

Sexually Transmitted Diseases Sourcebook, 2nd Edition

Basic Consumer Health Information about Sexually Transmitted Diseases, Including Information on the Diagnosis and Treatment of Chlamydia, Gonorrhea, Hepatitis, Herpes, HIV, Mononucleosis, Syphilis, and Others

Along with Information on Prevention, Such as Condom Use, Vaccines, and STD Education; And Featuring

a Section on Issues Related to Youth and Adolescents, a Glossary, and Resources for Additional Help and Information

Edited by Dawn D. Matthews. 538 pages. 2001. 0-7808-0249-7. $78.

"Recommended for consumer health collections in public libraries, and secondary school and community college libraries."
— American Reference Books Annual 2002

"Every school and public library should have a copy of this comprehensive and user-friendly reference book."
—Choice, Association of College & Research Libraries, Sep '01

"This is a highly recommended book. This is an especially important book for all school and public libraries."
—AIDS Book Review Journal, Jul-Aug '01

"Recommended reference source."
—Booklist, American Library Association, Apr '01

"Recommended pick both for specialty health library collections and any general consumer health reference collection."
—The Bookwatch, Apr '01

■

Skin Disorders Sourcebook

Basic Information about Common Skin and Scalp Conditions Caused by Aging, Allergies, Immune Reactions, Sun Exposure, Infectious Organisms, Parasites, Cosmetics, and Skin Traumas, Including Abrasions, Cuts, and Pressure Sores

Along with Information on Prevention and Treatment

Edited by Allan R. Cook. 647 pages. 1997. 0-7808-0080-X. $78.

". . . comprehensive, easily read reference book."
—Doody's Health Sciences Book Reviews, Oct '97

SEE ALSO Burns Sourcebook

■

Sleep Disorders Sourcebook

Basic Consumer Health Information about Sleep and Its Disorders, Including Insomnia, Sleepwalking, Sleep Apnea, Restless Leg Syndrome, and Narcolepsy

Along with Data about Shiftwork and Its Effects, Information on the Societal Costs of Sleep Deprivation, Descriptions of Treatment Options, a Glossary of Terms, and Resource Listings for Additional Help

Edited by Jenifer Swanson. 439 pages. 1998. 0-7808-0234-9. $78.

"This text will complement any home or medical library. It is user-friendly and ideal for the adult reader."
—American Reference Books Annual, 2000

"A useful resource that provides accurate, relevant, and accessible information on sleep to the general public. Health care providers who deal with sleep disorders patients may also find it helpful in being prepared to answer some of the questions patients ask."
—Respiratory Care, Jul '99

"Recommended reference source."
—Booklist, American Library Association, Feb '99

Sports Injuries Sourcebook, 1st Edition

Basic Consumer Health Information about Common Sports Injuries, Prevention of Injury in Specific Sports, Tips for Training, and Rehabilitation from Injury

Along with Information about Special Concerns for Children, Young Girls in Athletic Training Programs, Senior Athletes, and Women Athletes, and a Directory of Resources for Further Help and Information

Edited by Heather E. Aldred. 624 pages. 1999. 0-7808-0218-7. $78.

"While this easy-to-read book is recommended for all libraries, it should prove to be especially useful for public, high school, and academic libraries; certainly it should be on the bookshelf of every school gymnasium." —*E-Streams, Mar '00*

"Public libraries and undergraduate academic libraries will find this book useful for its nontechnical language." —*American Reference Books Annual, 2000*

Sports Injuries Sourcebook, 2nd Edition

Basic Consumer Health Information about the Diagnosis, Treatment, and Rehabilitation of Common Sports-Related Injuries in Children and Adults

Along with Suggestions for Conditioning and Training, Information and Prevention Tips for Injuries Frequently Associated with Specific Sports and Special Populations, a Glossary, and a Directory of Additional Resources

Edited by Joyce Brennfleck Shannon. 614 pages. 2002. 0-7808-0604-2. $78.

Stress-Related Disorders Sourcebook

Basic Consumer Health Information about Stress and Stress-Related Disorders, Including Stress Origins and Signals, Environmental Stress at Work and Home, Mental and Emotional Stress Associated with Depression, Post-Traumatic Stress Disorder, Panic Disorder, Suicide, and the Physical Effects of Stress on the Cardiovascular, Immune, and Nervous Systems

Along with Stress Management Techniques, a Glossary, and a Listing of Additional Resources

Edited by Joyce Brennfleck Shannon. 610 pages. 2002. 0-7808-0560-7. $78.

"I am impressed by the amount of information. It offers a thorough overview of the causes and consequences of stress for the layperson. . . . A well-done and thorough reference guide for professionals and nonprofessionals alike." —*Doody's Review Service, Dec '02*

Stroke Sourcebook

Basic Consumer Health Information about Stroke, Including Ischemic, Hemorrhagic, Transient Ischemic Attack (TIA), and Pediatric Stroke, Stroke Triggers and Risks, Diagnostic Tests, Treatments, and Rehabilitation Information

Along with Stroke Prevention Guidelines, Legal and Financial Information, a Glossary, and a Directory of Additional Resources

Edited by Joyce Brennfleck Shannon. 600 pages. 2003. 0-7808-0630-1. $78.

Substance Abuse Sourcebook

Basic Health-Related Information about the Abuse of Legal and Illegal Substances Such as Alcohol, Tobacco, Prescription Drugs, Marijuana, Cocaine, and Heroin; and Including Facts about Substance Abuse Prevention Strategies, Intervention Methods, Treatment and Recovery Programs, and a Section Addressing the Special Problems Related to Substance Abuse during Pregnancy

Edited by Karen Bellenir. 573 pages. 1996. 0-7808-0038-9. $78.

"A valuable addition to any health reference section. Highly recommended." —*The Book Report, Mar/Apr '97*

". . . a comprehensive collection of substance abuse information that's both highly readable and compact. Families and caregivers of substance abusers will find the information enlightening and helpful, while teachers, social workers and journalists should benefit from the concise format. Recommended." —*Drug Abuse Update, Winter '96/'97*

SEE ALSO *Alcoholism Sourcebook, Drug Abuse Sourcebook*

Surgery Sourcebook

Basic Consumer Health Information about Inpatient and Outpatient Surgeries, Including Cardiac, Vascular, Orthopedic, Ocular, Reconstructive, Cosmetic, Gynecologic, and Ear, Nose, and Throat Procedures and More

Along with Information about Operating Room Policies and Instruments, Laser Surgery Techniques, Hospital Errors, Statistical Data, a Glossary, and Listings of Sources for Further Help and Information

Edited by Annemarie S. Muth and Karen Bellenir. 596 pages. 2002. 0-7808-0380-9. $78.

Transplantation Sourcebook

Basic Consumer Health Information about Organ and Tissue Transplantation, Including Physical and Financial Preparations, Procedures and Issues Relating to Specific Solid Organ and Tissue Transplants, Rehabilitation, Pediatric Transplant Information, the Future of Transplantation, and Organ and Tissue Donation

Along with a Glossary and Listings of Additional Resources

Edited by Joyce Brennfleck Shannon. 628 pages. 2002. 0-7808-0322-1. $78.

"Recommended for libraries with an interest in offering consumer health information." — *E-Streams, Jul '02*

"This is a unique and valuable resource for patients facing transplantation and their families."
— *Doody's Review Service, Jun '02*

■

Traveler's Health Sourcebook

Basic Consumer Health Information for Travelers, Including Physical and Medical Preparations, Transportation Health and Safety, Essential Information about Food and Water, Sun Exposure, Insect and Snake Bites, Camping and Wilderness Medicine, and Travel with Physical or Medical Disabilities

Along with International Travel Tips, Vaccination Recommendations, Geographical Health Issues, Disease Risks, a Glossary, and a Listing of Additional Resources

Edited by Joyce Brennfleck Shannon. 613 pages. 2000. 0-7808-0384-1. $78.

"Recommended reference source."
— *Booklist, American Library Association, Feb '01*

"This book is recommended for any public library, any travel collection, and especially any collection for the physically disabled."
— *American Reference Books Annual, 2001*

■

Vegetarian Sourcebook

Basic Consumer Health Information about Vegetarian Diets, Lifestyle, and Philosophy, Including Definitions of Vegetarianism and Veganism, Tips about Adopting Vegetarianism, Creating a Vegetarian Pantry, and Meeting Nutritional Needs of Vegetarians, with Facts Regarding Vegetarianism's Effect on Pregnant and Lactating Women, Children, Athletes, and Senior Citizens

Along with a Glossary of Commonly Used Vegetarian Terms and Resources for Additional Help and Information

Edited by Chad T. Kimball. 360 pages. 2002. 0-7808-0439-2. $78.

■

Women's Health Concerns Sourcebook

Basic Information about Health Issues That Affect Women, Featuring Facts about Menstruation and Other Gynecological Concerns, Including Endometriosis, Fibroids, Menopause, and Vaginitis; Reproductive Concerns, Including Birth Control, Infertility, and Abortion; and Facts about Additional Physical, Emotional, and Mental Health Concerns Prevalent among Women Such as Osteoporosis, Urinary Tract Disorders, Eating Disorders, and Depression

Along with Tips for Maintaining a Healthy Lifestyle

Edited by Heather E. Aldred. 567 pages. 1997. 0-7808-0219-5. $78.

"Handy compilation. There is an impressive range of

diseases, devices, disorders, procedures, and other physical and emotional issues covered . . . well organized, illustrated, and indexed." — *Choice, Association of College and Research Libraries, Jan '98*

SEE ALSO *Breast Cancer Sourcebook, Cancer Sourcebook for Women, 1st and 2nd Editions, Healthy Heart Sourcebook for Women, Osteoporosis Sourcebook*

■

Workplace Health & Safety Sourcebook

Basic Consumer Health Information about Workplace Health and Safety, Including the Effect of Workplace Hazards on the Lungs, Skin, Heart, Ears, Eyes, Brain, Reproductive Organs, Musculoskeletal System, and Other Organs and Body Parts

Along with Information about Occupational Cancer, Personal Protective Equipment, Toxic and Hazardous Chemicals, Child Labor, Stress, and Workplace Violence

Edited by Chad T. Kimball. 626 pages. 2000. 0-7808-0231-4. $78.

"As a reference for the general public, this would be useful in any library." — *E-Streams, Jun '01*

"Provides helpful information for primary care physicians and other caregivers interested in occupational medicine. . . . General readers; professionals."
— *Choice, Association of College & Research Libraries, May '01*

"Recommended reference source."
— *Booklist, American Library Association, Feb '01*

"Highly recommended." — *The Bookwatch, Jan '01*

■

Worldwide Health Sourcebook

Basic Information about Global Health Issues, Including Malnutrition, Reproductive Health, Disease Dispersion and Prevention, Emerging Diseases, Risky Health Behaviors, and the Leading Causes of Death

Along with Global Health Concerns for Children, Women, and the Elderly, Mental Health Issues, Research and Technology Advancements, and Economic, Environmental, and Political Health Implications, a Glossary, and a Resource Listing for Additional Help and Information

Edited by Joyce Brennfleck Shannon. 614 pages. 2001. 0-7808-0330-2. $78.

"Named an Outstanding Academic Title."
— *Choice, Association of College & Research Libraries, Jan '02*

"Yet another handy but also unique compilation in the extensive Health Reference Series, this is a useful work because many of the international publications reprinted or excerpted are not readily available. Highly recommended." — *Choice, Association of College & Research Libraries, Nov '01*

"Recommended reference source."
— *Booklist, American Library Association, Oct '01*

Teen Health Series

Helping Young Adults Understand, Manage, and Avoid Serious Illness

Diet Information for Teens
Health Tips about Diet and Nutrition

Including Facts about Nutrients, Dietary Guidelines, Breakfasts, School Lunches, Snacks, Party Food, Weight Control, Eating Disorders, and More

Edited by Karen Bellenir. 399 pages. 2001. 0-7808-0441-4. $58.

"Full of helpful insights and facts throughout the book. . . . An excellent resource to be placed in public libraries or even in personal collections."
— *American Reference Books Annual 2002*

"Recommended for middle and high school libraries and media centers as well as academic libraries that educate future teachers of teenagers. It is also a suitable addition to health science libraries that serve patrons who are interested in teen health promotion and education." — *E-Streams, Oct '01*

"This comprehensive book would be beneficial to collections that need information about nutrition, dietary guidelines, meal planning, and weight control. . . . This reference is so easy to use that its purchase is recommended." — *The Book Report, Sep-Oct '01*

"This book is written in an easy to understand format describing issues that many teens face every day, and then provides thoughtful explanations so that teens can make informed decisions. This is an interesting book that provides important facts and information for today's teens." — *Doody's Health Sciences Book Review Journal, Jul-Aug '01*

"A comprehensive compendium of diet and nutrition. The information is presented in a straightforward, plain-spoken manner. This title will be useful to those working on reports on a variety of topics, as well as to general readers concerned about their dietary health." — *School Library Journal, Jun '01*

Drug Information for Teens
Health Tips about the Physical and Mental Effects of Substance Abuse

Including Facts about Alcohol, Anabolic Steroids, Club Drugs, Cocaine, Depressants, Hallucinogens, Herbal Products, Inhalants, Marijuana, Narcotics, Stimulants, Tobacco, and More

Edited by Karen Bellenir. 452 pages. 2002. 0-7808-0444-9. $58.

Mental Health Information for Teens
Health Tips about Mental Health and Mental Illness

Including Facts about Anxiety, Depression, Suicide, Eating Disorders, Obsessive-Compulsive Disorders, Panic Attacks, Phobias, Schizophrenia, and More

Edited by Karen Bellenir. 406 pages. 2001. 0-7808-0442-2. $58.

"In both language and approach, this user-friendly entry in the *Teen Health Series* is on target for teens needing information on mental health concerns." — *Booklist, American Library Association, Jan '02*

"Readers will find the material accessible and informative, with the shaded notes, facts, and embedded glossary insets adding appropriately to the already interesting and succinct presentation."
— *School Library Journal, Jan '02*

"This title is highly recommended for any library that serves adolescents and parents/caregivers of adolescents." — *E-Streams, Jan '02*

"Recommended for high school libraries and young adult collections in public libraries. Both health professionals and teenagers will find this book useful." — *American Reference Books Annual 2002*

"This is a nice book written to enlighten the society, primarily teenagers, about common teen mental health issues. It is highly recommended to teachers and parents as well as adolescents." — *Doody's Review Service, Dec '01*

Sexual Health Information for Teens
Health Tips about Sexual Development, Human Reproduction, and Sexually Transmitted Diseases

Including Facts about Puberty, Reproductive Health, Chlamydia, Human Papillomavirus, Pelvic Inflammatory Disease, Herpes, AIDS, Contraception, Pregnancy, and More

Edited by Deborah A. Stanley. 400 pages. 2003. 0-7808-0445-7. $58.

Health Reference Series